UNUSUAL OCCURRENCES AS CLUES TO CANCER ETIOLOGY

Proceedings of the 18th International Symposium of
The Princess Takamatsu Cancer Research Fund, Tokyo, 1987

UNUSUAL OCCURRENCES AS CLUES TO CANCER ETIOLOGY

Edited by
ROBERT W. MILLER, SHAW WATANABE,
JOSEPH F. FRAUMENI, JR., TAKASHI SUGIMURA,
SHOZO TAKAYAMA, and HARUO SUGANO

JAPAN SCIENTIFIC SOCIETIES PRESS, Tokyo
TAYLOR & FRANCIS LTD., London and Philadelphia

Published jointly by:
JAPAN SCIENTIFIC SOCIETIES PRESS
Hongo 6-2-10, Bunkyo-ku, Tokyo 113, Japan
ISBN 4-7622-1556-2
          and
TAYLOR & FRANCIS LTD.
4 John Street, London WCIN 2 ET, UK
ISBN 0-85066-459-4

Distributed in all areas outside Japan and Asia between Pakistan and Korea by TAYLOR & FRANCIS LTD.

Printed in Japan

Organizing Committee of the 18th International Symposium

Robert W. MILLER
    Division of Cancer Etiology, National Cancer Institute, Bethesda, Maryland
    20892, U.S.A.
Shaw WATANABE
    Epidemiology Division, National Cancer Center Research Institute, Tokyo 104,
    Japan
Joseph F. FRAUMENI, JR.
    Division of Cancer Etiology, National Cancer Institute, Bethesda, Maryland
    20892, U.S.A.
Takashi SUGIMURA
    National Cancer Center, Tokyo 104, Japan
Shozo TAKAYAMA
    National Cancer Center Research Institute, Tokyo 104, Japan
Haruo SUGANO
    Cancer Institute, Tokyo 170, Japan

Preface

Alert clinical observations have played an important role in providing clues to cancer etiology. The next step, epidemiologic study, helps to establish the causal relationship between specific causes and genetic and environmental factors. Laboratory research provides understanding of the mechanism involved in both carcinogenesis and normal biology, after developing information not previously available from animal experimentation.

The leaders in cancer research in Japan have been especially aware of the importance of clinical observation in cancer etiology, and have selected this topic in place of a mainstream through issue for the 18th International Cancer Symposium sponsored by the Princess Takamatsu Cancer Research Fund. In so doing, they have brought together more than two dozen clinicians who have made and followed through on observations that implicated certain chemicals, viruses, parasites, ionizing radiation in genetics in carcinogenesis. The result can see in this proceedings how ideas originated, were advanced, and led to new understanding of etiology, prevention and early detection. We hope this proceedings will serve as a guide to the future as well as a chronicle of the past.

Robert W. MILLER
Shaw WATANABE

Contents

Viruses and Other Microorganisms

Genetic and Other Host Factors

Contributors

George H. BARROWS
Department of Pathology, Saint Francis Medical Center, Hartford, Connecticut 06015, U.S.A.

Kåre BERG
Institute of Medical Genetics, University of Oslo, Blindern, Oslo 3, Norway

Henry FALK
Division of Environmental Hazards and Health Effects, Center for Environmental Health, Centers for Disease Control, Koger Center, Atlanta, Georgia 30333, U.S.A.

Joseph F. FRAUMENI, JR.
Division of Cancer Etiology, National Cancer Institute, Bethesda, Maryland 20892, U.S.A.

Richard A. GATTI
Department of Pathology, University California Los Angeles, School of Medicine, Los Angeles, California 90024, U.S.A.

David G. HARNDEN
Paterson Institute for Cancer Research, Christie Hospital & Holt Radium Institute, Withington, Manchester M20 9BX, England, UK

Clark W. HEATH, JR.
Bureau of Preventive Health Services, South Carolina Department of Health and Environmental Control, Columbia, South Carolina 29201, U.S.A.

Arthur L. HERBST
Department of Obstetrics and Gynecology, University of Chicago, Chicago, Illinois 60637, U.S.A.

Akihiro IGATA
Department of Virology, Faculty of Medicine, Kagoshima University, Kagoshima, Kagoshima 890, Japan

Yutaka INABA
Department of Hygiene, Juntendo University, School of Medicine, Bunkyo-ku, Tokyo 113, Japan

Isao ISHIKAWA
Division of Nephrology, Department of Internal Medicine, Kanazawa Medical University, Kahoku, Ishikawa 920–02, Japan

Marshall E. KADIN — Department of Pathology, Beth Israel Hospital, Boston, Massachusetts 02215, U.S.A.

Nanao KAMADA — Department of Internal Medicine, Research Institute for Nuclear Medicine and Biology, Hiroshima University, Minami-ku, Hiroshima 734, Japan

Hiroo KATO — Department of Epidemiology, Radiation Effects Research Foundation (RERF), Minami-ku, Hiroshima 732, Japan

Alfred G. KNUDSON, JR. — Fox Chase Cancer Center, The Institute for Cancer Research, Philadelphia, Pennsylvania 19111, U.S.A.

Masanori KURATSUNE — Nakamura Gakuen College, Jonan-ku, Fukuoka 814, Japan

Frederick P. LI — Division of Cancer Etiology, National Cancer Institute, Danna Farber Cancer Center, Boston, Massachusetts 02115, U.S.A.

Robert W. MILLER — Division of Cancer Etiology, National Cancer Institute, Bethesda, Maryland 20892, U.S.A.

Nancy E. MUELLER — Department of Epidemiology, Harvard School of Public Health, Boston, Massachusetts 02115, U.S.A.

Guy R. NEWELL — Department of Cancer Prevention, M. D. Anderson Hospital & Tumor Institute, University of Texas System Cancer Center, Houston, Texas 77030, U.S.A.

Yukio NISHIMOTO — Hiroshima Hospital of West Japan Railway Company, Higashi-ku, Hiroshima 732, Japan

Gregory T. O'CONOR — Department of Pathology, Loyola University Medical Center, Maywood, Illinois 60153, U.S.A.

David T. PURTILO — Department of Pathology & Microbiology, University of Nebraska Medical Center, Omaha, Nebraska 68105–1065, U.S.A.

Bracha RAMOT — Institute of Hematology, The Chaim Sheba Medical Center, Affiliated to the Tel-Aviv University, Sackler School of Medicine, Tel-Hashomer 52621, Israel

Haruo SUGANO — Cancer Institute, Toshima-ku, Tokyo 170, Japan

Takashi SUGIMURA — National Cancer Center, Chuo-ku, Tokyo 104, Japan

Sun SHIQUAN — Institute of Radiation Protection, Ministry of Nuclear Industry, Taiyuan, Shanxi, People's Republic of China

Shozo TAKAYAMA — National Cancer Center Research Institute, Chuo-ku, Tokyo 104, Japan

Hassan N. TAWFIK — Department of Pathology, National Cancer Institute, Cairo University, Cairo, Egypt

Margaret A. TUCKER — Division of Cancer Etiology, National Cancer Institute, Bethesda, Maryland 20892, U.S.A.

Shaw WATANABE — Epidemiology Division, National Cancer Center Research Institute, Chuo-ku, Tokyo 104, Japan

Opening Address

H.I.H. Princess KIKUKO TAKAMATSU

It has long been one of my delightful duties to deliver the opening address at the annual International Symposium held under the auspices of the Cancer Research Fund that bears my name. This year, however, to my deepest sorrow, I feel very differently, since my husband, Prince Takamatsu, passed away with lung cancer last February.

Under such pertinent circumstances, I do sincerely welcome everyone who has gathered here today to participate in the 18th International Symposium of the Princess Takamatsu Cancer Research Fund.

The title of this year's symposium is, "Unusual Occurrences as Clues to Cancer Etiology". Investigating unique factors associated with certain patients in order to detect the causes of cancer is a means by which the important milestone of removing these risk factors from everyday life can be reached, thereby preventing cancer. Each individual case encourages both research workers and clinicians in this regard.

The discovery of the means of preventing cancer, I believe to be of vital importance to people who wish to remain healthy throughout their natural life span.

I wish to express my sincere thanks to Dr. Robert Miller and Dr. Joseph Fraumeni, Jr., of the National Cancer Institute, U.S.A., for their valuable assistance as members of the committee organizing this symposium.

I now declare open the 18th International Symposium of the present series, with every confidence in its fruitful outcome.

APPROACHES TO UNUSUAL OCCURRENCES OF CANCER

UNUSUAL OCCURRENCES AS CLUES TO CANCER ETIOLOGY, R. W. MILLER ET AL. (EDS.),
JAPAN SCI. SOC. PRESS, TOKYO/TAYLOR & FRANCIS, LTD., PP. 3–12, 1988

NAKAHARA MEMORIAL LECTURE

Rare Events and Cancer Epidemiology

Robert W. MILLER

Clinical Epidemiology Branch, National Cancer Institute, Bethesda, Maryland 20892, U.S.A.

Abstract: Physicians who think epidemiologically are rare. A method is suggested for detecting their aptitude early in their career when help may be offered to make the most of their special talent.

Clusters geographically or in families may provide clues to cancer etiology. Clusters have been systematically thought by mapping cancer mortality in the US and independently in China. Case-control studies have revealed environmental exposure responsible for some of the clusters.

Clusters noted by alert clinicians or other astute observers have revealed most of the known environmental causes of human cancers. Genetic influence in carcinogenesis has been identified by studies of peculiar cancer occurrence, such as familial aggregation, multiple primary cancer or the occurrence of cancer with other diseases as, for example, congenital malformations and immunodeficiency disorders. Ethnic differences in cancer occurrence may be revealing. Thus, in Japan there is low frequency of B-cell lymphoma but high frequency of certain autoimmune diseases, as if inherent protection against one predisposes the other.

As a rule of thumb, the occurrence of three rare observations is not likely to be due to chance. Examples include ideal carcinoma in three persons with cystic fibrosis of the pancreas who survived to about 30 years of age, and the occurrence in Klinefelter's syndrome of germ cell tumor of the pineal—a neoplasm that has an unusually high frequency in Japan.

Finally, the history of discoveries concerning cancer etiology, an aspect of what Comroe has called "research on research", can point the way to new discoveries in the future.

I am greatly honored to present this lecture in memory of Dr. Nakahara. He and I met in 1973 at the third annual symposium sponsored by the Princess Takamatsu Cancer Research Fund. He was a man of great warmth and achievement. Among his achievements was the initiation of these symposia. Two topics we are discussing here that would have been of great interest to him are the importance of the lymphocyte in tumor resistance, which he studied almost 70 years ago, and the role of the host in resisting cancer.

At the age of 65, when he became the first Director of the Research Institute of the National Cancer Center, he appointed very active young scientists in their thirties as Division Chiefs. He later wrote that "they were, according to the standards of the Japanese bureaucratic circles, too young for [these] posts . . . " (*1*). They have since fully justified his confidence in them as they led the Institute to its present reputation as one of the best in the world.

The young, on their own without a leader such as Dr. Nakahara, sometimes make immensely insightful clinical observations. Perhaps this is the product of fresh minds, not yet in the habit of focusing in medicine on diagnosis and therapy, to the disadvantage of etiology. At this symposium we will hear how Dr. Janet K. Baum, while an intern in Ann Arbor found a series of women in whom oral contraceptives caused highly vascular, life-threatening hepatic adenomas. Japan has had a counterpart experience. In 1953, Dr. M. Miyanishi, an intern at Hiroshima University, curious as to why a man only 30 years of age had a bronchogenic carcinoma, learned that he had worked at a mustard-gas factory for one year during the war. More than 100 cases of respiratory-tract cancer have now been traced to this exposure.

The Instinct to Think Etiologically

Some people have a flair to think etiologically, and do it throughout their lives. For them such thinking is a quirk of mind that cannot be suppressed. It causes one to note, for example, that the direction of stripes in a necktie provides a clue to its place of origin. Those with stripes descending from left to right as one faces the wearer, are usually made in the United States. The others, with stripes from right to left, are usually from Asia or Europe.

In the United States people with this turn of mind can be found in business, where market research can make them rich, in journalism where investigative reporting makes news, in detective work where it can help make arrests, or in politics where sampling voters and adjusting to their interests can help win elections.

By contrast with these occupations, medicine has only a small pool of susceptibles from which to draw observational scientists. My impression is that pool is larger in Japan and China than in western countries, perhaps related to culture and tradition. In all countries more susceptibles need to be identified early in their medical careers and given an opportunity to develop and apply their talent. Surely a test to detect this capability can be devised for students who are in medical school or who plan to apply.

A general appraisal of research potential may lie in an educational plan developed by the Department of Human Genetics at the Medical College of Virginia (*2*). McKusick's book, Mendelian Inheritance in Man (*3*), was used as a source of disease entities, and each of the 168 first-year medical students was assigned one entry to bring up to date through library research. The student had to prepare an entry for the volume in the same way that McKusick's group does for each new edition. Through this assignment, the students learned early how to use the library (the librarian was forewarned), and their aptitude for uncovering new information could be evaluated. The first class that undertook this task entered medical school in 1984. It will be interesting to see if the performance of this exercise, given at the outset of medical school, relates to career choices made after graduation. So far, at the end of two years, the students have scored 13 points higher on Part 1 of the National Board Examinations than the average for students at the school in the past seven years. The authors noted that if this talent could be harnessed for the 16,000 students who enter U.S. medical schools each year, they could rewrite their textbooks annually (4).

Time-space Clusters

Etiologic observations made clinically can concern environmental exposures, host susceptibility or interactions between the two. At this symposium we will hear about examples of each. Virtually all human carcinogens (and teratogens) were first recognized by astute clinicians, who reported on occupational or other time-space clusters. Since 1975 maps of cancer mortality by small geographic areas within a country have led to recognition of clusters to which attention had not been drawn by local physicians. A new chapter in human environmental carcinogenesis is being written as a result. It is remarkable that similar maps were made during the Cultural Revolution in the People's Republic of China (5, 6). In neither country was it known that the same study was in progress on the other side of the world.

Cancers due to viruses are being increasingly recognized by the occurrence of geographic clusters, some of them involving rare cell types—adult T cell leukemia and juvenile laryngeal papillomatosis, for example (7). Some viral cancers are epidemic, such as hepatocellular carcinoma attributed to infection with hepatitis B virus. On the basis of such etiologic relationships first recognized through the occurrence of a cluster, vast new understanding of carcinogenesis is coming from laboratory research.

Physical agents have also been identified as carcinogens through a concentration of cases in particular subgroups of the population. Ionizing radiation was found to be a leukemogen and a skin carcinogen in early radiation workers. Soon after, a cluster of cases of osteosarcoma was found in radium-dial painters, among whom a far less well known excess of carcinoma arising from the lining of the mastoid or paranasal sinuses has also developed (8). The induction of this rare cancer has been attributed to radium deposited in the underlying bone and its disintegration to radon gas, which is trapped within the sinus and serves as a contiguous long-term source of radiation. This rarity is not likely to be encountered again, but by referring to it here, perhaps familiarity with its occurrence can be extended.

No one would have predicted that certain forms of asbestos can cause cancer. Because clusters of bronchogenic carcinoma were observed among asbestos workers, and largely because a cluster of cases of mesothelioma was noted in South Africa among persons whose homes were near open-pit mines, the inert looking fibers are now known to induce cancer if the length is greater than 5 μm and the diameter is less than 0.25 μm (9). Thus the carcinogenicity of asbestos is due to its physical properties, placing it as a physical carcinogen in the same category as ionizing radiation and ultra-violet light.

Astute observers have identified families in which the asbestos worker polluted his home with dust from his clothing. Wives and children developed mesothelioma decades later (*10, 11*). Chisolm has referred to such instances as "fouling one's own nest (*12*)".

A cluster of particular interest in Japan involves a benign disorder, subacute necrotizing lymphadenitis, which concentrates in Hokkaido, with the greatest frequency in women who are 20–34 years of age (*13*). Many more cases have been reported there than in the rest of the world, except perhaps for Korea. In leafing through a compendium of abstracts in English of Korean medical articles published in 1985 I found one that mentioned 15 cases studied immunologically at Kyung Hee University (*14*), which is in a suburb of Seoul. This large number may well signify the presence of a cluster there, which could provide an opportunity for parallel studies to those in Japan.

Genetics of Cancer

Clues to genetic influences on disease occurrences have also been identified by alert clinicians. Usually the first step is delineation of a syndrome. In 1957 Elena Boder and Richard Sedgwick separated ataxia-telangiectasia (AT) from a tangle of telangicctatic and neurological diseases, and published their findings unobtrusively in the University of Southern California Medical Bulletin (*15*). Once the syndrome was delineated, a flood of new information followed about this disorder and others that predispose to lymphoma.

The high proportion of presentations at this symposium on lymphoma was unintentional. It attests to the variety of information that has been developed about this form of neoplasia, beginning with clinical observations. From such human models of disease for which no animal models are yet known, has come important new knowledge about carcinogenesis.

Environmental and Genetic Interactions

Skin cancer exemplifies the interaction between genetics and environmental exposures. This neoplasm develops excessively in albinos because of their lack of pigmentation, in xeroderma pigmentosum because of a defect in the repair of DNA, and in epidermodysplasia verruciformis because of hypersusceptibility to infection with human papilloma virus types 5 and 8 in particular (*16*). These interactions, first recognized clinically, opened new avenues of laboratory research through which understanding of normal as well as abnormal biology is being defined. Dr. "George" Wu, the former Director of the Cancer Institute in Beijing has referred to the link between clinical observation and laboratory research as the "Bridge of Heaven."

Ethnic Differences

Insufficient attention is being paid to cancers that are rare in certain ethnic groups. Among these rarities are Ewing's sarcoma in non-whites, testicular cancer in Japanese and Blacks, and acute lymphocytic leukemia in black children (*17*).

TABLE 1. Incidence per Million of Four Childhood Cancers, U.S. and Japan Compared

Cancer	U.S. Whites[a]		Kanagawa Pref.[b]	
	No.	%	No.	%
Neuroblastoma	347	8.7	138	8.2
Wilms' tumor	319	7.7	66	3.9
Retinoblastoma	122	3.3	118	6.9
Liver cancer	54	1.4	41	2.4

[a] Surveillance, Epidemiology and End Results Program, NCI, 1972–1983. [b] Kanagawa Prefecture Childhood Cancer Registry, 1972–1982.

Knudson has suggest that the polymorphisms involved in the resistant ethnic groups are less mutable than those in susceptible groups (U.S.-Japan Workshop on the Genetics of Human Cancer, March 23–25, 1987) (*18*). At the same workshop, through the use of population-based registries in each country, another difference in cancer rates was uncovered, which may have the same explanation: the incidence of Wilms' tumor among U.S. white children is twice as common as in Japan, whereas retinoblastoma is twice as common in Japan (Table 1). Wilms' tumor is thought to have a relatively constant rate worldwide (*19*), so Japan is unique, insofar as we now know. High rates for retinoblastoma have previously been noted in Israel, India and Pakistan, among other nations (*17*). Perhaps mutability of the gene locus varies considerably by ethnic group.

Two earlier workshops in this series concerned differences between the U.S. and Japan in the occurrence of lymphocytic diseases (*13, 20*). Chronic lymphocytic leukemia is rare in Japanese, as well as in Chinese and Koreans, as compared with U.S. Whites, among whom 30 percent of adult leukemia is of this type. In Japan nodular lymphoma accounts for only 10 percent of lymphoma as compared with 44 percent among U.S. Whites (*13*). In Japan there is what appears to be a reciprocal relationship between certain lymphomas and autoimmune disease: systemic lupus erythematosus (SLE), Hashimoto's thyroiditis and Takayasu's aortitis. These diseases are 2–3 times more common in Japanese than in U.S. Whites (*13*). A similar reciprocal relationship has previously been noted by Purtilo and Sullivan (*21*) in the U.S. male preponderance of lymphoma and the marked female preponderance of SLE (9:1). They suggested that an X-linked immunoregulatory gene protects females against lymphoma but predisposes them to SLE and other autoimmune disorders. The same explanation may apply to the reciprocal relationship between these diseases in U.S. Whites and Japanese.

How many Unusual Occurrences Are Needed?

The first case may be sufficient, as illustrated by respiratory cancer among mustard-gas workers in Japan. My rule of thumb, though, is that three pairs of rare occurrences in a short period of time signals a real association, as in vinyl chloride workers who developed angiosarcoma of the liver, women on oral contraceptives who developed liver neoplasia, or children with the fetal hydantoin syndrome who developed neuroblastoma. It is puzzling that after the "rule of three" was satisfied in 1980 concerning the occurrence of neuroblastoma in the fetal hydantoin syndrome (*22*), no further cases have come to notice.

Recently, there has been an increasing flow of reports concerning teratomas of the mediastinum in Klinefelter's syndrome (*23*). In the general population the neoplasm also occurs in the testis, retroperitoneum and pineal area, but in Klinefelter's syndrome germ cell tumors occur mainly in the mediastinum. Why in this location is a puzzle. Four germ cell tumors have been reported in or near the pineal of patients with Klinefelter's syndrome (*24, 25*), two of them in Japan (*25, 26*). The rule of three would be fulfilled if a third case were found in Japan. It may be easy to ascertain additional cases because in Japan pineal germ cell tumors occur about 12 times more often than they do elsewhere (*27*). Routine buccal smears for Barr bodies in males with these tumors would indicate the presence of an extra X chromosome, characteristic of Klinefelter's syndrome. Such a study would be simple and informative, and may lead to further understanding of the genesis of this neoplasm and its high frequency in Japan.

Our most recent application of the rule of three concerns a particular cancer in patients with cystic fibrosis (CF) of the pancreas. As more of these patients survive to adulthood, adenocarcinoma of the ileum has affected three of them at 29–34 years of age (*28–30*). The causal relationship between CF and the neoplasm is supported by past observations that celiac disease, in which steatorrhea also occurs, also has an increased risk of adenocarcinoma of the small intestine, not of the ileum but of the jejunum (*31*). These findings are important with regard to early detection of the neoplasm in CF, and new understanding of intestinal carcinogenesis. Specifically, why does steatorrhea cause cancer in the small intestine, a site seldom affected by malignancy?

Physicians Are Not the only Clinical Etiologists

Astute etiological observations have been made by a variety of non-physicians. We had a wonderful clerk in our Branch who discovered several unusual occurrences of cancer while abstracting and cataloging medical records at the Los Angeles Children's Hospital in the early 1960s. The most remarkable was a family in which one child had a brain tumor and a sibling had a meningomyelocoele. The clerk was intrigued by this sibship concurrence of a neoplasm and a birth defect involving the same organ system, so she searched all over Los Angeles for the medical records of the family members. She found that in four generations eight members had had brain tumors, due, it was later found, to neurofibromatosis without the usual external manifestations (*32*). Multiple tumors, thought to be neurofibromas were seen on a myelogram of one affected member (P. Wright, personal communication). A sequel to the story is that still another member of the family developed a brain tumor, which came to my notice when a volunteer at the hospital mentioned to me that she had assisted a child that day who was the ninth member of a family to develop a brain tumor (personal communication from my mother, who was the volunteer).

In Lin County, China, there is a high frequency of esophageal cancer. To detect the cancer early, a vigorous health education program was mounted, so the people were well acquainted with the earliest symptoms. When a barefoot doctor asked a peasant if he or anyone in his family had difficulty in swallowing he said, no, but his chickens did. In this way it was found that there was a parallel occurrence in chickens. Eventually 152 affected chickens were collected by mail carriers and brought to the center where esophageal cancer was being studied (*33*).

In California five workers at a factory that made the pesticide, dibromochloropropane (DBCP) were unable to father children and suspected that an occupational exposure was responsible. Their physicians discounted the possibility, so the men took their own semen samples to a laboratory where oligospermia or azoospermia was found (*34*).

It will be noted that the foregoing observations were made by an astute clerk, by an alert peasant and by the patients themselves. It is a good idea when a peculiarity in cancer occurrence is seen, to ask the patient what he or she thinks the explanation might be.

Research on Research

For this symposium each speaker was asked to begin with a brief history as to how the subject to be presented first came to mind. How did it unfold and grow? Too seldom is this information recorded. Perhaps it is considered a personal aside, insufficiently detached for the annals of science. Comroe, an outstanding cardiopulmonary physiologist, may be as well remembered for his historical contributions toward the end of his life as for his scientific contributions over half a century. He published the historical essays as a collection in a volume with the subtitle, "Insights into Medical Discovery" (*35*). It is a wonderful book, published at cost, which tells how key research ideas often had their seeds and roots in seemingly obscure basic research. Prior to this, he and Dripps (*36*) formulated a list of the ten most outstanding clinical advances in cardiopulmonary medicine by consulting leaders in the field. Open heart surgery headed the list. Comroe and Dripps then traced the origin and development of the research required before the procedure could be performed. It included understanding the circulation of blood, the discovery of anesthesia, invention of the EKG, the discovery of heparin, and the development of techniques for cardiac catheterization and angiocardiography. Comroe and Dripps referred to their analyses as "research on research," and disdained anecdotal accounts. Comroe's collected essays, a by-product of his formal historical research, *are* anecdotal, however, and in the aggregate are filled with insights into medical discovery. It will be interesting to see if the historical parts of the presentations at this symposium are a step in the same direction.

What Rare Events May Provide Clues to Cancer Etiology?

From the presentations at this symposium we can see that a variety of rare events may provide clues to cancer etiology. The rarity may be in the cancer, as, for example, mesothelioma due to asbestos, or hepatic angiosarcoma due to vinyl chloride. Or the exposure may be unusual, as illustrated by mustard-gas, which causes cancer of the respiratory tract, or atomic radiation which causes a variety of cancers.

Family aggregation may be etiologically informative whether the cancer is of the same type or certain diverse types, as in the Li-Fraumeni syndrome. Multiple primary cancers, such as osteosarcoma in patients with retinoblastoma, provide the opportunity to extend laboratory investigations for one cancer to the others with which it occurs excessively.

Rare diseases associated with cancer have been a rich source of new information not only with respect to the biology of cancer but also normal function, as in lymphoma among patients with congenital immunodeficiency disorders or in aniridia with Wilms' tumor. Rare laboratory observations may be etiologically important, as exemplified by the chomosomal abnormalities recently found in lipomas.

Geographic clustering has emerged in the past decade as a basis for case-control studies that can lead to environmental carcinogens, such as oral cancer from snuff-dipping among southern U.S. women and urinary bladder cancer among chemical workers living in Salem County, New Jersey.

Finally, among the rare events that provide clues to cancer etiology is the alert clinician, whose contributions are exemplified in the presentations made at this symposium.

REFERENCES

1. Nakahara, W. A pilgrim's progress in cancer research, 1918 to 1974: autobiographical essay. Cancer Res., *34*: 1767–1774, 1974.
2. Bodurtha, J. N., Townsend J. I., Proud, V. K., and Nance, W. E. Updating McKusick: An educational exercise for medical students. Am. J. Med. Genet., *24*: 505–511, 1986.
3. McKusick, V. A. Mendelian Inheritance in Man, sixth ed., Johns Hopkins Univ. Press, Baltimore, 1983.
4. Bodurtha, J. N., Verbin, S., Papp, K. K., and Nance, W. E. Recent innovations in human genetics education. The curricularization of McKusick, Am. J. Human Genet., *41*: 304–305, 1987.
5. Editorial Committee, Atlas of Cancer Mortality in the People's Republic of China, China Map Press, Beijing, 1980.
6. Li, F. P. and Shiang, E. Cancer mortality in China. J. Natl. Cancer Inst., *65*: 217–221, 1980.
7. Klein, G. (ed.), Viral Oncology, 842 pp., Raven Press, New York, 1980.
8. Littman, M. S., Kirsh, I. E., and Keane, A. T. Radium-induced malignant tumors of the mastoid and paranasal sinuses. Am. J. Roentgenol., *131*: 773–785, 1978.
9. Wagner, J. C. Mesothelioma and mineral fibers. Cancer, *57*: 1905–1911, 1986.
10. Anderson, H. A., Lilis, R., Baum, S. M., Fischbein, A. S., and Selikoff, I. J. Household contact asbestos: neoplastic risk. Ann. N. Y. Acad. Sci., *271*: 311–323, 1976.
11. Li, F. P., Lokich, J., Lapey, J., Neptune, W. B., and Wilkins, E. W., Jr. Familial mesothelioma after intense asbestos exposure at home. JAMA, *240*: 467, 1978.
12. Chisolm, J. J. Fouling one's own nest. Pediatrics, *62*: 614–617, 1978.
13. Kadin, M. E., Berard, C. W., Nanba, K., and Wakasa, H. Lymphoproliferative diseases in Japan and western countries. Hum. Pathol., *14*: 745–772, 1983.
14. Lee, W. H., Yang, M. H., and Lee, C. K. An immunopathological study of necrotizing lymphadenitis. Kyung Hee Univ. Med. J., *9*: 17–26, 1984 (cited in Med. Abstr. Korea, *12*: 72–73, 1985).

15. Boder, E. and Sedgwick, R. P. Ataxia-telangiectasia. A familial syndrome of progressive cerebellar ataxia, oculocutaneous telangiectasia and frequent pulmonary infection. Univ. So. Calif. Med. Bull., *9*: 15–27, 1957.

16. Lutzner, M. A. Papillomaviruses and neoplasia in man. Monogr. Pathol., *27*: 126–170, 1986.

17. Miller, R. W. Ethnic differences in cancer occurrence: genetic and environmental influences with particular reference to neuroblastoma. *In;* J. J. Mulvihill, R. W. Miller, and J. F. Fraumeni, Jr. (eds.), Genetics of Human Cancer, pp. 1–14, Raven Press, New York, 1977.

18. Li, F. P. and Takebe, H. Genetics of human cancer: meeting report. Unpublished.

19. Innis, M. D. Nephroblastoma: possible index cancer of childhood. Med. J. Aust., *1*: 18–32, 1972.

20. Miller, R. W., Gilman, P. A., and Sugano, H. Meeting highlights: differences in lymphocytic diseases in the United States and Japan. J. Natl. Cancer Inst., *67*: 739–740, 1981.

21. Purtilo, D. T. and Sullivan, J. L. Immunological bases for superior survival of females. Am. J. Dis. Child., *133*: 1251–1253, 1979.

22. Allen, R. W., Jr., Ogden, B., Bentley, F. L., and Jung, A. L. Fetal hydantoin syndrome, neuroblastoma, and hemorrhagic disease in a neonate. JAMA, *244*: 1464–1465, 1980.

23. Nichols, C. R., Heerema, N. A., Palmer, C., Loehrer, P. J., Williams, S. D., and Einhorn, L. H. Klinefelter's syndrome associated with mediastinal germ cell neoplasms. J. Clin. Oncol., *5*: 1290–1294, 1987.

24. Ellis, S. J., Crockard, A. and Barnard, R. O. Klinefelter's syndrome, cerebral germinoma, Chiari malformation, and syrinx: a case report. Neurosurgery, *18*: 220–222, 1986.

25. Ahagon, A., Yoshida, Y., Kusuno, K., and Uno, T. Suprasellar germinoma in association with Klinefelter's syndrome. J. Neurosurg., *58*: 136–138, 1983.

26. Oki, S., Nakao, K., Kuno, S., and Imura, H. A case of Klinefelter's syndrome associated with hypothalamic-pituitary dysfunction caused by an intracranial germ cell tumor. Endocrinol. Jpn., *34*: 145–151, 1987.

27. Araki, C. and Matsumoto, S. Statistical reevaluation of pinealoma and related tumors in Japan. J. Neurosurg., *30*: 146–149, 1969.

28. Redington, A. N., Spring, R., and Batten, J. C. Adenocarcinoma of the ileum presenting as non-traumatic clostridial myonecrosis in cystic fibrosis. Br. Med. J., *290*: 1871–1872, 1985.

29. Roberts, J. A., Tullet, W. M., Thomas, S. StJ., Galloway, D., and Stack, B.H.R. Bowel adenocarcinoma in a patient with cystic fibrosis. Scott. Med. J., *31*: 109, 1986.

30. Siraganian, P. A., Swender, P. T., and Miller, R. W. Adenocarcinoma of the ileum in cystic fibrosis. Lancet *ii*: 1158, 1987.

31. Nielson, S.N.J. and Wood, L. E. Adenocarcinoma of the jejunum in association with nontropical sprue. Arch. Pathol. Lab. Med., *110*: 822–824, 1986.

32. Lee, D. K. and Abbott, N. L. Familial central nervous system neoplasia. Case report of a family with von Recklinghausen's neurofibromatosis. Arch. Neurol., *20*: 154–160, 1969.

33. Miller, R. W. Cancer epidemics in the People's Republic of China. J. Natl. Cancer Inst., *60*: 1195–1203, 1978.

34. Miller, R. W. Areawide chemical contamination: lessons from case histories. JAMA, *245*: 1548–1551, 1981.

35. Comroe, J. H., Jr. Retrospectroscope. Insights into Medical Discovery, 182 pp., Von

Gehr Press, Menlo Park, Calif., 1977.

36.   Comroe, J. H., Jr. and Dripps, R. D. Scientific basis for the support of biomedical science. Science, *192*: 105–111, 1976.

KEYNOTE LECTURE

Etiologic Insights from Cancer Mapping

Joseph F. Fraumeni, Jr.

Epidemiology and Biostatistics Program, National Cancer Institute, Bethesda, Maryland 20892, U.S.A.

Abstract: In the 1970s the epidemiology program at the U.S. National Cancer Institute made a systematic effort to identify cancer clustering by analyzing patterns of mortality at the county level, where the population is small enough to be relatively homogeneous, yet large enough to provide reliable data and stable rates. When the mortality rates for the period 1950–69 were plotted in a series of computer-generated color-coded maps, there arose a surprising number and variety of geographic patterns. This review describes how leads to the causes of several cancers have been generated and explored through a progression of descriptive and correlational studies, followed by analytical studies to determine reasons for the elevated risks in certain areas of the country. For example, the high lung cancer rates among men in some coastal areas were related mainly to asbestos exposures in shipyard work, while the elevated oral cancer rates among women in the rural south were linked to the use of smokeless tobacco (snuff).

A recent update of cancer maps covering the period 1970–80 revealed geographic patterns resembling those in the earlier atlas, but with a tendency toward greater uniformity of rates around the country. Yet some new high-risk areas emerged, such as elevated rates of lung and oral cancers among women in Florida and along the Pacific coast, which seemed correlated with smoking habits, and high rates of non-Hodgkin's lymphoma among men in central areas that may be associated with agricultural exposure to herbicides.

Our experience suggests that cancer mapping on a small-area scale is a useful strategy for formulating and pursuing leads to environmental and lifestyle determinants of cancer. In other countries also, the mapping approach has helped to stimulate and target research into the origins of cancer and the means of prevention.

In the mid-1970s, the epidemiology group at the National Cancer Institute prepared an atlas of cancer mortality in the U.S. that plotted cancer death rates at a county level using computer-mapping techniques (*1*). Previous surveys had revealed some geographic patterns by region and state, but the variation seemed rather limited and predictable on the basis of demographic factors (*e.g.*, the degree of urbanization). At the time attention centered on the striking international variation in cancer occurrence and the dramatic changes in risk among migrant populations that indicated the importance of environmental determinants (*2*), suggesting that a large fraction of cancer may be preventable. Although the variation in cancer occurrence within the U.S. was much smaller than the global differences, we wondered whether mapping cancer mortality using relatively small areas such as counties might help to identify unusual patterns or high-risk areas that would escape notice when larger geographic units were examined.

In planning this effort, we were impressed that many of the first clues to cancer etiology came from clinical observations of unusual case clusters that could be traced to a particular exposure. This was the situation, for example, with liver angiosarcoma related to vinyl chloride, mesothelioma to asbestos, and vaginal cancer to prenatal DES exposure. It was possible for alert clinicians to identify these clusters, because they involved tumors that were rare in the general population. The detection of clustering of the common tumors seemed to require a more systematic approach, which we thought might be taken using the county mortality system, particularly in view of the availability of U.S. mortality statistics over many years.

The Mapping Project

Our geographic studies involved a step-wise approach. After obtaining mortality data from the National Center for Health Statistics, and population data from the Census Bureau, we prepared a directory of age-adjusted rates for various cancers by sex and race at the county level for the 20-year period from 1950 through 1969 (*3*). Next, a series of computer-generated color-coded atlases were published, the first involving cancer mortality in the white population for the period of 1950–69 (*1*); the second reporting the corresponding patterns in the nonwhite population (*4*); and the third showing maps for non-neoplastic diseases, especially those related to cancer either by predisposition or by sharing of risk factors (*5*). While the directory of county-by-county rates may have seemed to be an ordinary compilation of cancer statistics, the visualization of geographic patterns by color mapping served to bring the information to life. The maps revealed a surprising number and variety of geographic patterns, including clusters of high-rate areas, or so-called "hot spots," which stimulated not only scientific interest but also public and political concern (*6, 7*).

A series of descriptive and correlational studies was undertaken to characterize the tumors in more detail and to generate hypotheses about possible risk factors. Next, in collaboration with other research groups, we embarked upon field studies in various parts of the country with unusually high mortality rates. These studies usually took the case-control approach in which individuals with and without a particular cancer were interviewed in an effort to uncover environmental or lifestyle factors that might be responsible for the high rates in certain areas (*8*).

Recently, we published an atlas updating the mortality data through 1980 for the white population, with emphasis on the changing distribution of cancer during the 30-year time span (*9*). For each form of cancer, maps were shown for three decades (1950s, 1960s, and 1970s) along with a trend map depicting the percent change in mortality over time. To obtain more stable numbers, we used state economic areas, which represent counties or groups of counties with similar sociodemographic characteristics. While most cancers showed a trend toward a more uniform distribution of rates, some new patterns emerged in the 1970s that have enhanced the opportunities for further research into cancer etiology. This report briefly reviews the patterns for selected cancers, using information from the new atlas, and suggests some explanations based on studies prompted by the earlier maps.

All Cancers

The maps for all cancers combined in males and females revealed consistently high rates in urban areas of the northeast and around the Great Lakes, and in southern Louisiana. In the trend map, the rates in other parts of the country have risen more rapidly, suggesting a more even geographic distribution of cancer. It is likely that this trend reflects an increasing homogeneity of American lifestyles, including smoking and dietary habits, although some effect may result from greater uniformity in diagnostic measures and standardization of death certificate practices, a wider distribution of improved medical care and survival rates, and greater mobility of the population.

Lung Cancer

The maps for lung cancer have attracted particular attention. Among males, the mortality rates in the 1950s and 1960s were high in urban areas of the north and in certain seaboard areas of the south, especially along the southeast Atlantic and Gulf coasts (Fig. 1). The excess in urbanized areas appeared consistent with patterns of smoking, although occupational exposures seemed involved to some extent. Case-control studies in coastal areas of Georgia (10), Virginia (11), and northeast Florida (12) revealed an elevated risk of lung cancer associated with shipbuilding, especially during World War II, with asbestos exposure appearing to be the major hazard. However, the risk was not limited to any single trade within the industry, such as insulators or pipecoverers, who actually handle asbestos. In some areas the risk affected men who worked a relatively brief period in plants that closed soon after the war. There was also a synergistic interaction between shipyard employment and tobacco smoking, with the risk for former shipyard workers who smoked heavily being 20 times higher than for non-smokers who had never been employed in the industry. This finding is consistent with the multiplicative effect characteristically observed when asbestos exposures are combined with smoking. The etiologic role of asbestos was also suggested by a parallel cluster of mesothelioma detected among residents of coastal Virginia, with three-fourths of the cases working in shipyards (13). Most were heavily exposed to asbestos as pipecoverers and insulators, but other trades with lighter exposures were reported also. It is interesting that among five women with mesothelioma in the area, four were married to shipyard workers, indicating the spread of asbestos beyond the workplace.

The high rates of lung cancer among males along the Gulf coast appear to

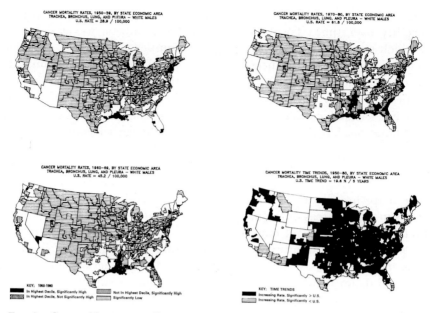

FIG. 1.   Geographic patterns of lung cancer mortality among white males, by decade and trend analysis according to state economic area, 1950–80.

have a different explanation. In a case-control study in southern Louisiana, there was an excess risk among the Cajun population, mainly due to smoking practices, including the heavy use of hand-rolled cigarettes (14). During the 1970s, the lung cancer rates declined in the northeast and became more pronounced in the south, both in rural and urban counties. Also, the high-rate cluster in Louisiana extended inland along the Mississippi River.

Among females, the rates for lung cancer have risen more sharply than in males, reflecting the accelerated use of cigarettes among women in the past 20 to 30 years. The maps for females shown in Fig. 2 were not remarkable until the 1970s when aggregations of high mortality were seen in Florida and along the mid-Atlantic and Pacific coasts, as the rates rose more rapidly in those areas than in the rest of the country. The contribution of smoking patterns to these geographic variations is suggested by the higher proportion of ever smokers and current smokers among female controls along the West Coast (e.g., Seattle and San Francisco) compared to other areas involved in our population-based case-control studies of certain cancers (e.g., the national bladder cancer study of 1977–78).

Nasal Cancer

Mortality rates for cancers of the nasal cavity and sinuses are about 1/100th of those for lung cancer, with no obvious clustering on the maps for either sex. Since an excess risk of nasal cancer had been reported among furniture makers in England but not in the U.S., we carried out a correlational study among the male population of furniture-industry counties. An elevated mortality from nasal cancer was found in these areas, while the rates for most other cancers were at or below expected values

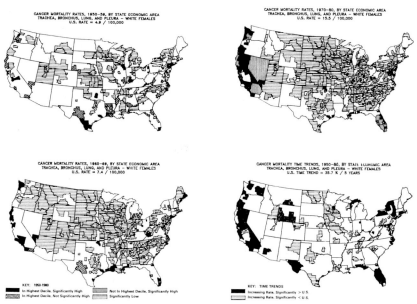

FIG. 2. Geographic patterns of lung cancer mortality among white females, by decade and trend analysis according to state economic area, 1950–80.

(15). This finding indicates the potential for correlational studies to detect occupational clustering not apparent on the maps. To pursue this lead, we conducted a case-control interview study of nasal cancer in the high-exposure areas of North Carolina and Virginia (16). Employment in the furniture industry was not associated with squamous cell carcinomas, but it increased the risk of the less common adenocarcinomas by 5-fold. In both sexes, heavy cigarette smokers showed a 2- to 3-fold excess risk, mainly for squamous cell cancers, the first time that smoking has been linked to cancer of the nasal passages. Among females, a 2-fold increased risk was associated with work in the textile industry, consistent with the results of other studies (17).

Oral Cancer

Special interest has centered on the maps for cancer of the oral cavity and pharynx. Among males, the rates were consistently high in the urban northeast and other metropolitan areas. This pattern appeared to correspond with levels of alcohol consumption and tobacco smoking, the major risk factors for this cancer. Preliminary results from a recent population-based case-control study indicate that the risks of oral-pharyngeal cancer among smokers and drinkers were multiplicative, rising to 35-fold among those who daily consumed two or more packs of cigarettes and more than four alcoholic drinks. Because of the large study size, it was possible to implicate smoking and drinking among subjects exposed to one but not the other factor. However, combined exposures to smoking and drinking were shown to account for about three-fourths of all oral-pharyngeal cancer in the U.S.

Among females, however, the rates for oral cancer were highest in rural counties of the south. In a case-control study conducted among North Carolina females, we found that the elevated rates could be explained by the long-standing habit of dipping snuff, *i.e.*, placing finely ground smokeless tobacco between the gum and cheek (*18*). The risk of oral cancer associated with the chronic use of snuff among non-smokers was 4-fold, but it reached nearly 50-fold for cancers arising on the gum and buccal mucosa, tissues in direct contact with the tobacco. The responsible carcinogen is unknown, but high levels of nitrosamines have been identified in snuff and in the saliva of snuff users. Because of concerns about the recent popularity of smokeless tobacco among young people in the U.S., the epidemiologic findings helped to stimulate public health and legislative measures to warn the public about the dangers of this habit and to regulate advertising practices.

In the 1970s, the rates of oral cancer among women declined somewhat in the rural south, while high-rate areas appeared along the Pacific and Florida coasts. This newly-emerging pattern resembles that for female lung cancer, suggesting the influence of cigarette smoking on both cancers.

Esophageal Cancer

Although alcohol potentiates the effects of tobacco smoke on cancers of the esophagus, oral cavity, and larynx, it is unclear why the risks for esophageal cancer in the U.S. are so much higher among blacks than whites, especially black males in urban areas. Their rates are especially high in Washington, D.C., exceeding the national level for black males by over 2-fold and for white males by 7-fold. In a case-control study in Washington, D.C., the dominant risk factor among black males was alcohol consumption, which overwhelmed a smaller influence of smoking (*19*). In addition, an effect was associated with nutritional deficiency, even after adjusting for alcohol intake and socioeconomic status (*20*). The dietary deficiency appeared broadly based and could not be narrowed down to any particular food class or micronutrient.

A cluster of high rates for esophageal cancer was also found among black men from the eastern part of South Carolina, especially in rural areas. Preliminary analysis suggests again that alcohol is the major factor, particularly the use of home-brewed (moonshine) whiskey, with dietary deficiencies contributing to the risk.

Stomach Cancer

The early maps for stomach cancer in males and females showed excessive mortality primarily in rural counties of the north central region, which appeared correlated with the concentration of high-risk ethnic groups from northern Europe (*21*). This cluster is less apparent in the 1970s. A similar aggregation in certain southwestern states seemed related to the excess risk among Hispanic groups. In a study in southern Louisiana, where the rates are particularly high in blacks, dietary factors were important. Higher risks were associated with the intake of smoked foods, homemade sausages and home-cured meats, while fruits and vitamin C appeared to be protective (*22*).

Colorectal Cancer

International correlations and migrant studies have suggested that dietary factors are important in the development of colon and rectal cancers. In the U.S., there is a north-south gradient of colon cancer, with rates in both sexes being about 50% higher in northern areas, partly due to the elevated risks of urban populations with high socioeconomic levels (*23*). The patterns for rectal cancer are similar, suggesting risk factors in common with colon cancer. It is interesting that lower rates in the south prevail even in areas attracting large numbers of retirees from the north. Is this a reversal of the pattern for colon and rectal cancers described among population groups migrating from low- to high-risk areas? Preliminary data from a case-control study in Florida retirement communities suggest there is no rapid reduction in risk of colorectal cancer, but the younger the age at migration, the lower the risk (*24*). Further research is needed to determine what aspect of the southern environment, lifestyle, or diet may be protective. It is noteworthy that the geographic differentials have diminished over time as more areas in the south display rising mortality rates than in the north.

Another opportunity for studying colon cancer is provided by an outlier from the usual geographic pattern, that is, a cluster of rural agricultural counties with high rates in eastern Nebraska (*25*). In a case-control study, the elevated risk of colon cancer was primarily among persons of Czechoslovakian background, an ethnic group predominating in the study area. High-fat diets, derived from meat and dairy products, and beer drinking appeared to contribute to the risk, but the numbers of subjects in our study were too small to draw firm conclusions.

Pancreas Cancer

For pancreas cancer, the amount of geographic variation was less evident than for most other tumors (*26*). Nevertheless, among males, clusters of high-rate areas were seen in the urban northeast and in Louisiana and the Mississippi delta area. A case-control study in Louisiana revealed elevated risks associated with smoking and also provided leads to dietary risk factors prevalent in the Cajun population (*27*). Most conspicuous were increased risks associated with the use of pork products and with deficiencies of fruit consumption.

Renal Cancer

Ethnic factors contributed also to the high death rates for kidney cancer in the north central parts of the U.S., although the geographic differential has declined over time as rates in the south have risen more rapidly than in the north. In Minnesota, a case-control study of renal adenocarcinoma, which comprises 85% of renal cancer, revealed an elevated risk associated with German or Scandinavian background (*28*). The ethnic associations seemed to be partly explained by dietary factors, as indicated by a high intake of traditional meat and pickled-smoked foods and by a relation to obesity, especially in females. In addition, cigarette smokers showed an excess risk of about 60% overall, surpassing 2-fold among heavy smokers. A parallel study of renal pelvis cancers in the area revealed a surprising 6- to 7-fold excess risk among cigarette smokers, reaching 11-fold among heavy smokers, plus increased risks related to certain occupational exposures (*e.g.*, coal or natural gas, mineral or cutting oils), and to heavy use of phenacetin-containing analgesic drugs (*29*).

Bladder Cancer

The distribution of bladder cancer was striking, with rates in males being particularly high in the northeast and in urban areas around the Great Lakes (*30*). A large case-control study in several parts of the U.S. suggested that 22% of the risk in males is attributable to occupational factors. In some areas, such as New Jersey, associations were found with chemical and petrochemical exposures (*31, 32*). A new finding was a significant 50% excess risk of bladder cancer in men employed as truck drivers or deliverymen, with a positive trend associated with increasing duration of employment (*33, 34*). Occupational risks were more pronounced in urban areas and extended to other groups exposed to motor exhausts, such as taxicab and bus drivers. This association is stimulating research to clarify whether components of motor exhausts, including nitro-polycyclic-aromatic-hydrocarbons (*e.g.*, nitro-pyrenes), are involved in bladder carcinogenesis.

In females, the maps for bladder cancer did not show the peculiarities seen in males, except for elevated rates in rural areas of New York and northern New England. Based on preliminary results from a case-control study in New Hampshire and Vermont, this pattern may result from work of both sexes in the textile and leather industries, where dyes containing aromatic amines were used.

Breast Cancer

The geographic patterns of breast cancer resembled those for colon cancer, with most low rates in the south and high rates in the northeast, especially in urban areas. Like colon cancer, the north-south differences have diminished over time, as rates have risen in many areas of the south, including rural areas of Appalachia. When the geographic patterns were analyzed by age group, only postmenopausal women (*i.e.*, 55+ years) showed a northern predominance, suggesting that environmental or lifestyle exposures have a greater impact at older ages, while the rates for premenopausal women (22–44 years) were distributed almost uniformly across the country (*35*).

Cervix Cancer

A pattern different from breast cancer was seen for cervical cancer. High rates were scattered throughout the south, with the heaviest concentration in Appalachia, which correlates with the tendency of this tumor to affect rural women in the lower socioeconomic classes (*36*). Rates in the north remained low except for parts of New England. Although mortality has declined substantially throughout the country, the rates in several midwestern states decreased less rapidly, so that in the 1970s a cluster of relatively high rates appeared in the midwest as well as Appalachia. Further studies are needed to clarify the origins and natural history of invasive cervical cancer in these areas, with emphasis on the impact of screening programs.

Prostate Cancer

Although geographic variation for prostate cancer is limited, some clustering of high-rate areas has persisted in the northeastern and north central states, particularly in rural areas. Over time, mortality has remained generally stable, except for some clustering of areas with rising rates in Florida and California. Correlational analyses have suggested that ethnic factors may influence the distribution of this cancer (37), but further investigation is needed into the origins of this common but poorly understood cancer.

Non-Hodgkin's Lymphoma

In both sexes, the rates for non-Hodgkin's lymphoma have been generally low in the south and elevated in various metropolitan centers and in coastal areas of California (38). Over time, there has been an upward trend in mortality rates, notably in central areas of the country. In Kansas, where high rates emerged among males in the 1970s, a case-control study indicated that men exposed to herbicides more than 20 days per year had a 6-fold increased risk of non-Hodgkin's lymphoma relative to non-farmers (39). The risk was elevated primarily among men exposed to phenoxyacetic acids (2-4, D), which are not likely to be contaminated by dioxin. Further studies are underway to clarify the risk of lymphoma among agricultural and other workers exposed to pesticides.

Skin Cancer

For melanoma in both sexes, a striking southern predominance has persisted over time, with high mortality rates mainly in the southeast and south central regions. This pattern is consistent with the effects of sunlight exposure on the distribution of melanoma (40). For other skin cancers, the mortality patterns are similar, despite the low case-fatality rates of basal and squamous cell carcinomas. Since non-melanoma skin cancers are not reported routinely to cancer registries, special surveys were conducted during the 1970s in conjunction with ground measurements of ultraviolet (UV) radiation. The gradient with UV exposure in the U.S. was steeper for squamous cell carcinoma than basal cell carcinoma, while the relation of melanoma incidence to UV exposure was less clear-cut (41). This pattern for melanoma is consistent with evidence suggesting that intermittent rather than chronic exposures are important, along with host-susceptibility factors including dysplastic nevi.

Comments

Since Percivall Pott described scrotal cancer among chimney sweeps in 1775, etiologic insights have often come from case clusters occurring in small groups of people. Since clustering of common tumors is not obvious through clinical experience, surveillance systems using routinely collected cancer statistics may be useful. Our experience suggests that aggregations of cancer on a small-area scale may provide leads to environmental or lifestyle risk factors, although one must be cautious about fluctuations in diagnosis, reporting, survival time, migration and mobility. While U.S. mortality statistics have the advantage of nationwide coverage for a substantial period of time, the patterns are less informative for cancers with favorable survival rates and problems in classification. More helpful in these instances are the population-based incidence data from the Surveillance, Epidemiology and End Results (SEER) program of NCI (*42*). Although the SEER program provides information on about 12% of the U.S. population since the early 1970s, the patterns of cancer incidence and survival complement the mortality data and greatly expand the opportunities for epidemiologic study.

Publication of the U.S. cancer maps in the 1970s was soon followed by similar atlases from several other countries. Most remarkable have been the cancer maps of China (*43*), which have stimulated a number of analytical studies in high-risk areas, including intervention trials to evaluate the preventive impact of vitamin and mineral supplementation for certain cancers (*e.g.*, of the esophagus). Recently, in Scandinavian countries where national cancer registries are located, atlases based on incidence data have been useful in identifying high-risk communities, particularly for tumors that are not well represented in mortality statistics.

Although clinicians and experimentalists have long provided important leads for epidemiological testing, the atlases from various countries illustrate the value of developing national statistical resources as surveillance systems to generate and explore hypotheses about the causes of cancer and other diseases as well. In recently updating the U.S. cancer maps, we also found utility in the periodic monitoring of geographic patterns. Although spatial variations for particular tumors usually persist over time, there has been a tendency toward greater uniformity of rates around the country, so that opportunities to pursue existing geographic leads should not be delayed. Most intriguing are the new high-risk areas appearing for certain cancers (*e.g.*, lung and oral cavity in females, non-Hodgkin's lymphoma in males), which also deserve prompt investigation in hopes of detecting and controlling emergent carcinogenic hazards.

REFERENCES

1.   Mason, T. J., McKay, F. W., Hoover, R., Blot, W. J., and Fraumeni, J. F., Jr. Atlas of Cancer Mortality for U.S. Counties: 1950–69, DHEW publ. No. (NIH) 75–780, U.S. Government Printing Office, Washington, D.C., 1975.

2.   Haenszel, W. M. and Kurihara, M. Studies of Japanese migrants. I. Mortality from cancer and other diseases among Japanese in the United States. J. Natl. Cancer Inst., *40*: 43–68, 1968.

3. Mason, T. J. and McKay, F. W. U.S. Cancer Mortality by County: 1950–1969, DHEW publ. No. (NIH) 74–615, U.S. Government Printing Office, Washington, D.C., 1974.

4. Mason, T. J., McKay, F. W., Hoover, R., Blot, W. J., and Fraumeni, J. F., Jr. Atlas of Cancer Mortality among U.S. Nonwhites: 1950–69, DHEW publ. No. (NIH) 76–1204, U.S. Government Printing Office, Washington, D.C., 1976.

5. Mason, T. J., Fraumeni, J. F., Jr., Hoover, R., and Blot, W. J. An Atlas of Mortality from Selected Diseases, DHEW publ. No. (NIH) 81–2397, U.S. Government Printing Office, Washington, D.C., 1981.

6. Blot, W. J. and Fraumeni, J. F., Jr. Geographic epidemiology of cancer in the United States. In: D. Schottenfeld and J. F. Fraumeni, Jr. (eds.), Cancer Epidemiology and Prevention, pp. 179–193, W. B. Saunders, Philadelphia, 1982.

7. Fraumeni, J. F., Jr. The face of cancer in the United States. Hosp. Practice, 18: 81–96, 1983.

8. Fraumeni, J. F., Jr. Etiologic clues from cancer mapping in the United States. Gann Monogr. Cancer Res., 33: 171–179, 1987.

9. Pickle, L. W., Mason, T. J., Howard, N., Hoover, R., and Fraumeni, J. F., Jr. Atlas of U.S. Cancer Mortality among Whites: 1950–1980, DHHS publ. No. (NIH) 87–2900, U.S. Government Printing Office, Washington, D.C., 1987.

10. Blot, W. J., Harrington, J. M., Toledo, A., Hoover, R., Heath, C. W., Jr., and Fraumeni, J. F., Jr. Lung cancer after employment in shipyards during World War II. N. Engl. J. Med., 299: 620–624, 1978.

11. Blot, W. J., Morris, L. E., Stroube, R., Tagnon, I., and Fraumeni, J. F., Jr. Lung and laryngeal cancers in relation to shipyard employment in coastal Virginia. J. Natl. Cancer Inst., 65: 571–575, 1980.

12. Blot, W. J., Davies, J. E., Brown, L. M., Nordwall, C. W., Buiatti, E., Ng, A., and Fraumeni, J. F., Jr. Occupation and the high risk of lung cancer in northeast Florida. Cancer, 50: 364–371, 1982.

13. Tagnon, I., Blot, W. J., Stroube, R. B., Day, N. E., Morris, L. E., Peace, B. B., and Fraumeni, J. F., Jr. Mesothelioma associated with the shipbuilding industry in coastal Virginia. Cancer Res., 40: 3875–3879, 1980.

14. Pickle, L. W., Correa, P., and Fontham, E. Recent case-control studies of lung cancer in the United States. In: M. Mizell and P. Correa (eds.), Lung Cancer: Causes and Prevention, pp. 101–115, Verlag Chemie International, Inc., Deerfield Beach, Fla., 1984.

15. Brinton, L. A., Stone, B. J., Blot, W. J., and Fraumeni, J. F., Jr. Nasal cancer in U.S. furniture industry counties. Lancet, 2: 628, 1976.

16. Brinton, L. A., Blot, W. J., Becker, J. A., Winn, D. M., Browder, J. P., Farmer, J. C., Jr., and Fraumeni, J. F., Jr. A case-control study of cancers of the nasal cavity and paranasal sinuses. Am. J. Epidemiol., 119: 896–901, 1984.

17. Brinton, L. A., Blot, W. J., and Fraumeni, J. F., Jr. Nasal cancer in the textile and clothing industries. Br. J. Ind. Med., 42: 469–474, 1985.

18. Winn, D. M., Blot, W. J., Shy, C. M., Pickle, L. W., Toledo, A., and Fraumeni, J. F., Jr. Snuff dipping and oral cancer among women in the southern United States. N. Engl. J. Med., 304: 745–749, 1981.

19. Pottern, L. M., Morris, L. E., Blot, W. J., Ziegler, R. G., and Fraumeni, J. F., Jr. Esophageal cancer among black men in Washington, D. C. I. Alcohol, tobacco, and other risk factors. J. Natl. Cancer Inst., 67: 777–783, 1981.

20. Ziegler, R. G., Morris, L. E., Blot, W. J., Pottern, L. M., Hoover, R., and Fraumeni, J. F., Jr. Esophageal cancer among black men in Washington, D. C. II. Role of nu-

trition. J. Natl. Cancer Inst., *67*: 1199–1206, 1981.

21. Hoover, R. N., Mason, T. J., McKay, F. W., and Fraumeni, J. F., Jr. Cancer by county: New resource for etiologic clues. Science, *189*: 1005–1007, 1975.

22. Correa, P., Fontham, E., Pickle, L. W., Chen, V., Lin, X., and Haenszel, W. Dietary determinants of gastric cancer in southern Louisiana inhabitants. J. Natl. Cancer Inst., *75*: 645–654, 1985.

23. Blot, W. J., Fraumeni, J. F., Jr., Stone, B. J., and McKay, F. W. Geographic patterns of large bowel cancer in the United States. J. Natl. Cancer Inst., *57*: 1225–1231, 1976.

24. Ziegler, R. G., Devesa, S. S., and Fraumeni, J. F., Jr. Epidemiologic patterns of colorectal cancer. *In;* V. T. DeVita, Jr., S. Hellman, and A. S. Rosenberg (eds.), Important Advances in Oncology 1986, pp. 209–232, J. B. Lippincott, Philadelphia, 1986.

25. Pickle, L. W., Greene, M. H., Ziegler, R. G., Toledo, A., Hoover, R., Lynch, H. T., and Fraumeni, J. F., Jr. Colorectal cancer in rural Nebraska. Cancer Res., *44*: 363–369, 1984.

26. Blot, W. J., Fraumeni, J. F., Jr., and Stone, B. J. Geographic correlates of pancreas cancer in the United States. Cancer, *42*: 373–380, 1978.

27. Falk, R. T., Pickle, L. W., Fontham, E. T., Correa, P., and Fraumeni, J. F., Jr. Lifestyle risk factors for pancreatic cancer in Louisiana: A case-control study. Am. J. Epidemiol., in press.

28. McLaughlin, J. K., Mandel, J. S., Blot, W. J., Schuman, L. M., Mehl, E. S., and Fraumeni, J. F., Jr. A population-based case-control study of renal cell carcinoma. J. Natl. Cancer Inst., *72*: 275–284, 1984.

29. McLaughlin, J. K., Blot, W. J., Mandel, J. S., Schuman, L. M., Mehl, E. S., and Fraumeni, J. F., Jr. Etiology of cancer of renal pelvis. J. Natl. Cancer Inst., *71*: 287–291, 1983.

30. Blot, W. J. and Fraumeni, J. F., Jr. Geographic patterns of bladder cancer in the United States. J. Natl. Cancer Inst., *61*: 1017–1023, 1978.

31. Schoenberg, J. B., Stemhagen, A., Mogielnicki, A. P., Altman, R., Abe, T., and Mason, T. J. Case-control study of bladder cancer in New Jersey. I. Occupational exposures in white males. J. Natl. Cancer Inst., *72*: 973–981, 1984.

32. Zahm, S. H., Hartge, P., and Hoover, R. The national bladder cancer study: Employment in the chemical industry. J. Natl. Cancer Inst., *79*: 217–222, 1987.

33. Silverman, D. T., Hoover, R. N., Albert, S., and Graff, K. M. Occupation and cancer of the lower urinary tract in Detroit. J. Natl. Cancer Inst., *70*: 237–245, 1983.

34. Silverman, D. T., Hoover, R. N., Mason, T. J., and Swanson, G. M. Motor exhaust-related occupations and bladder cancer. Cancer Res., *46*: 2113–2116, 1986.

35. Blot, W. J., Fraumeni, J. F., Jr., and Stone, B. J. Geographic patterns of breast cancer in the United States. J. Natl. Cancer Inst., *59*: 1407–1411, 1977.

36. Hoover, R., Mason, T. J., McKay, F. W., and Fraumeni, J. F., Jr. Geographic patterns of cancer mortality in the United States. *In;* J. F. Fraumeni, Jr. (ed.), Persons at High Risk of Cancer: An Approach to Cancer Etiology and Control, pp. 343–360, Academic Press, New York, 1975.

37. Blair, A. and Fraumeni, J. F., Jr. Geographic patterns of prostate cancer in the United States. J. Natl. Cancer Inst., *61*: 1379–1384, 1978.

38. Cantor, K. P. and Fraumeni, J. F., Jr. Distribution of non-Hodgkin's lymphoma in the United States between 1950 and 1975. Cancer Res., *40*: 2645–2652, 1980.

39. Hoar, S. K., Blair, A., Holmes, F. F., Boysen, C. D., Robel, R. J., Hoover, R., and Fraumeni, J. F., Jr. Agricultural herbicide use and risk of lymphoma and soft-tissue

sarcoma. JAMA, *256*: 1141–1147, 1986.

40. Scotto, J., Fears, T. R., and Fraumeni, J. F., Jr. Solar radiation. *In;* D. Schottenfeld and J. F. Fraumeni, Jr. (eds.), Cancer Epidemiology and Prevention, pp. 254–276, W. B. Saunders, Philadelphia, 1982.

41. Scotto, J. and Fraumeni, J. F., Jr. Skin (other than melanoma). *In;* D. Schottenfeld and J. F. Fraumeni, Jr. (eds.), Cancer Epidemiology and Prevention, pp. 996–1011, W. B. Saunders, Philadelphia, 1982.

42. Young, J. L., Jr., Percy, C. L., Asire, A. J., Berg, J. W., Cusano, M. M., Gloeckler, L. A., Horm, J. W., Lourie, W. I., Jr., Pollack, E. S., and Shambaugh, E. M. Cancer incidence and mortality in the United States 1973–77. Natl. Cancer Inst. Monogr., *57*: 1–5, 1981.

43. Li, J. Y., Liu, B. Q., Li, G. Y., Chen, Z. J., Sun, X. D., and Rong, S. D. Atlas of cancer mortality in the People's Republic of China: An aid for cancer control and research. Int. J. Epidemiol., *10*: 127–133, 1981.

UNUSUAL OCCURRENCES AS CLUES TO CANCER ETIOLOGY, R. W. MILLER ET AL. (EDS.),
JAPAN SCI. SOC. PRESS, TOKYO/TAYLOR & FRANCIS, LTD., PP. 27–35, 1988

Investigation of Cancer Case Clusters: Possibilities and Limitations

Clark W. Heath, Jr.

South Carolina Department of Health and Environmental Control, Columbia, South Carolina 29201, U.S.A.

Abstract: Discovery of meaningful biologic events through investigation of individual cancer case clusters is limited by the greater likelihood that any given cluster, otherwise unspecified, will be a random event and by restrictions arising from the necessarily retrospective nature of any studies undertaken. In the face of long and variable latencies, it is difficult to document potential oncogenic exposures and to estimate dosage. Since case numbers are usually small, statistical assessments may have only limited value. This, however, encourages greater attention to be given to case features and clinical details from which patterns of case associations within clusters can occasionally be seen. When similar epidemiologic case patterns are repeatedly encountered in different cluster situations (as was apparent with parish and school associations, reviewed here, in several communities in the United States), some biologic basis for such case clustering may be suspected. Similar suspicions are aroused when additional cases of rare cancer are observed in community settings to which case clustering has already drawn attention.

The earliest account of a cancer case cluster, as far as I am aware, appeared in 1890 in the German literature (*1*). The report described two cases of acute leukemia in Kiev, Russia. The first case was a 17 year old boy whose illness began in February 1889 and who died a month later. The second case was a 32 year old man who worked as a hospital ward attendant and who helped to provide hospital care for the first patient. This man became ill in late April 1889, two months after the onset of the first case, and he died two weeks later. Both cases ran similar fulminant courses with bleeding, fever, and rapidly enlarging spleens. The blood of each must have been plainly leukemic to the naked eye (the principal form of leukemia then recognizable). White cell counts exceeded 300,000 cells per cubic mm., as gauged by white cell/red cell volume ratios of 1/7 and 1/9. The author of the report speculated about infectious causation, given the time-space closeness of the two cases and the apparent similarity between leukemic leukemia and leukocytosis.

From that beginning, there have developed over ensuing years, and especially since 1960, a great variety of observations, methodologies and speculations, all under the general rubric of "case clustering." The field is no longer the domain just of leukemia and cancer, but it encompasses other conditions such as chronic neurologic disorders and birth defects, conditions where causes are obscure and latency is often variable. The focus of etiologic concern has also expanded. From a principal interest in infectious agents, attention has increasingly shifted, since the early 1970's, to chemical and physical environmental causes.

At the same time, the field has come to involve not merely time-space closeness but forms of case clustering defined by other parameters of closeness: time only, space only, or case features quite independent of time and space. A prominent example of non-time/non-space clustering was the reported instance of Hodgkin disease occurring in persons who attended school together but who only later, at different times and places, developed tumor (2).

As clinical-epidemiologic descriptions of particular case clusters have appeared, they have soon been followed by statistical efforts, often entire statistical methodologies, to define the extent to which case clustering may occur beyond chance expectation within differing parameters of case closeness (3–8). The results of these statistical studies have, on the whole, shown little if any general tendency for cancer cases, and leukemia/lymphoma cases in particular, to come in clusters. However, since such assessments may not always detect clustering in disease settings where etiology is known and where some form of case aggregation is predictable (infectious diseases especially), interest continues in studying case clusters as a possible source of etiologic information.

In this paper, I wish to focus not on the statistical aspects of cluster assessment, but on the clinical-epidemiologic process of assessing individual time-space clusters, how such assessments may yield biologic clues, and where their limitations lie. To do this I shall describe and comment upon a selection of individual case cluster studies with which I was concerned between 1960 and 1975 in work with colleagues in the U.S. Public Health Services (Centers for Disease Control). For most of that time, a major mission was to help in national efforts to learn more about possible infectious or viral causes of leukemia. Field investigations of varying intensity were conducted in a wide variety of case cluster situations, perhaps 20 or 30 a year. The majority of these concerned leukemia or lymphoma among children. Our conscious decision to focus on childhood disease was based on the greater epidemiologic simplicity of childhood events as well as presumptions of shorter and hence more well defined latency.

More often than not, the case clusters we examined showed no particular epidemiologic features to distinguish the cases involved from non-clustered cases, other than their mere time-space closeness. Those occasional situations which did attract our particular interest, however, seem now in retrospect to have displayed one or more of three qualities:

1. The cases involved shared epidemiologic features which could not reasonably be expected of randomly selected cases and which seemed compatible with biologically meaningful etiologic ideas;

2. Epidemiologic features were similar to those observed in studies of earlier clusters; and

3. Excessive local incidence of disease continued after epidemiologic investigations began.

Epidemiologic Associations

The 1960 study of childhood leukemia occurrence in Niles, Illinois, illustrates the finding of shared case features beyond mere time-space closeness (9). In this suburban town (population about 20,000), eight cases of childhood leukemia occurred over a three-year span (1957–60). This number of cases represented about a five-fold increase above expected incidence and above rates observed at the same time in neighboring towns. Beyond excess incidence for the town as a whole, however, investigation revealed that seven of the eight cases were from Roman Catholic families belonging to the town's principal Catholic parish. Three of these seven patients were students at the parish school at the time of illness onset, and the remaining four had one or more older siblings attending that school. Survey information showed that 59% of children in the town were from families belonging to the parish, and 33% were from families with one or more children attending the school. Three public grade schools and two junior high schools served the community.

Case occurrence seemed also linked to an unusual pattern of rheumatic-like illness diagnosed at the same time in parish school children. One of these patients later developed Hodgkin disease. In addition, investigation of other causes of childhood mortality in the town showed an excess in neonatal deaths caused by various forms of congenital heart disease.

The association with rheumatic illness, coupled with an apparently discrete clustering of case onsets within two particular school years (1957–8 and 1959–60) suggested some form of short-latency infectious etiology. To explore this idea further, we conducted a questionnaire survey regarding past childhood illness experience in the community. The survey suggested some disparity in infectious incidence over the years between parish-school-associated children and other children, particularly with respect to chickenpox, measles and rubella in 1956 (this being in the days before widespread immunization against childhood infections). Survey results, however, were obviously limited by the small size of the population and by their retrospective nature, and so the idea that common infections might trigger leukemic illness in particular settings remained theoretical. A later statistical study in North Carolina based on age, seasonality and sibling sequences, proposed a similar mechanism with respect to the etiology of childhood lymphocytic leukemia (10). Here again, however, small case numbers limited pursuit of the concept.

Recurrent Epidemiologic Patterns

Finding the same epidemiologic case pattern in one case cluster that was seen earlier in another is a further type of evidence which encourages particular attention to be given to a particular cluster. Following the observation in Niles, Illinois, of cases focused on a particular community school, several later cluster investigations elsewhere yielded similar findings. Four of these studies are summarized below as examples.

Kendall Park, New Jersey: In this residential community (population about 10,000), six cases of acute leukemia were observed in persons under age 20 over a 13 year period (1957–69; expected incidence about two cases). All of the four most recent cases (three in 1968 and one in 1965) occurred in Roman Catholic families from which one or more children attended the community's one parochial parish school. About a third of the community were Catholic. The community was served in all by four elementary schools: the parochial school, enrolling about 500 students, and three public schools enrolling about 1,500. Two additional childhood cases were recognized in former residents of the community, one diagnosed in 1968 and the other in early 1969. Both families belonged to the Catholic parish and had children attending the parish school at the time when they lived in the town. One of the cases occurred in a child with Down syndrome. These two families had moved from the community 30 and 31 months prior to onset of leukemic symptoms. The majority of cases were between one and six years of age (six of eight). Various social relationships existed among some of the families but none seemed to link all or most of the cases except for the recent association with the particular parish and school. No other unusual disease patterns were identified in the course of the community investigation.

Middletown, Connecticut: From 1950 through 1969, eight cases of acute leukemia occurred in children in this town of about 32,000 residents. Although this overall incidence was not increased over what might be expected for childhood leukemia/lymphomas in a town this large (about 9 cases, age 0–14), the three most recent cases were diagnosed over a six month period in 1969, and all six cases since 1957 had occurred in families belonging to one of five Roman Catholic parishes in the town. The town as a whole was about 40% Catholic. Three of the five parishes were geographically based (including the parish with which recent case occurrence was associated), and all three were about equal in terms of population and geography. The six cases since 1957, therefore, had appeared in a population subset which accounted for only about 10% of the total community (expected incidence about 0.5 case). One additional childhood acute leukemia case was recognized in a family which had moved from the town a year before their child became ill. That family was Catholic and had lived in the same parish area with the same parish affiliations as the other six case families. Incidence of other childhood tumors in the town was also reviewed. The only two cases identified (cases of hepatoblastoma and Wilms' tumor diagnosed in 1967 and 1969) both occurred in Roman Catholic families living in the same parish area as the leukemia cases and attending the same parish.

Beyond the association of childhood cancer with the particular parish, it was striking that the three most recent cases of leukemia had occurred in children who were attending the same public elementary school at their time of diagnosis. That school was one of two serving the particular parish area, and one of nine overall in the town (one parochial and eight public). Each school enrolled about 500 students. No unusual patterns were noted in a review of adult leukemia/lymphoma incidence in the town.

Dubois, Pennsylvania: Three cases of lymphoma were diagnosed in young boys (ages 7, 11 and 14) over a six month period in the winter and spring of 1969–70 in this small western Pennsylvania town (population about 10,000) (Table 1). Review of childhood cancer incidence since 1960 identified only one other case, acute leu-

TABLE 1. Leukemia and Lymphoma, Age 0–19, Dubois, Pennsylvania, 1960–1970

Case characteristics	Case number			
	1	2	3	4
Age at diagnosis, race, sex	14WF	14WM	7WM	11WM
Date of symptom onset	June 1964	July 1969	January 1970	March 1970
Date of diagnosis	January 1965	November 1969	January 1970	April 1970
Diagnosis	Acute stem cell leukemia	Reticulum cell sarcoma	Lymphosarcoma progressing to acute lymphatic leukemia	Lymphosarcoma with marrow infiltration
Family church affiliation	Lutheran	St. Catherine	St. Catherine	St. Catherine
School attendance at onset	Public school	Public school (St. Catherine 1966–1967)	St. Catherine	St. Catherine
History of chickenpox	Unknown	Unknown	Sibs, spring 1970; not patient	Patient and sibs, Dec. 1963 and Dec. 1969

kemia in a 14 year old girl diagnosed in 1965. Overall, for this 11 year period, these four cases about equalled expected incidence of childhood leukemia/lymphoma for the town. The obvious clustering of cases in 1969–70, however, together with certain clinical and epidemiologic features of these three most recent cases, made the situation unusual. Of the three recent cases, the first was diagnosed as reticulum cell sarcoma, the second as mediastinal lymphosarcoma progressing to acute leukemia, and the third as mediastinal lymphosarcoma with bone marrow infiltration.

Epidemiologically, the three recent cases were found all to have occurred in Roman Catholic families which belonged to one of three parishes in the Dubois area. The town's population was about 25% Catholic, of whom about 60% attended that one parish. The two most recent patients also attended the parish parochial school at the time of their illness onsets, one in second grade, the other in sixth grade. The third patient had attended that same school three years before. The town and its surrounding school district contain a total of 20 elementary and junior high schools. The parish school attended by the two most recent patients enrolled about 300 students, and all other schools about 5,000 students.

Of particular note was the observation that during the school year (1969–70) in which the three recent cases were diagnosed, a sizable chickenpox epidemic occurred in many of the Dubois area schools, coinciding with the onset of illness in the two most recent cases. A questionnaire survey in the school district during the following school year indicated that this epidemic was particularly severe in the parish school and that cases there tended to occur early in the epidemic (during the late fall of 1969) rather than in the more usual pattern of late winter and early spring.

Of the two most recent lymphoma patients, the first had not had chickenpox before and did not develop the disease during the epidemic, although his two younger siblings did, albeit late in the epidemic after their brother's lymphoma was diagnosed. The second patient, together with his four siblings, had typical varicella in late December 1969, some three months before the onset of symptoms related to his lymphoma. This event was distinctly unusual since the patient and his three older siblings had already been well documented by history to have had chickenpox six years before.

Orange, Texas: In 1960, three cases of acute leukemia were diagnosed in two to three year old children living in this small southeastern Texas city (population about 25,000) (*11*). Expected incidence was estimated at about 0.4 case per year for children under age 15; these three cases were the only ones diagnosed in children in the town from 1956 through 1961. All three patients lived in the same residential area about a half mile apart, but without any apparent links in community activities. Of particular concern in the town was the occurrence at the same time of a cluster of births associated with congenital heart disease. Six such infants were born to Orange residents between December 1960 and October 1961. Their diagnoses included a variety of complex abnormalities of septa, chambers and great vessels, with or without tracheo-esophageal fistulae and other organ abnormalities. The father of one of these babies was found to have chronic granulocytic leukemia in October 1961. The six birth defect families lived scattered throughout the town. No links with the leukemia families were found with respect to community affiliations or activities.

This association of a childhood leukemia case cluster with a congenital heart disease cluster in the same community at the same time was of course reminiscent of the earlier observations made in Niles, Illinois. Similarly, the observations regarding school and parish affiliations among cases in Kendall Park, Middletown and Dubois also remind one of case features in Niles. In a general sense such findings, coupled with suggestive associations in Niles regarding childhood infection patterns, and more specifically so regarding chickenpox occurrence in Dubois, raise the idea that acute communicable disease patterns within community subpopulations may on occasion relate etiologically to childhood cancer occurrence.

Continued Excess Case Occurrence

The third type of observation in cluster studies which can particularly suggest that the observed clustering may have a biologic basis is the obvious one whereby the disease in question continues to appear in the population under study with the same unusual frequency or pattern that has already been observed. An obvious and dramatic example of such recurrent cancer patterns was the continued appearance of hepatic angiosarcoma in vinyl chloride polymerization workers in Louisville, Kentucky (*12*). Occasionally, but not often, this sort of continued observation has been made in studies of community cancer clusters. To a limited degree this was studied in a followup investigation regarding the Niles, Illinois, situation, although sustained case surveillance in that small suburban community, where urban medical care pat-

TABLE 2.   Leukemia and Lymphoma, Age 0–19, Niles, Illinois, 1956–1969

Community segment	Number of cases			
	1956–1961		1962–1969	
	Observed	Expected	Observed	Expected
Parish families[a]	8	0.6	4	1.0
All other families	1	1.4	5	2.9
Total	9	2.0	9	3.9

[a] Families attending the parish church and with children attending the parish school.

terns are complex and populations are mobile, was difficult. Data were assembled from mortality and hospital sources through 1969, and case family interviews were conducted to determine community affiliations. Nine cases of leukemia/lymphoma occurred in Niles residents under age 20 from 1962 through 1969 (Table 2). Four of these cases (two cases of acute lymphocytic leukemia and two Hodgkin disease) occurred in families which belonged to the parish and used the parish school, and five were in other town groups (three acute lymphocytic leukemia and one lympho-sarcoma). From estimates of changes in population sizes within the community over this time period, it was estimated that these cases represented about a two-fold increase over expected incidence overall, with the excess being somewhat greater in the parish group (an observed-expected ratio of 4.0) than in the remainder. This suggestion of continued excess childhood cancer occurrence in the parish group is of course limited by the small numbers involved and the underlying difficulty of data collection.

Winchester, Virginia: A clear example of continued disease occurrence in a case cluster setting is provided by observations made regarding cases of Burkitt tumor which were diagnosed during the early 1970's in the northwestern Virginia town of Winchester (*13*). In September 1971, two such cases were diagnosed in that town in young boys age 15 and nine. Both cases presented as peri-tonsillar tumors with symptom onset a month earlier. The two boys lived on the same street three houses apart in a new subdivision. They were not acquainted and did not share community activities, despite living close together. Over the five year period 1967–71, six other cases of childhood leukemia/lymphoma were diagnosed in the town (four acute leukemia and two reticulum cell sarcoma). These cases showed no spatial clustering and no associations with the two Burkitt tumors, although they represented a distinctly greater number than expected incidence (2.6 cases). In September 1975 a third case of Burkitt tumor was diagnosed in another young boy (age 8) who lived in the same subdivision as the two earlier patients, although about a half mile away. The child's illness began with pharyngitis in late July 1975 and was followed by a persistent and enlarging cervical mass. There were no known community contacts with the two earlier cases or their families. All three boys had attended the same neighborhood school, but at quite different times. Antibodies against Epstein-Barr virus were present in low titer in one boy but absent in another.

Recurrence of this rare tumor in this small community after attention was drawn to the initial case cluster strongly suggests that the sequence of events represents more than just a chance case aggregation. What the underlying biologic process might be is unclear, beyond the sense that it may belong in the area of acute infectious agents. Soon after Burkitt tumor came to be widely recognized in Africa, reports of time-space clustering among such cases in Uganda were not uncommon, and this seemed to be a distinct feature of the disease (*14, 15*). Later, however, evidence of clustering became increasingly difficult to confirm, especially in other parts of Africa (*16, 17*). The reason for this discrepancy in epidemiologic behavior remains unclear.

Limitations

The investigation of individual cancer clusters is obviously an inefficient process. By whatever parameters clustering is judged—time-space clustering or otherwise—it is obvious that chance aggregations occur. Since, with the possible exception of Burkitt tumor, not much tendency for clustering beyond chance levels can be expected, it follows that most case clusters investigated will be of the chance variety unless some process of selection is applied. It seems logical therefore to give preference to rare and homogeneous diagnoses as well as to case groups in young persons where latencies may be shorter and epidemiologic variables less diverse.

Even where one encounters a cluster that appears to have biologically meaningful features, the severely retrospective nature of the investigation, given long and variable latencies, will almost always leave one in a position where one can only hypothesize, but rarely demonstrate, an underlying biologic process. Where questions of environmental chemical or radiation exposure are raised, and particularly in the face of the intense public concern which such issues arouse, there is often the temptation to read more into potential exposures than may really exist, both in terms of extent of exposure and in terms of dosage. At best, such case investigations can only raise hypotheses. It is not clear that any such hypotheses have as yet been convincingly established, at least from the viewpoint of time-space cancer clustering in communities.

The numerical aspects of cluster investigations are also frustrating since, almost by definition, small case numbers are involved. The role of statistical assessment is therefore limited, especially in the face of the usual self-selection which governs cluster recognition and which curtails the traditional process of testing for statistical significance. This does, however, encourage greater reliance on close clinical and epidemiologic investigation of individual cases. Conceivably, this may be a blessing in disguise since the true promise of cluster studies, limited though they are in overall potential, may well lie in the degree to which clear and detailed observations can be made regarding the particular cases which make up the cluster.

ACKNOWLEDGMENTS

I wish to express appreciation to the following medical-epidemiologic colleagues for their help over the years in investigating the various cluster situations discussed in this paper: Thomas M. Brown, Jr., Glyn G. Caldwell, Shanklin B. Cannon, Ronald H. Goldenson, Charles M. Janeway, Joel A. Krackow, John M. Leonard, Peter McPhedran, Dennis M. O'Connor, Jeffrey G. Rosenstock, James M. Veasey and Leo Zelkowitz.

REFERENCES

1. Obrastzow. Zwei Fälle von acuter Leukämie. Deutsche Med. Woch., *16*: 1150–1153, 1890.
2. Vianna, N. J., Greenwald, P., Brady, J., Polan, A. K., Dwork, A., Mauro, J., and Davies, J. N. Hodgkin's disease: cases with features of a community outbreak. Ann. Intern. Med., *77*: 169–180, 1972.
3. Knox, G. Epidemiology of childhood leukaemia in Northumberland and Durham. Br. J. Prev. Soc. Med., *18*: 17–24, 1964.
4. Mantel, N. The detection of disease clustering and a generalized regression approach. Cancer Res., *27*: 209–220, 1967.
5. Evatt, B. L., Chase, G. A., and Heath, C. W., Jr. Time-space clustering among cases of acute leukemia in two Georgia counties. Blood, *41*: 265–272, 1973.

6. Smith, P. G. and Pike, M. C. Case clustering in Hodgkin's disease: a brief review of the present position and report of current work in Oxford. Cancer Res., *34*: 1156–1160, 1974.

7. Zack, M. M., Jr., Heath, C. W., Jr., Andrews, M. D., Grivas, A. S., and Christine, B. W. High school contact among persons with leukemia and lymphoma. J. Natl. Cancer Inst., *59*: 1343–1349, 1977.

8. Greenwald, P., Rose, J. S., and Daitch, P. B. Acquaintance networks among leukemia and lymphoma patients. Amer. J. Epidemiol., *110*: 162–177, 1979.

9. Heath, C. W., Jr. and Hasterlik, R. J. Leukemia among children in a suburban community. Am. J. Med., *34*: 796–812, 1963.

10. Spiers, P. S. and Quade, D. On the question of an infectious process in the origin of childhood leukemia. Biometrics, *26*: 723–738, 1970.

11. Heath, C. W., Jr., Manning, M. D., and Zelkowitz, L. Case clusters in the occurrence of leukaemia and congenital malformations. Lancet, *2*: 136–137, 1964.

12. Creech, J. L., Jr. and Johnson, M. N. Angiosarcoma of liver in the manufacture of polyvinyl chloride. J. Occup. Med., *16*: 150–151, 1974.

13. Levine, P. H., Sandler, S. G., Komp, D. M., O'Conor, G. T., and O'Connor, D. M. Simultaneous occurrence of "American Burkitt's Lymphoma" in neighbors. New Engl. J. Med., *288*: 562–563, 1973.

14. Pike, M. C., Williams, E. H., and Wright, B. Burkitt's tumour in the West Nile District of Uganda 1961–5. Br. Med. J., *2*: 395–399, 1967.

15. Morrow, R. H., Pike, M. C., and Smith, P. C. Burkitt's lymphoma: a time-space cluster of cases in Bwamba County of Uganda. Br. Med. J., *1*: 491–492, 1971.

16. Brown, T. M., Jr. and Heath, C. W., Jr. Time-space clustering among cases of Burkitt's tumor. Cancer Res., *34*: 1216–1218, 1974.

17. Siemiatycki, J., Brubaker, G., and Geser, A. Space-time clustering of Burkitt's lymphoma in East Africa: analysis of recent data and a new look at old data. Int. J. Cancer, *25*: 197–203, 1980.

CHEMICALS AND RADIATION

Vinyl Chloride-induced Hepatic Angiosarcoma

Henry FALK

Centers for Disease Control, Center for Environmental Health and Injury Control, Atlanta, Georgia 30333, U.S.A.

Abstract: In early 1974, an alert plant physician reported the occurrence of several cases of the otherwise rare hepatic angiosarcoma (HAS) at a single polyvinyl chloride (PVC) production facility in Louisville, Kentucky (U.S.A.). Upon further investigation, the relative risk for HAS at this plant appeared to be approximately 5,000, strongly indicating a causal relationship with some factor at the plant. Epidemiologic studies at this and other PVC polymerization plants identified vinyl chloride monomer (VCM) as the causative agent. Experimental studies reported in early 1974 confirmed VCM as a hepatic carcinogen capable of producing HAS and other tumors.

Follow-up epidemiologic studies revealed that: 1) HAS is the end stage of a progressive liver disease consisting of hepatocytic and sinusoidal cell hyperplasia, sinusoidal dilatation, and hepatic fibrosis; 2) over 100 cases of VCM-induced HAS have occurred worldwide; and 3) an increased risk of lung cancer has been reported in some cohort studies of PVC polymerization workers, although this outcome may be related to PVC dust or factors other than VCM.

A national study of HAS in the United States identified 3 other causes of HAS: Thorotrast, inorganic arsenic, and androgenic-anabolic steroids. Of 168 cases found to occur during 1964 through 1974, 42 cases (25%) were associated with the 4 known etiologic agents, while 126 cases (75%) were of unknown etiology.

In early 1974, John Creech and Maurice Johnson, Louisville plant physician and corporate medical director, respectively, of the B. F. Goodrich Company, reported the first cluster of hepatic angiosarcoma (HAS) cases in polyvinyl chloride (PVC) polymerization workers (*1*). Because of the rarity of this tumor in the general population (approximately 27/year in the United States at that time), this alert clinician noted the first case with interest, sensed concern when the second case appeared, and understood quickly that something important had happened when the third case in several years was diagnosed. In his words, it was like seeing several patients in a row with red, white, and blue spots on their nose—whatever the cause, which was still uncertain, the problem was hard to miss. Indeed, a rough relative risk calculation very early in the investigation, based on the first 4 cases of hepatic angiosarcoma that had occurred, suggested a relative risk of approximately 5,000, an almost astronomical figure.

Within several weeks, investigations undertaken by the U.S. Public Health Service and others confirmed the diagnosis of HAS, showed that a non-malignant liver disease consisting of hepatic fibrosis and portal hypertension was also occurring among the same workers, and identified vinyl chloride monomer (VCM) as the cause (2). Dr. Creech, the alert physician, or surgeon in this case, had also noticed the strawberry-like appearance of the liver capsule, caused by irregular, patchy fibrosis, in the PVC polymerization workers, yet another clue that something unusual had happened.

The impact of this discovery on the public and the scientific community was dramatic. 1) A seemingly innocuous substance to which hundreds of thousands of workers had been exposed over a period of several decades was suddenly transformed into an apparently potent carcinogen producing a rapidly fatal (usually within 3 months) malignancy. 2) Convincing evidence of the carcinogenicity of VCM arrived so swiftly from both human epidemiologic and animal experimental data that emergency regulations were enacted with minimal delay. 3) The widespread uses of VCM in consumer products and its general release into the environment were abruptly stopped as the general public became fearful of potential long-term effects. 4) Scientific investigations proceeded rapidly to unravel the pathogenesis and other aspects of the disease.

Vinyl Chloride-induced Liver Disease and Angiosarcoma

There are three phases in PVC production: VCM production, PVC polymerization, and PVC fabrication. The largest number of workers is in the multitude of PVC fabricating plants, while historically exposures to VCM were dramatically higher (up to levels effectively producing anesthesia) in the PVC polymerization process. Occasional case reports, or small clusters of cases, in VCM production or PVC fabrication workers have been reported (3), but in the most recent review of occupational cases worldwide the great majority of cases are still in polymerization workers (4, 5). Cases of HAS from environmental exposures have also been sporadically reported, but no sustained increase has yet been noted. The worldwide register of VCM-related cases maintained by Stafford and Bennett of ICI Chemicals (England) suggests that cases may have peaked in the mid to late 1970's (maximum of 11 HAS deaths/year) and may be declining by the mid 1980's, with 125 VCM-related HAS deaths worldwide by the end of 1986. Of 130 incident cases in this register, the U.S.A. had 36, West Germany 31, France 21, UK 12, Canada 10, and the remainder distributed mainly among other European countries. Two were reported from Japan.

Prior to 1974, VCM was treated by many as an almost inert substance; it was in fact used as the proverbial "inert substance" or propellant in aerosol cans (*e.g.*, hair spray). In retrospect, should we have anticipated this problem before its clinical

TABLE 1.   Chronology of PVC Production and Health Risks

1942	Start of commercial PVC production in U.S.
1949	Earliest references to AOL and hepatic effects
1966–7	Detailed description of AOL
1960's	Reports of hepatomegaly
1971	First report of experimental carcinogenicity
1972–3	Detailed description of hepatotoxicity
1974	First cluster of HAS

appearance? Should the alert epidemiologist have seen this coming before the alert clinician diagnosed the cases?

VCM has actually caused 2 unusual diseases, HAS and acroosteolysis. Dr. Creech said that people will always remember him for the VCM/HAS association, but that was easy to spot. The more difficult was recognizing the VCM-induced cases of acroosteolysis, which he and his associates had described earlier. The classic appearance of acroosteolysis includes the following triad: Raynaud's phenomenon, scleroderma-like lesions on the hands and forearms, and lytic lesions of the terminal phalanges of the fingers (6). Occasionally, systemic manifestations have been observed (radiographic changes in the patella, sacroiliac joint, and terminal phalanges of the feet). More recently vascular changes in the digital arteries of the hand were found to accompany acroosteolysis. For a number of years it was thought that this disease was caused by external, manual contact with VCM/PVC, unrelated to systemic absorption and without systemic effects. In any event, early references to acroosteolysis and vague hepatic effects started over 20 years prior to 1974 (Table 1); and detailed descriptions of acroosteolysis and hepatotoxicity appeared in the late 1960's and early 1970's (7). Experimental carcinogenicity, albeit at very high doses, was reported in 1971, but in the skin, lungs, and bones of the rat, rather than in its liver (8).

Part of the answer for the delay in recognizing the dangers of vinyl chloride is that investigators underestimated the hepatotoxicity of VCM because it was a different type of hepatotoxin rather than the weak hepatotoxin it appeared to be. Detailed review of liver pathology in vinyl chloride workers by Popper *et al.* elucidated the progression of VCM-induced liver disease (9). The earliest stage consists of combined hyperplasia of both the hepatocytes and the sinusoidal cells, with sinusoidal dilatation and excess reticulin surrounding the sinusoids. The hyperplastic sinusoidal cells progress to increasing atypia and ultimately HAS; the sinusoidal dilatation may progress, occasionally to the extent of peliosis hepatis, and increased fibrous deposition leads to hepatic fibrosis and portal hypertension. In VCM-exposed workers hepatocellular carcinoma only rarely develops, but in experimental animals increasing hepatocyte atypia leading to hepatocellular carcinoma is more often seen. What is not seen in workers until late stages and then secondary to the above are the signs of hepatocellular injury measured by the standard liver function tests (Table 2). As a result, the silent progression of serious hepatotoxicity could have been misconstrued as less serious hepatotoxicity.

When the natural course of vinyl chloride-induced hepatotoxicity was fully

TABLE 2. VCM-induced *vs.* Classic Hepatotoxicity

VCM-induced hepatotoxicity:
relatively silent progression
not detected early by standard liver function tests
effective screening tests lacking
least common of all causes of hepatotoxicity
various parts of spectrum seen with VCM, Thorotrast, arsenic, and steroids
(androgenic-anabolic and contraceptive)
Classic hepatotoxicity:
clinical signs and symptoms appear early
hepatic effects noted by enzyme changes, and other readily available laboratory tests
many clinical screening tests are used
wide array of hepatotoxins have been identified

described, there were actually no readily available, easily applied, or fully effective screening tests for detecting the early stages of the disease. A variety of approaches have been used, including liver scans, grey-scale ultrasonography, indocyanine green and bile acid clearances, *in vivo* capillary microscopy, and most simply the presence of persistent, multiple liver function test abnormalities.

Causal Agents of Hepatic Angiosarcoma

The discovery of VCM-induced HAS raised many new questions. For example, vinyl chloride was actually the third identified cause of HAS. German vintners in the 1940's and 1950's who had previously been heavily exposed to inorganic arsenical pesticides had been reported to have high rates of HAS. In addition, Thorotrast recipients in Portugal and other parts of the world (*e.g.*, Denmark, Germany, Japan) had been shown to have high rates of HAS, as well as hepatocellular carcinoma and cholangiocarcinoma. (Thorotrast is a colloidal suspension of thorium dioxide, used primarily in the late 1920's and 1930's for liver-spleen scans; it unfortunately remains in the liver and radioactively decays, releasing alpha particles, well beyond the life span of the recipient.) An intriguing question was whether this rare tumor with three known causal agents, but the bulk of cases still considered as idiopathic, had other identifiable etiologies.

A case-finding effort utilizing a variety of methods (Table 3) identified 168 cases in the U.S. during the years 1964–1974 (*10*). An interesting observation for those who study rare tumors was that in addition to the large number of cases of HAS not identified on the death certificate as HAS, 50% of cases reported on the death certificate as HAS turned out to be misdiagnosed, *i.e.*, false positives. HAS cases occurred at a younger age than other reported sarcomas of the liver, and even in the non-VCM, non-apparently occupational-induced cases a striking male preponderance was seen starting in the 30–39 year old age group. Extensive case investigations showed 7% related to VCM, 12% to Thorotrast, 4% to arsenic (mostly in the form of large doses of Fowler's Solution for the treatment of asthma or other conditions), and 4 cases (2%) associated with the use of androgenic-anabolic steroids. A matched death certificate case-control study did not reveal any other occupational factors associated with HAS; 75% of the cases were still considered idiopathic.

TABLE 3.   HAS Case Solicitation Methods 1964–1974, U.S. (CDC)

A mailing to all U.S. pathologists
Separate mailings to State epidemiologists, tumor registries, and tumor referral centers
Death certificate review of Code 197.8
Files of Armed Forces Institute of Pathology (AFIP)
Studies of VCM/PVC plants
Medical journal announcements
Previously published cases

Detailed pathology review showed the pathologic appearance of cases for the different causal agents and for the idiopathic cases to be identical.

The relatively large number of Thorotrast-induced cases was surprising, since almost none had previously been reported in the U.S. The review of 26 U.S. cases showed that most had received the Thorotrast during carotid arteriography (54%) or hepatolienography (35%). Of interest was the apparent rising number of cases related to low-dose procedures occurring after prolonged latent periods (11). This suggested the possibility of a second, and larger, wave of VCM-induced cases among workers with lesser exposures at some time in the future; so far there is no evidence that this is happening.

Most intriguing were the 4 cases of HAS associated with androgenic-anabolic steroids (12). Limited FDA data on androgenic-anabolic steroid use suggested a very low probability of even 1 such case occurring. We postulated as a result that these cases served as a link between the type of hepatic disorders seen after VCM (or arsenic and Thorotrast) exposure and that seen after exposure to contraceptive and anabolic steroids. The common feature would be the precursor stages, usually not recognized by clinical laboratory tests and consisting of areas of hyperplasia of hepatocytes and sinusoidal cells and of sinusoidal dilatation. This common precursor lesion could then lead potentially to hepatic adenoma, carcinoma, peliosis, and angiosarcoma, with the frequency of these outcomes differing for each of the causal agents. The androgenic-anabolic steroids served as the link, because they had been reported to induce all of these outcomes, i.e., adenoma, carcinoma, peliosis, and, with our report, HAS. Since our report in 1979, occasional cases of VCM-associated hepatocellular carcinoma (13) and oral contraceptive-associated peliosis and, rarely, HAS have been reported (14). The clinical overlap, however, is not impressive even if there is conceivably a single spectrum for these hepatic disorders.

PVC Polymerization Worker Cohort Studies

Another question that arose with the discovery of VCM-induced HAS was whether VCM-exposed workers would turn out to be similar to experimental animals in whom a variety of tumors, including non-hepatic angiosarcomas as well as tumors of other organs, develop. To answer this question a number of cohort studies of PVC polymerization workers have been conducted in different parts of the world. The National Institute of Occupational Safety and Health (NIOSH), Centers for Disease Control (CDC) conducted one such study in four PVC polymerization plants, following workers through 1973 (15).

Before describing this study, let me point out some of the limitations of our study, which apply to many of the other studies as well (*16*). 1) The PVC polymerization industry was born in the 1940's; most of the new workers started while still very young. Even in 1973, most had hardly lived into their 50's and, therefore, still had not passed through the age of peak cancer occurrence. It is perhaps too early to see the full spectrum of disease that may occur in these groups. 2) Most of the cohort studies have a relatively small number of deaths among workers with prolonged exposure and latency. This diminishes the ability to detect findings. 3) Most studies have had difficulty, due to lack of past measurements, in precisely quantifying past exposure to VCM, PVC dust, and other chemicals used in the polymerization process (*e.g.*, other monomers used with VCM to make copolymers).

In the NIOSH/CDC study a total of 1,294 workers with at least 5 years of exposure and 10 years since last exposure to VCM were studied. Thirty-five malignant neoplasms were observed with only 23.5 expected (SMR=149; $p<0.05$). No other statistically significant increases were seen. When all malignant neoplasms were subdivided by site, the only statistically significant increase was for biliary and liver cancer (7 Obs. *vs.* 0.6 Exp.; SMR=1,155; $p<0.01$). This increase was entirely due to HAS. Nonsignificant increases were seen for brain and CNS cancer (3 Obs. *vs.* 0.9 Exp.), respiratory system cancer (12 Obs. *vs.* 7.7 Exp.) and lymphatic and hematopoietic system cancer (4 Obs. *vs.* 2.5 Exp.). At a higher cut-off for latency (≥ 15 years), brain and CNS cancer (3 Obs. *vs.* 0.6 Exp.) and respiratory system cancer (11 Obs. *vs.* 5.7 Exp.) became statistically significant at $p<0.05$.

In summary, the cohort studies are definitive with regard to increases in HAS; there are enough inconsistencies between studies and difficulties from small numbers that more investigation is needed before definitive conclusions are reached on the other tumor types mentioned. In our study (NIOSH/CDC) we became intrigued by the lung cancer increase for two reasons: 1) among the initial cases there appeared to be an altered histologic distribution with a greater than expected proportion of large cell undifferentiated cases, and 2) the lung cancer cases appeared to have worked more heavily in areas with exposure to PVC dust rather than VCM (*17*). Subsequently, cases of pneumoconiosis secondary to PVC dust exposure were reported. Nevertheless, this association is still tenuous, and needs further study in groups whose exposures to VCM, PVC dust, and other chemicals are clearly defined.

Toxicology

Toxicologic studies indicate that 1) HAS is linked to the amount of VCM metabolized rather than to the VCM concentration, 2) reactive intermediates, particularly the epoxide (chloroethylene oxide) formed by oxidative metabolism of the carbon/carbon double bond, are most likely the carcinogenic agent, 3) the short-lived metabolites are formed in the hepatocytes but are carcinogenic in the adjacent sinusoidal cells to which they migrate presumably because these cells have less detoxification potential, and 4) the reactive metabolites covalently bond to macromolecules such as DNA.

Another series of questions stimulated by the discovery of VCM-induced HAS related to the carcinogenic potential of the array of chemicals structurally similar to VCM. Many experimental and epidemiologic studies have since been initiated to study compounds such as vinyl bromide, acrylonitrile, chloroprene, vinylidene chloride, trichloroethylene, and tetrachloroethylene.

Surveillance of Rare Tumors

To go back to my earlier question, what could the alert epidemiologist have done to anticipate or detect this problem before it was diagnosed by the alert clinician? First, surveillance of rare, or marker, tumors such as HAS (or mesothelioma) is most useful when the system covers the entire population—otherwise, important geographic patterns or clusters may be missed. Second, it is extremely time-consuming and requires too much effort to consider national reporting or surveillance individually for each of these marker tumors; it would be ideal to have a single system which would simultaneously collect data on a broad variety of rare, marker tumors. It is not inconceivable to think of such a system. CDC is currently instituting a pilot surveillance system to collect computerized pathologic information and other data from all cases seen by selected medical examiners—eventually this pilot system will be expanded to provide broad coverage of cases seen by medical examiners. Sooner or later, similar computerized data should probably exist for all autopsies and biopsies and surveillance of data from pathologists should be conceivable. Third, a systematic approach to analyzing epidemiologic and experimental data should identify rare tumors of interest to study. HAS, *e.g.*, would have been of interest even before the association with VCM was known for the following reasons: a) the higher male: female ratio and earlier age of appearance than that for all other hepatic sarcomas; b) the previously noted human causative agents (Thorotrast and arsenic); and c) the large number of experimental chemicals that induce HAS in animals. In summary, surveillance for rare, marker tumors might provide unique opportunities for epidemiologic and pathogenetic studies of occupational and environmental carcinogens. Setting up such a systematic or centralized approach will not be easy.

REFERENCES

1. Creech, J. L., Jr. and Johnson, M. N. Angiosarcoma of liver in the manufacture of polyvinyl chloride. J. Occup. Med., *16*: 150–151, 1974.
2. Thomas, L. B., Popper, H., Berk, P. D., Selikoff, I., and Falk, H. Vinyl chloride-induced liver disease—From idiopathic portal hypertension (Banti's syndrome) to angiosarcomas. N. Engl. J. Med., *292*: 17–22, 1975.
3. Maltoni, C., Clini, C., Vicini, F., and Masina, A. Two cases of liver angiosarcoma among polyvinyl chloride (PVC) extruders of an Italian factory producing PVC bags and other containers. Am. J. Ind. Med., *5*: 297–302, 1984.
4. Forman, D., Bennett, B., Stafford, J., and Doll, R. Exposure to vinyl chloride and angiosarcoma of the liver: A report of the register of cases. Br. J. Ind. Med., *42*: 750–753, 1985.
5. Bennett, B. Personal communication. Feb. 1987.
6. Wilson, R. H., McCormick, W. E., Tatum, C. F., and Creech, J. L. Occupational acroosteolysis—Report of 31 cases. JAMA, *201*: 577–581, 1967.

7. Lange, C. E., Juhe, S., Stein, G., and Veltman, G. So-called vinyl chloride disease: Is it an occupational systemic sclerosis? Int. Arch. Occup. Environ. Health, *32*: 1–32, 1974.
8. Viola, P. L., Bigotti, A., and Caputo, A. Oncogenic response of rat skin, lungs, and bones to vinyl chloride. Cancer Res., *31*: 516–522, 1971.
9. Popper, H., Thomas, L. B., Telles, N. C., Falk, H., and Selikoff, I. J. Development of hepatic angiosarcoma in man induced by vinyl chloride, Thorotrast, and arsenic. Am. J. Pathol., *92*: 349–376, 1978.
10. Falk, H., Herbert, J., Crowley, S., Ishak, K. J., Thomas, L. B., Popper, H., and Caldwell, G. G. Epidemiology of hepatic angiosarcoma in the United States, 1964–1974. Environ. Health Perspect., *41*: 107–113, 1981.
11. Falk, H., Telles, N. C., Ishak, K. G., Thomas, L. B., and Popper, H. Epidemiology of Thorotrast-induced hepatic angiosarcoma in the United States. Environ, Res., *18*: 65–73, 1979.
12. Falk, H., Thomas, L. B., Popper, H., and Ishak, K. G. Hepatic angiosarcoma associated with androgenic-anabolic steroids. Lancet, *ii*: 1120–1124, 1979.
13. Evans, D., Williams, W. J., and Kung, I. T. Angiosarcoma and hepatocellular carcinoma in vinyl chloride workers. Histopathology, *7*: 377–388, 1983.
14. Forbes, A., Portmann, B., Johnson, P., and Williams, R. Hepatic sarcomas in adults: A review of 25 cases. Gut, *28*: 668–674, 1987.
15. Waxweiler, R. J., Stringer, W., Wagoner, J. K., Jones, J., Falk, H., and Carter, C. Neoplastic risk among workers exposed to vinyl chloride. Ann. N.Y. Acad. Sci., *271*: 40–48, 1976.
16. Salmon, A. G. Vinyl chloride: The evidence for human carcinogenicity in different target organs. Br. J. Ind. Med., *42*: 73–74, 1985.
17. Waxweiler, R. J., Smith, A. H., Falk, H., and Tyroler, H. A. An epidemiologic investigation of an excess lung cancer risk in workers at a synthetic chemical plant. Environ. Health Perspect., *41*: 159–165, 1981.

Steroid Related Neoplasia in Human Liver

George H. Barrows,[*1] E. Truman Mays,[*2] and
William M. Christopherson[*3]

*Departments of Pathology, Saint Francis Medical Center and University of Connecticut, Hartford, Connecticut 06105,[*1] Department of Surgery, University of Kentucky, Lexington 40534, Kentucky,[*2] and Department of Pathology, University of Louisville, Louisville, Kentucky 40292,[*3] U.S.A.*

Abstract: Prior to the early 1970's, benign liver neoplasms were among the rarest of tumors. The seemingly rapid increase, especially in young females ingesting oral contraceptives, as well as the catastrophic presentation of many of the tumors resulting from liver rupture and hemoperitoneum, stimulated studies by several investigators. In the Liver Tumor Registry at the University of Louisville, we have examined the histologic material, and finalized the data on 227 tumors, the majority in young women. With few exceptions, they had used oral contraceptives or were either pregnant or immediately post-partum and presumably in a hyperestrogenic state. There have been 82 hepatocellular adenomas (HCA), 105 cases of focal nodular hyperplasia (FNH), and 31 hepatocellular carcinomas.

The hepatocellular carcinomas occurred in non-cirrhotic livers, and 14 of the 31 cases were of a distinct, but rare type, polygonal cell carcinoma with lamellar fibrosis. While it seems reasonable to believe steroids play a role in adenomas and in FNH it is less certain that they produce hepatocellular carcinomas since malignant liver tumors are not uncommon in this age group without the use of oral contraceptives. With an estimated 50 million women either currently using or who have used oral contraceptives the risk must be very slight.

Prior to the use of oral contraceptives, only a few reports of benign liver tumors had been made. The first recorded association between steroid administration and hepatic neoplasia was made by Caroli *et al.* in 1953 in a patient who had developed hepatocellular carcinoma after estrogen administration (*1*). In 1971, Bernstein and co-workers (*2*) described a young patient with Fanconi's anemia treated with oxymethalone. A number of similar case reports have been made but only a few have developed metastasis (*3*). Histologic review of similar lesions has revealed the majority to be benign with structure similar to tumors associated with contraceptive steroids. The first case of a hepatic neoplasm occurring in contraceptive steroid users was reported in 1972 by Horvath *et al.* (*4*). In 1973, Davis and coworkers were first to note the occurrence of spontaneous rupture and hemoperitoneum in young females (5). Contraceptive history was not reported in these women, but one patient was pregnant. The association of hepatic neoplasia with oral contraceptive usage became widely publicized after Baum et al. reported seven cases of benign liver tumors in oral contraceptive users (6). This publication led to a flurry of case reports describing benign hepatic tumors associated with oral contraceptive use. Many of these lesions were referred to as "benign hepatomas" without critical evaluation of the histology. Mays et al. (7) were the first to provide a detailed description of a specific lesions, focal nodular hyperplasia (FNH), associated with oral contraceptives. The lesions had distinctive vascular changes which the authors suggested might play a role in pathogenesis. A number of other liver tumors including "hamartomas" (8), hepatocellular adenoma (HCA) (9), and hepatoblastoma (10) were reported during the next few years. These findings raised concern that the continued widespread use of "the pill" might spawn an increase in benign liver lesions associated with complications (11).

A dramatic clinical triad of liver tumor, abdominal pain and hemorrhagic shock from tumor rupture was found in many early case reports (9, 12, 13). With more extensive analysis, this appeared to be a complication of a minority of tumors (14).

The majority of lesions have been benign; however, there have also been reports of malignant liver tumors associated with contraceptive use. In 1973, Hermann and David (16) reported a "well differentiated hepatoma" which had ruptured. In 1975 Christopherson and associates (13) documented a hepatocellular carcinoma with extensive vein invasion in a woman taking oral contraceptives. Additional cases of hepatocellular carcinoma have been reported (17–19). As with the benign lesions, this may represent the coincidental reporting of an accumulation of cases rather than an actual increase in incidence. An uncommon type of hepatocellular carcinoma, eosinophilic glassy cell hepatoma (20), was frequently seen in patients taking contraceptive steroids (15). Since hepatocellular carcinoma is much more common than benign liver neoplasia, its actual association with steroids remains questionable.

Vascular abnormalities have been associated with steroid use. Extensive vascular lesions have been described in the liver and mesenteric vessels of patients taking contraceptive steroids (21–24). Vascular changes and peliosis hepatis within the adjacent liver have been associated with steroid related hepatic neoplasms (7, 25, 26). Angiosarcoma has also been reported in association with sex steroid usage (27, 28) but appears to be a rare event.

Reviews of the pertinent literature to 1976 have been published by Sturtevant (29) and Klatskin (30). Several investigators have published studies on large series of liver lesions associated with contraceptive steroids. Nime and associates (26) completed a multi-institution study of 94 cases in 1979. Nissen et al. studied 90 cases of hepatic neoplasms related to contraceptive use (14) referred to a registry at University of California in Irvine.

Since the initial reports of Baum et al., we have maintained a registry for steroid related liver tumors to allow systematic review of histologic and clinical features of these uncommon lesions. Descriptions of the clinical findings and pathology in these cases have been published over the past 12 years (15, 31). This study presents an

TABLE 1. Tumor Types

	Number	
Focal nodular hyperplasia	105	(46.3%)
Hepatocellular adenoma	82	(36.1%)
Hepatocellular carcinoma	31	(13.7%)
Unclassified	9	(3.9%)

anthology of the findings from these cases and review of current status of these steroid related liver tumors.

Material

The histologic material and case histories of over two hundred twenty-five liver neoplasms related to steroid use have been accessioned between 1973 and 1986. Cases have been referred by pathologists and clinicians from many institutions over a large geographic area. A uniform set of histologic criteria have been used to define the lesion. Histologic material was reviewed in all cases to verify the diagnosis and assure proper classification. As much clinically related data as possible have been collected regarding the patient's age, predisposing factors, medications, physical and laboratory findings. Three major types of liver neoplasia have been associated with sex steroid use: focal nodular hyperplasia, hepatocellular adenoma, and hepatocellular carcinoma (Table 1).

Physical Findings

Forty percent of the benign liver tumors were discovered fortuitously during evaluation for other diseases or routine surgery. Eighteen percent of the patients with benign lesions had presentation with hematoperitoneum in the setting of hemorrhagic shock and 24% had abdominal pain. A mass was noted on physical exam in only 25% of patients with benign liver lesions. Epigastric pain without hemoperitoneum occurred in nearly 25% of patients with both FNH and HCA. This finding was often associated with intratumor hemorrhage.

Three of 23 (13%) of patients with hepatocellular carcinoma presented with hemoperitoneum and an additional nine (39%) complained of abdominal pain. A single patient with hepatocellular carcinoma presented with icterus. This patient had advanced disease and was terminal.

Laboratory Evaluation

Laboratory findings were evaluated in detail from the first 100 patients accessioned (31). Liver function tests were usually within normal limits except for occasional elevated alkaline phosphatase. Evidence of anemia was sometimes present, but unless related to hematoperitoneum, no distinct alteration of hematologic parameters occurred. In several cases of hepatocellular carcinoma, carcinoembryonic antigen (CEA) was positive but in keeping with other studies (32), there was no consistent elevation of tumor markers including alpha-fetoprotein. This is in contrast to the usual finding of abnormal liver function tests and elevated serum marker studies associated with hepatocellular carcinoma (*33, 34*). When performed, liver scan, selective arteriography, and computed axial tomography usually revealed a tumor mass which sometimes was vascular and other times avascular. The imaging studies were particularly valuable in follow-up, when the tumors were not completely removed surgically.

Gross Characteristics of the Lesions

The right lobe of the liver was involved three times as often as the left in keeping with the larger mass of this lobe. A small percentage of patients with multiple tumors had both lobes involved. The benign tumors varied in size, shape, and appearance, but had some consistent findings. Adenomas tended to be larger, ranging size from 1 to 22 cm while focal nodular hyperplasia was 2 to 15 cm. Both FNH and HCA occurred embedded within the liver parenchyma or as pedunculated growths. In some cases, the pedunculated tumors were mistaken for ovarian tumors on pelvic examination.

The classic gross appearance of HCA was different from that of FNH. Adenomas were usually softer with a cut surface varying from light yellow to dark brown. Sectioning usually revealed a variegated appearance in adenomas due to necrosis, hemorrhage or bile staining. Adenomas also lacked the large fibrous septa and central scar which characterize focal nodular hyperplasia.

While most descriptions of HCA stress encapsulation, among the cases seen in association with contraceptive steroids, encapsulation was often absent. This was particularly true when multiple tumors occurred. Tumors from patients with no history of steroid exposure were more likely to have encapsulation. This raises the possibility that some adenomas associated with steroid use may represent a form of monomorphic hyperplasia rather than true adenoma.

Focal nodular hyperplasia was usually non-encapsulated. Typically, FNH has a central scar with radiating septa and a coarsely nodular appearance. It should be noted that a great variety of gross appearances of both lesions was observed. The presence or absence of encapsulation was not a reliable criterion to distinguish between the two.

Hemorrhage and necrosis were present in focal nodular hyperplasia but, more frequently, in hepatocellular adenoma associated with contraceptive steroid use. Intratumor hemorrhage occurred in several unruptured tumors of both types. Hemorrhage was also observed in adenomas of some women not exposed to exogenous steroids.

Multiple Tumors

Most patients with benign tumors had solitary nodules. However, a minority of patients with adenoma had multiple nodules (Table 2). When multiple adenomas were present there was usually a dominant mass with smaller nodules in close proximity. Some of the smaller lesions probably represented adenomatous hyperplasia

TABLE 2. Incidence of Multiple Tumors Focal Nodular Hyperplasia *vs.* Adenoma

Number	Focal nodular hyperplasia	Hepatocellular adenoma
2–3	15.3%	16.9%
4–5	3.1	2.8
>5	2.0	4.2
Total	20.4%	23.9%

and not true neoplasms. When FNH was multiple, two to five masses were present of similar size. Two patients who continued to use oral contraceptives developed second tumors separated by an interval of several years.

Age of Patients

All patients were young, averaging 30 years, in keeping with the age group most frequently using contraceptive steroids. The mean age and age distribution for FNH, HCA, and hepatocellular carcinoma were similar (Table 3).

TABLE 3. Mean Ages and Range of Contraceptive Steroid Associated Liver Tumors

Type	Mean age	Range
Focal nodular hyperplasia	30	20–52
Adenoma	31.6	14–55
Hepatocellular carcinoma	26.5	17–47
Unclassified	34.2	27–47

Steroid Exposure

Over 60% of the women with benign tumors had documented oral contraceptive usage for varying periods (Table 4). A few patients had lesions associated with conjugated estrogens, were pregnant or were immediately post-partum. One patient had an ovarian thecoma which was presumed to be functional. Definitive information regarding the type of oral contraceptive used was available in over 50% of cases. Although there was a preponderance of cases associated with mestranol this was also the drug most frequently used in contraceptives during the study period. A significant number of patients had used ethynyl-estradiol roughly proportional to the marketing patterns of the period. In the United Kingdom, where mestranol and ethynyl estradiol were used with equal frequency, nearly 50% of patients with similar

TABLE 4. Steroid Exposure in Patients with Benign Liver Tumors

Months	Patients
>12	5%
12–35	14
36–71	27
72–95	18

lesions had used preparations containing ethynyl estradiol. The mean duration of oral contraceptive use was over six years, with 80 to 85% of women using these preparations for over three years. In some cases there was an interruption for pregnancy and frequently the patients used more than one brand of contraceptive. As the dosage of steroids in oral contraceptives has decreased there has been a decline in the number of case reports of these lesions (20).

Nearly 75% of patients with hepatocellular carcinoma had used contraceptive steroids. An additional 10% had used conjugated equine estrogen. Steroid usage was not documented in the remaining 15%.

Microscopic Appearance

The two major types of benign tumors could be readily classified by the histologic features in most cases. Focal nodular hyperplasia has a distinctive appearance readily distinguishable from adenoma. Detailed histologic descriptions of the lesions have been presented in previous studies (15, 31). Alpha-1 antitrypsin inclusions were found in HCA, FNH, and hepatocellular carcinoma, but these markers were not related to corresponding phenotypic alpha-1 antitrypsin deficiency (35).

The reproducibility of these histologic features has been confirmed by Nime et al. (26). It is interesting to note that these workers reclassified all "hamartomas" to either focal nodular hyperplasia or adenoma. When focal nodular hyperplasia is small and inactive, the presence of mature fibrosis and lack of proliferative activity may account for the original diagnosis of "hamartoma". These lesions were often seen in patients who had discontinued contraceptive use several years prior to resection of the tumor.

Vascular Changes in Association with Benign Lesions

Characteristic vascular changes were often present in the hepatic arteries and veins of the contraceptive steroid associated liver tumors. The branches of the hepatic artery and portal veins had combinations of intimal and smooth muscle proliferation with vascular enlargement, occlusive intimal thickening and at times obstructive thrombosis. In some cases these changes led to areas of infarction of the parenchymal tissue served by the vessels. Peliosis hepatis and hepatic sinusoidal dilatation were also observed in a few instances. Other investigators have noted similar vascular changes. Klatskin (30) reported peliosis hepatis and medial hypertrophy of arterioles in a large review of hepatic tumors in women using contraceptive steroids. Nime et al. (26) found intimal and medial changes in 40% of focal nodular hyperplasia and 45% of hepatocellular adenomas associated with oral contraceptives. These changes were also present in 20 to 27% of patients in whom FNH and HCA occurred in the absence of contraceptive steroids. Using a system of grading, these investigators also documented increased severity of intimal and medial lesions among contraceptive users. Whether these changes are causally related to the benign hepatic neoplasms or steroids remains unclear. Contraceptive steroids have been reported in association with mesenteric vessel lesions (21–24) in addition to hepatic neoplasia. Vascular lesions similar to those found in the patients with contraceptive related

TABLE 5.   Comparison of Findings

	Pain	Hemoperitoneum	Mass	Incidental
FNH (n=98)	24.5%	9.2%*	16.3%*	46.9%*
HCA (n=71)	24.0	31.0*	36.6*	5.6*

* $p<0.001$ by Chi square

TABLE 6.   Findings in Hepatocellular Adenoma *vs.* Historic Controls

Clinical finding	Steroids	No steroids[a]	p value
Hemoperitoneum	31%	15%	<0.001
Hepatomegaly	37	37	N.S.
Pain	24	20	N.S.

[a] After Klatskin *Gastroenterology, 73*: 386–394, 1977

TABLE 7.   Findings in Focal Nodular Hyperplasia *vs.* Historic Controls

Clinical finding	Steroids	No steroids[a]	p value
Hemoperitoneum	9%	0.4%	<0.001
Hepatomegaly	6	12	N.S.
Pain	24	7	<0.001

[a] After Klatskin *Gastroenterology, 73*: 386–394, 1977

tumors have been seen in experimental animals receiving large doses of contraceptive steroids (*37, 38*).

The presence of these distinctive vascular lesions is of importance since the small number of deaths associated with these benign lesions has been primarily related to hemorrhage and shock from spontaneous rupture of these lesions (*11, 14, 15*). The occurrence of intrabdominal hemorrhage was significantly higher for women who had hepatocellular adenoma (Table 5). The reasons for increased occurrence of hemorrhage and rupture may be related to the larger, more friable architecture in these lesions or more rapid growth. While a change in incidence of these benign liver lesions has not been definitively substantiated with the advent of oral contraceptive use, the frequency of acute hemorrhage in reported cases does appear increased with respect to historically reported cases (Tables 6 and 7).

Hepatocellular Carcinoma

The diagnosis of hepatocellular carcinoma was reserved for those cases with nuclear anaplasia, abnormal mitotic activity, and evidence of vascular invasion. Fourteen of thirty one cases in this series were of a distinctive subtype, alternately called "eosinophilic glassy cell hepatocellular carcinoma" (*20*), or "polygonal cell type with fibrous stroma" (*39, 40*). This variant of hepatocellular carcinoma has distinctive eosinophilic polygonal cells with planar collagen lamella separating the nodules. Survival with this lesion was prolonged but all patients succumbed with the longest survivor living 39 months (*41*). While this lesion was seen with uncommon frequency in the present series, an investigative study regarding the incidence of glassy cell hepatoma subtype concluded that the association of this lesion with contraceptive steroids is due to its frequent occurrence in the age group at risk and not the use of contraceptive steroids *per se* (*42*).

"Well differentiated carcinomas" or "minimal deviation hepatomas" have been reported (*43*). These lesions have usually been downgraded to hepatocellular adenomas on review (*15, 26*). The presence of occasional mitoses and nuclear size variation may raise concern regarding the potential behavior of hepatocellular adenomas. In the face of orderly development and absence of nuclear anaplasia these features do not serve as basis for classification as malignant. Experience to date suggests that most of these lesions will behave in a benign fashion.

Predisposing Factors for Liver Oncogenesis

The presence of cirrhosis is a well established predisposing factor in the development of hepatic neoplasia (*36*). The liver tumors associated with contraceptive use in this series occurred in young women without any evidence of cirrhosis or liver damage (*15*). Alpha-1 antitrypsin deficiency is also associated with an increased risk for development of hepatoma. Although alpha-1 antitrypsin serves as a tumor marker for most contraceptive related tumors, alpha-1 antitrypsin phenotypes of most patients examined were normal (*35*). Hepatitis B virus antigen has also been associated with increased risk for development of hepatocellular carcinoma (*44*). While there are no systematic studies regarding this marker, the absence of cirrhosis or recognizable histologic evidence of hepatitis in the uninvolved liver of these patients makes this agent an unlikely influence. Likewise no other agents known to be associated with hepatic neoplasia (*45–49*) have been reported with liver neoplasia related to steroids.

Role of Contraceptive Steroids in Hepatic Neoplasia

The strongest implication of contraceptive steroids as a causative factor in benign liver tumors comes from their frequent association with these neoplasms and regression of these neoplasms after withdrawal of all steroid medications (*13, 50, 51*). Rapid growth of pre-existing benign liver lesions has also been reported during pregnancy (*52*). The development of hepatocellular carcinoma after hepatocellular adenoma and, less commonly, focal nodular hyperplasia has been reported in rare instances. Because malignant transformation is extremely uncommon, there is no clear relationship of hepatocellular carcinoma to steroid use or pre-existing benign liver neoplasia. Experimental evidence of steroid oncogenesis have given conflicting results. Lesions similar to those in humans have been seen in experimental animal studies (*38, 53, 54*). The initial studies for screening showed an increase in benign liver tumors, but very large concentrations of steroids were employed in a strain of mice prone to develop spontaneous liver neoplasms. No significant increase of tumor initiation has been documented to date (*55, 56*). Contraceptive steroids have been shown to be non-mutagenic in *in-vitro* (Ames test) experiments (*57*). Activity by contraceptive agents as promoters of neoplasia have been reported in several studies (*55, 56*). The dosages employed in these studies were much larger than those used in oral contraceptives, particularly the most recent formulations (*59*). It is also possible that contraceptive steroids influence liver neoplasia indirectly by alteration of the normal hormonal milieu (*60, 61*) or that secondary hormonal changes such as prolactin elevation (*62*) play a role in the development of these lesions. Conversely it has been suggested that the presence of elevated female sex steroids in cirrhosis may be the reason for the increased frequency of hepatocellular carcinoma observed in this condition (*63*).

The known mechanism of steroids in target tissue requires the presence of steroid receptor proteins for transport of the steroids to the nucleus. Estrogen receptor proteins have been identified in steroid related neoplasia (*64–66*). However, the concentration of these hormone receptors has been low and often less than the unaffected liver surrounding the lesion (*64*). The presence of androgen receptor has recently been related to hepatocellular carcinoma (*67, 68*). Since the concentration of receptor protein in hepatocellular carcinoma has been elevated above that found in normal liver it may be more closely linked to the development of neoplasia. One hypothesis proposes a common path of activation of liver hormone receptor proteins by a shared gene locus which is altered by hepatitis B virus (*69*).

CONCLUSIONS

The uncommon association of liver neoplasia and contraceptive steroids has been supported by anecdotal reporting of case series. There seems to be, an as of yet undocumented, and rather recent decline in liver tumor occurrence in young women which we believe will continue. This is quite possibly related to the decrease in both estrogen and progesterone content of currently used birth control pills. There has certainly been no evidence of recent increases in these lesions despite the continuing exposure of over 50 million women to oral contraceptives. There is now strong evidence that oral contraceptive steroid usage decreases the risk of serious neoplasms in other organs (*70*). The increased frequency of liver neoplasms is outweighed by the observed decrease in other neoplasms. Thus, the collective risk of all types of neoplasms with steroid usage appears minimal. Of greater importance is an awareness of the medical community of the clinical behavior of these lesions and the ability to classify them so that they may be properly managed. The studies relating this uncommon occurrence of liver neoplasms have been of benefit in providing insight to the mechanisms of liver neoplasia and interaction of other drugs with the liver.

ACKNOWLEDGMENT
The authors thank Ms. Tammy Kuchinski for help with preparation of the manuscript.

REFERENCES

1. Caroli, J., Paraf, A., Charbonnier, A., and Vallin, J. Implantations d'oestrogenese apparement suivies d'un cancer primitif du foie. Rev. Int. Hepatol., *3*: 497, 1953.
2. Bernstein, M. S., Hunter, R. L., and Yachnin, S. Hepatoma and peliosis hepatis developing in a patient with Fanconi's anemia. N. Engl. J. Med., *284*: 1135–1136, 1971.

3. Farrell, C. C., Joshua, D. E., Uren, R. F., Baird, P. S., Perkins, K. W., and Kronenberg, H. Androgen induced hepatoma. Lancet, *i*: 430–432, 1975.

4. Horvath, E., Kovacs, K., and Ross, R. C. Ultrastructural findings in a well-differentiated hepatoma. Digestion, *7*: 74–82, 1972.

5. Davis, J. B., Schenken, J. R., and Zimmerman, O. Massive hemoperitoneum from rupture of benign hepatocellular adenoma. Surgery, *73*: 181–187, 1973.

6. Baum, J. K., Holtz, F., Bookstein, J. J., and Klein, E. W. Possible association between benign hepatomas and oral contraceptives. Lancet, *ii*: 926–929, 1973.

7. Mays, E. T., Christopherson, W. M., and Barrows, G. H. Focal nodular hyperplasia of the liver-possible relationship to oral contraceptives. Am. J. Clin. Pathol., *61*: 735–746, 1974.

8. O'Sullivan, J. P. and Wilding, R. P. Liver hamartomas in patients on oral contraceptives. Br. Med. J., *3*: 7–10, 1974.

9. Albritton, D. R., Tompkins, R. K., and Longmire, W. P., Jr. Hepatic cell adenoma: a report of four cases. Ann. Surg., *180*: 14–19, 1974.

10. Meyer, P., LiVolsi, V. A., and Cornog, J. L. Hepatoblastoma associated with an oral contraceptive. Lancet, *ii*: 1387, 1974.

11. Rooks, J. B., Howard, H. W., Ishak, K. G., Strauss, L. T., Greenspan, J. R., and Paganini, A. Epidemiology of hepatocellular adenoma. JAMA, *242*: 644–648, 1979.

12. Antoniades, K. and Brooks, C. E., Jr. Hemoperitoneum from liver cell adenoma in a patient on oral contraceptives. Surgery, *77*: 137–139, 1975.

13. Christopherson, W. M., Mays, E. T., and Barrows, G. Liver tumors in women on contraceptive steroids. Obstet. Gynecol., *46*: 221–223, 1975.

14. Nissen, E. D., Kent, D. R., and Nissen, S. E. Role of oral contraceptive agents in the pathologenesis of liver tumors. *In;* K. Lapis and J. V. Johannessen (eds.), Liver Carcinogenesis, pp. 61–84, Hemisphere Publishing, Washington, 1979.

15. Christopherson, W. M., Mays, E. T., and Barrows, G. H. Liver tumors in young women: a clinical pathologic study of 201 cases in the Louisville registry. Progr. Surg. Pathol., *2*: 187–205, 1980.

16. Hermann, R. E. and David, T. E. Spontaneous rupture of the liver caused by hepatoma. Surgery, *74*: 715–718, 1974.

17. Forman, D., Doll, R., and Peto, R. Trends in mortality from carcinoma of the liver and use of oral contraceptive steroids. Br. J. Cancer, *48*: 349–354, 1983.

18. Henderson, B. E., Preston-Martin, S., Edmonson, H. A., Peters, R. L., and Pike, M. C. Hepatocellular carcinoma associated with use of oral contraceptives. Br. J. Cancer, *48*: 437–440, 1983.

19. Neuberger, J., Forman, D., Doll, R., and Williams, R. Oral contraceptives and hepatocellular carcinoma. Br. Med. J., *292*: 1355–1357, 1986.

20. Christopherson, W. M. Possible etiologic factors for some malignant hepatic tumors. *In;* J. R. Strohlein and M. M. Romsdahl, (eds.), Gastrointestinal Cancer, pp. 257–269, Raven Press, New York, 1981.

21. Brennan, M. F., Clarke, A. M., and Macbeth, W. A. Infarctions of the midgut associated with oral contraceptives. N. Engl. J. Med., *279*: 1213–1214, 1968.

22. Hoyumpa, A. M., Schiff, L., and Helfman, E. L. Budd-Chiari syndrome in women taking oral contraceptives. Am. J. Med., *50*: 137–140, 1971.

23. Irey, N. S., Manion, W. C., and Taylor, H. B. Vascular lesions in women taking oral contraceptives. Arch Pathol., *89*: 1–8, 1970.

24. Irey, N. S. and Norris, H. J. Intimal vascular lesions associated with female reproductive steroids. Arch Pathol., *96*: 227–234, 1973.

25. Nissen, E. D. and Kent, D. R. Liver tumors and oral contraceptives. Obstet. Gynecol.,

46: 460–467, 1975.

26. Nime, F. and Pickren, J. W., Vana, J., Aronoff, B. L., Baker, H. W., and Murphy, G. P. The histology of liver tumors in oral contraceptive users observed during a national survey by the American College of Surgeons Commission on Cancer. Cancer, *44*: 1481–1489, 1979.

27. Falk, H., Thomas, L. B., Popper, H., and Ishak, K. G. Hepatic angiosarcoma associated with androgenic-anabolic steroids. Lancet, *ii*: 1120–1123, 1979.

28. Hoch-Ligeti, C. Angiosarcoma of the liver associated with diethylstilbestrol. JAMA, *240*: 1510–1511, 1978.

29. Sturtevant, F. M. Oral Contraceptives and Liver Tumors, Williams and Wilkins, Baltimore, 1979.

30. Klatskin, G. Hepatic tumors: possible relationship to use of oral contraceptives. Gastroenterology, *73*: 386–394, 1977.

31. Christopherson, W. M. and Mays, E. T. Liver tumors and oral contraceptives: experience with the first one hundred registry patients. J. Natl. Cancer Inst., *58*: 176–182, 1977.

32. Neuberger, J., Nunnerley, H. B., Davis, M., Portman, B., Laws, J. R., and Williams, R. Oral contraceptive-associated liver tumours: occurrence of malignancy and difficulties in diagnosis. Lancet, *i*: 263, 1980.

33. Chlebowski, R. T., Tong, M., and Weissman, J. Hepatocellular carcinoma: diagnostic and prognostic features in North American patients. Cancer, *53*: 2701–2706, 1984.

34. Nagasue, N., Yukaya, H., Hamada, T., Hirose, S., Kanashima, R., and Inokuchi, K. The natural history of hepatocellular carcinoma. A study of 100 untreated cases. Cancer, *54*: 1461–1465, 1984.

35. Palmer, P. E., Christopherson, W. M., and Wolfe, H. J. Alpha-1-antitrypsin, protein marker in oral contraceptive-associated liver tumors. Am. J. Clin. Pathol., *68*: 736–739, 1977.

36. Edmondson, H. A. Atlas of tumor pathology: tumors of the liver and intrahepatic bile ducts. Armed Forces Inst. Pathol. Fascicle., *25*: 193–206, 1956.

37. Almen, T., Hartel, M., Nylander, G., and Olivercronah, J. The effect of estrogen on the vascular endothelium and its possible relation to thrombosis. Surg. Gynecol. Obstet., *140*: 938–940, 1975.

38. Barrows, G. H., Christopherson, W. M., and Drill, V. A. Liver lesions and oral contraceptive steroids. Toxicol. Environ. Health, *3*: 219–230, 1977.

39. Peters, R. L. Pathology of hepatocellular carcinoma. *In;* K. Okuda and R. L. Peters (eds.), Hepatocellular Carcinoma, pp. 107–168, John Wiley, New York, 1976.

40. Berman, M. M., Libbey, N. P., and Foster, J. H. Hepatocellular carcinoma: polygonal cell type with fibrous stroma: an atypical variant with a favorable prognosis. Cancer, *46*: 1448–1455, 1980.

41. Christopherson, W. M. "Case 16" *In;* F. Vellios (ed.), Seminar: Obstetric and Gynecologic Pathology, pp. 127–132, ASCP Press, Chicago, 1978.

42. Goodman, Z. D. and Ishak, K. G. Hepatocellular carcinoma in women: probable lack of etiologic association with oral contraceptive steroids. Hepatology, *2*: 440–444, 1982.

43. Galloway, S. J., Casarella, W. J., and Lattes, R. Minimal deviation hepatoma. Am. J. Roentgenol. Radium Med., *125*: 184–192, 1975.

44. Zuckerman, A. J. Role of hepatitis B virus in primary liver cancer. *In;* K. Lapis and J. V. Johannessen (eds.), Liver Carcinogenesis, pp. 105–110, Hemisphere Publ., Washington, D. C., 1979.

45. Kiely, J. M., Titus, J. L., and Orvis, A. L. Thorotrast-induced hepatoma presenting as hyperparathyroidism. Cancer, *31*: 1312–1314, 1973.

46. Makk, L., Delorme, F., Creech, J. L., Ogden, L. L., Fadell, E. H., and Songster, C. L. Clinical and morphological features of hepatic angiosarcoma in vinyl chloride workers. Cancer, *37*: 149–163, 1976.

47. Nakashima, T., Okuda, K., Kojiro, M., Sakamoto, K., Kubo, Y., and Shimokawa, Y. Primary liver cancer coincident with Schistosomiasis Japonica. A study of 24 necropsies. Cancer, *36*: 1483–1489, 1975.

48. Toth, B. Hepatocarcinogenesis by hydrazine mycotoxins of edible mushrooms. *In;* K. Lapis and J. V. Johannessen (eds.), Liver Carcinogenesis, pp. 23–32, Hemisphere Publ., Washington, D. C., 1979.

49. Linsell, C. A. Environmental chemical carcinogens and liver cancer. *In;* K. Lapis and J. V. Johannessen (eds.), Liver Carcinogenesis, pp. 173–181, Hemisphere Publ., Washington, D. C., 1979.

50. Emerson, G. B., Nachtnebel, V. L., Penkava, R. R., and Rothenberg, J. Oral contraceptive associated liver tumors. Lancet, *i*: 219–230, 1979.

51. Edmondson, H. A., Reynolds, T. F., Henderson, B., and Benton, B. Regression of liver cell adenomas associated with oral contraceptives. Ann. Intern. Med., *86*: 180–182, 1977.

52. Kent, D. R., Nissen, E. D., Facog, E. D., Nissen, S. E., and Ziehm, D. J. Effect of pregnancy on liver tumor associated with oral contraceptives. Obstet. Gynecol., *51*: 148–151, 1977.

53. Schardein, J. L., Kaump, D. H., Woosley, E. T., and Jellema, M. M. Long term toxicologic and tumorigenesis studies on an oral contraceptive agent in albino rats. Toxicol. Appl. Pharmacol., *16*: 10, 1970.

54. Committee on The Safety Of Medicine, Carcinogenicity tests of oral contraceptives. Her Majesty's Stationary Office, London, 1972.

55. Wanless, I. R. and Medline, A. Role of estrogens as promoters of hepatic neoplasia. Lab. Invest., *46*: 313–320, 1982.

56. Yager, J. D. and Yager, R. Oral contraceptive steroids as promoters of hepatocarcinogenesis in female Sprague-Dawley rats. Cancer Res., *40*: 3680–3685, 1980.

57. Lang, R. and Redmann, U. Nonmutagenicity of some sex hormones in the Ames salmonella/microsome mutagenicity test. Mutat. Res., *67*: 361–365, 1979.

58. Reuber, M. D. Influence of hormones on *n*-2-fluorenyldicatamide induced hyperplastic hepatic nodules in rats. J. Natl. Cancer Inst., *43*: 445–451, 1969.

59. Dickey, R. P., Chihal, H. J., and Peppler, R. D. Estrogen potencies of three new low-dose oral contraceptives. Am. J. Obstet. Gynecol., *125*: 976–979, 1976.

60. Malt, R. A., Galdabini, J. J., and Jeppsson, B. W. Abnormal sex-steroid milieu in young adults with hepatocellular carcinoma. World J. Surg., *7*: 247–252, 1983.

61. Rosner, W., Aden, D. P., and Khan, M. S. Hormonal influences on the secretion of steroid-binding proteins in human hepatoma derived cell line. Clin. Endocrinol. Metab., *59*: 806–808, 1984.

62. Buckley, A. R., Putnam, C. W., and Russell, D. H. Prolactin is a tumor promoter in rat liver. Life Sci., *37*: 2569–2575, 1985.

63. Johnson, P. J. Sex hormones and the liver. Clin Sci. *66*: 369–376, 1984.

64. Barrows, G. H., Christopherson, W. M., Mays, E. T., and Reese, D. Estrogen and progesterone receptor status of benign liver tumors. Am. J. Clin. Pathol., *75*: 872–873, 1981.

65. Bojar, H., Petzinna, D., Brolsch, C., and Staib, W. Steroid receptor status of focal-nodular hyperplasia of the human liver. Klin. Wochenschr., *62*: 446–450, 1984.

66. Iqbal, M. J., Wilkinson, M. L., Johnson, P. J., and Williams, R. Sex steroid receptor proteins in foetal, adult and malignant human liver tissue. Br. J. Cancer, *48*: 791–796, 1983.
67. Nagasue, N., Yukaya, H., and Ogawa, Y. Androgen receptors in hepatocellular carcinoma and surrounding parenchyma. Gastroenterology, *89*: 643–647, 1985.
68. Ohnishi, S., Murakami, T., Moriyama, T., Mitamura, K., and Imawari, M. Androgen and estrogen receptors in hepatocellular carcinoma and in the surrounding noncancerous liver tissue. Hepatology, *6*: 440–443, 1986.
69. Dejean, A., Bougueleret, L., Grazeschik, K., and Tiollais, P. Hepatitis B virus DNA integration in a sequence homologous to v-34b-A and steroid receptor genes in a hepatocellular carcinoma. Nature, *372*: 70–72, 1986.
70. Stubblefield, P. Oral contraceptives and neoplasia. J. Reprod. Med., *29*: 524–528, 1984.

UNUSUAL OCCURRENCES AS CLUES TO CANCER ETIOLOGY, R. W. MILLER ET AL. (EDS.),
JAPAN SCI. SOC. PRESS, TOKYO/TAYLOR & FRANCIS, LTD., PP. 61–66, 1988

A Cohort Study on Mortality of "Yusho" Patients:
A Preliminary Report

Masanori Kuratsune,[*1] Masato Ikeda,[*2] Yoshikazu Nakamura,[*3]
and Tomio Hirohata[*3]

*Nakamura Gakuen College and Nakamura Gakuen Junior College, Fukuoka 814, Japan,[*1] Department of Clinical Epidemiology, Institute of Industrial Ecological Sciences, University of Occupational and Environmental Health, Kitakyushu 807, Japan,[*2] and Department of Public Health, Faculty of Medicine, Kyushu University, Fukuoka 812, Japan[*3]*

Abstract: In 1968, a mass food poisoning (Yusho) occurred in western Japan involving more than 1,850 people, the majority of whom were residents of Fukuoka and Nagasaki prefectures. The poisoning is now understood to have been caused by ingestion of a commerical brand of rice oil contaminated with polychlorinated derivatives of biphenyls, dibenzofurans, quaterphenyls, and some other related compounds. The number of deaths seen among 1,761 victims (887 males and 874 females) from the date of official registration as Yusho up to the end of 1983 was compared with the expected number of deaths which was calculated on the basis of the national age, sex, and cause-specific death rates. Neither significantly increased nor significantly decreased mortality was seen among overall causes of death in males and females. A significant excess mortality was seen for malignant neoplasms at all sites in males but not in females. Neither significantly increased nor decreased mortality was seen for cancer of the esophagus, stomach, rectum and colon, pancreas, breast, and uterus. For cancer of the liver, however, a considerably increased mortality was seen in both males and females but the excess was statistically significant only in males. It was also notable that such increased mortality due to liver cancer was seen mainly among the patients living in Fukuoka prefecture but not at all among those in Nagasaki prefecture which approximate the Yusho patients in Fukuoka prefecture in number. Deaths from chronic liver diseases and liver cirrhosis were also found to be increased in both sexes but the increase was not statistically significant.

Early in October 1968, an epidemic of a strange disease characterized by severe acne-like eruptions was reported in Fukuoka, Nagasaki, and other prefectures in western Japan. Epidemiologic and chemical investigations demonstrated that the epidemic was caused by ingestion of a commercial brand of rice oil contaminated with a complex mixture of polychlorinated biphenyls (PCBs), polychlorinated dibenzofurans (PCDFs), polychlorinated quaterphenyls (PCQs) and other related compounds (*1–4*). Figure 1 shows the chemical structures of these compounds and

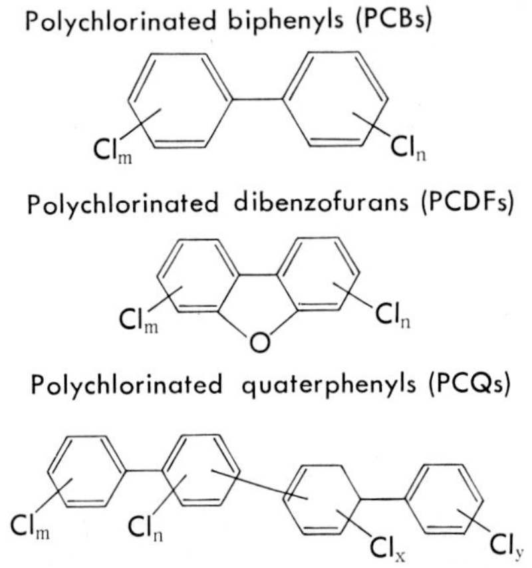

Polychlorinated biphenyls (PCBs)

Polychlorinated dibenzofurans (PCDFs)

Polychlorinated quaterphenyls (PCQs)

FIG. 1. Chemical structure of chlorinated hydrocarbons.

TABLE 1. Concentration of PCBs and Related Compounds in Samples of Toxic Rice Oil

Compound	No. of samples	Concentration (ppm)
Polychlorinated biphenyls (PCBs)	3	830, 900, 1,030[a]
Polychlorinated dibenzofurans (PCDFs)	3	5, 4, 5[a]
Polychlorinated quaterphenyls (PCQs)	2	705, 950[b]

[a] Ref. 5. [b] Ref. 6.

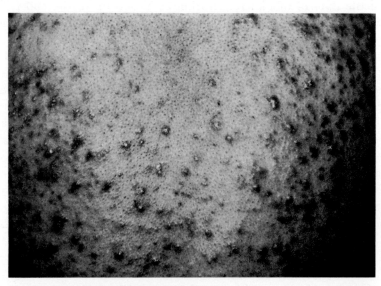

FIG. 2. Dermal lesions of Yusho patients.

Table 1 their concentration in the toxic rice oil consumed by patients. The disease was clinically diagnosed as chloracne and named "Yusho" which literally means "oil disease" in Japanese (Fig. 2).

The most notable manifestations of Yusho are dermal lesions such as comedo formation, acneform eruptions, hyperpigmentation, and hyperkeratosis (7). Peculiar ocular lesions such as swelled meibomian glands filled with yellow infarct-like material and pigmentation of the conjunctiva were also notable (8, 9). Most patients complained of various neurological symptoms such as headache, numbness of the limbs (10) and cough with sputum production for a prolonged period of time (11). Contrary to our expectation, patients showed few abnormalities of the liver in gross appearance or in liver function tests, but a marked proliferation of the smooth endoplasmic reticulum and a distinct reduction of the rough endoplasmic reticulum were noted by electron microscopy of liver biopsy specimens from one patient (12). During the 19 years since the poisoning, the above lesions have been very slow to improve and no complete recovery seems to have been attained yet in quite a few patients, as indicated by the fact that the subcutaneous adipose tissue samples from patients examined even 16 years after the onset of illness still contained, on average, 207 ppb of PCQs, which is more than 100 times the control level (13).

Cohort Analysis of Deaths

Analysis of deaths among the Yusho patients is important not only for better understanding of the health effects of prolonged exposure to these highly persistent man-made chlorinated hydrocarbons, but also for better health care. A cohort analysis was therefore made of the deaths (14).

The total number of patients officially registered as Yusho by the end of 1983

TABLE 2. Observed and Expected Numbers of Deaths and O/E Ratio by Cause of Death

Cause of death	Male			Female		
	Ob-served	Expected	O/E	Ob-served	Expected	O/E
All	79	66.13	1.19	41	48.90	0.84
Tuberculosis	1	1.26	0.79	0	0.50	0.00
Malignant neoplasms	33	15.51	2.13**	8	10.55	0.76
Esophagus	1	0.77	1.30	1	0.18	5.45
Stomach	8	5.69	1.40	0	3.26	0.00
Rectum, sigmoid colon, and anus	1	0.63	1.60	0	0.46	0.00
Liver	9	1.61	5.59**	2	0.66	3.04
Pancreas	1	0.71	1.41	1	0.46	2.18
Lung, trachea, and bronchus	8	2.45	3.26**	0	0.85	0.00
Breast	0	0.01	0.00	1	0.66	1.46
Uterus				1	0.58	1.71
Leukemia	1	0.45	2.23	0	0.32	0.00
Diabetes	1	0.75	1.34	0	0.69	0.00
Heart diseases	10	9.46	1.06	9	7.65	1.18
Hypertensive diseases	0	1.20	0.00	0	1.39	0.00
Cerebrovascular diseases	8	14.61	0.55	5	12.03	0.42*
Pneumonia and bronchitis	3	3.17	0.95	0	2.33	0.00
Gastric and duodenal ulcer	0	0.73	0.00	1	0.34	2.96
Chronic liver diseases and cirrhosis	6	2.26	2.65	2	0.73	2.74
Nephritis, nephrotic syndrome and nephrosis	0	0.79	0.00	2	0.71	2.81
Accidents	5	4.66	1.07	2	1.32	1.52

* $p < 0.05$, ** $p < 0.01$.

was 1,821. Information on name, date of birth, sex, address, and date and place of registration was obtained from the Ministry of Health and Welfare and the vital status of the registrants at the end of 1983 was confirmed by health departments of municipalities where they lived or still live; copies of the death certificates for decedents were also collected by these departments. Underlying causes of deaths seen before 1979 were assigned according to the 8th revision of ICD and deaths in 1979 and thereafter according to the 9th revision of ICD. Excluding 9 patients who had been officially registered as Yusho after death and 51 who were lost to follow-up, 1,761 patients (887 males and 874 females) were followed from the date of official registration to the end of 1983, the average duration of follow-up being about 11 years. The number of deaths during the observation period was compared with the expected number of deaths which was calculated by applying the national age, sex, and cause-specific death rates in 1970, 1975, and 1980 to the person-years at risk.

As shown in Table 2, the total number of deaths observed was 120, 79 males and 41 females. Male deaths were slightly more than expected but the difference was not statistically significant while females had fewer than expected, though again the difference was not statistically significant. Neither significantly elevated nor lowered mortality was seen for tuberculosis, diabetes, heart diseases, hypertensive diseases, pneumonia and bronchitis, gastric and duodenal ulcer, kidney diseases, or accidents. Deaths from cerebrovascular diseases were less than expected in both sexes, but significantly so only in females.

For deaths from cancer at all sites, a significantly increased mortality was seen in males but not in females. Neither significantly increased nor decreased mortality was seen for cancer of the esophagus, stomach, rectum and colon, pancreas, breast, and uterus, or leukemia. A significantly increased mortality was observed for cancer of the respiratory system in males but not in females.

For cancer of the liver (155, according to the 9th revision of ICD), 9 male deaths and 2 female deaths were observed and investigation of the clinical records of these decedents which is now in progress has so far demonstrated that at least 5 of them were from hepatoma. A marked excess of these deaths was observed in males, with an O/E (observed/expected) ratio as high as 5.59, and a less marked excess (O/E ratio=3.04) was also seen in females; the excess was statistically significant, however, only in males. Since about 45% and 40% of the patients are residents of Fukuoka and Nagasaki prefectures, respectively, where liver cancer is known to be the highest in the nation, an additional analysis was made by calculating expected number of deaths on the basis of liver cancer death rates in these prefectures instead of using the national average death rates. Again, a significantly increased mortality was observed in males (observed=9, expected=2.34, O/E ratio=3.85, $p<0.01$) but not in females (observed=2, expected=0.79, O/E ratio=2.53). In view of the long latent period common in the development of cancer, cancer cases which occurred soon after poisoning can hardly be regarded as having been caused by the poisoning alone. Excluding such cases, 4 deaths from liver cancer among males which occurred in Fukuoka prefecture more than 9 years after the onset of poisoning were compared with the corresponding expected number of deaths calculated from the male death rates there for this cancer. Again, a statistically significant excess mortality was seen (observed=4, expected=1.04, O/E ratio=3.85, $p<0.05$). Furthermore, not only deaths from liver cancer, but also deaths from chronic liver diseases and cirrhosis were found to be slightly increased in both males and females, although the increase was not statistically significant. Investigation of medical records has so far revealed that 2 of the 9 decedents from liver cancer had been infected with HB virus and only one had been a heavy drinker of alcohol.

The above findings suggest that the poisoning might have caused liver cancer at least in male patients. However, it seems still too early to draw any definite conclusion on this issue, because, as mentioned, contrary to the experience in Fukuoka prefecture, no excess death from liver cancer was seen in either male or female patients in Nagasaki prefecture where approximately the same number as in Fukuoka prefecture developed Yusho. Such a markedly uneven geographical distribution of deaths can hardly be explained by exposure to the toxic rice oil alone. Our findings should not be disregarded, however, because the hepatocarcinogenicity of PCBs in animals has been well documented (15, 16).

REFERENCES

1. Kuratsune, M., Yoshimura, T., Matsuzaka, J., and Yamaguchi, A. Epidemiologic study on Yusho, a poisoning caused by ingestion of rice oil contaminated with a commercial brand of polychlorinated biphenyls: Environ. Health Perspect. Exp. Issue, 5: 119–128, 1972.

2. Nagayama, J., Kuratsune, M., and Masuda, Y. Determination of chlorinated dibenzofurans in Kanechlors and 'Yusho Oil'. Bull. Environ. Contamin. Toxicol., 15: 9–13, 1976.

3. Miyata, H., Murakami, Y., and Kashimoto, T. Studies on the compounds related to PCB (VI). Determination of polychlorinated quaterphenyl (PCQ) in Kanemi rice oil caused the "Yusho" and investigation on the PCQ formation. J. Food Hyg. Soc., 19: 417–425, 1978.

4. Kashimoto, T., Miyata, H., Takayama, K., and Ogaki, J. Levels of PCDDs, coplanar PCBs and PCDFs in patients with Yusho and the causal oil by HR-GC. HR-MS. Fukuoka Acta Med., 78: 325–336, 1987 (in Japanese).

5. Nagayama, J., Masuda, Y., and Kuratsune, M. Chlorinated dibenzofurans in Kanechlors and rice oils used by patients with Yusho. Fukuoka Acta Med., 66: 593–599, 1975.

6. Yamaguchi, S. and Masuda, Y. Quantitative analysis of polychlorinated quaterphenyls in Yusho oil by high performance liquid chromatography. Fukuoka Acta Med., 76: 132–136, 1985 (in Japanese).

7. Urabe, H. and Asahi, M. Past and current dermatological status of Yusho patients. Environ. Health Perspect., 59: 11–15, 1985.

8. Ikui, H., Sugi, K., and Uga, S. Ocular signs of chronic chlorobiphenyls poisoning (Yusho). Fukuoka Acta Med., 60: 432–439, 1969 (in Japanese).

9. Kohno, T. and Ohnishi, Y. Ocular manifestations and polychlorinated biphenyls in the tarsal gland contents of Yusho patients. Fukuoka Acta Med., 76: 244–247, 1985 (in Japanese).

10. Nagamatsu, K. and Kuroiwa, Y. Electroencephalographical studies on 20 patients with chlorobiphenyl poisoning. Fukuoka Acta Med., 62: 157–158, 1971 (in Japanese).

11. Nakanishi, Y., Shigematsu, N., Kurita, Y., Matsuba, K., Kanegae, H., Ishimaru, S.,

and Kawazoe, Y. Respiratory involvement and immune status in Yusho patients. Environ. Health Perspect., *59*: 31–36, 1985.

12. Hirayama, C., Irisa, T., and Yamamoto, T. Fine structural changes of the liver in a patient with chlorobiphenyl intoxication. Fukuoka Acta Med., *60*: 455–461, 1969 (in Japanese).

13. Ohgami, T., Nonaka, S., Yoshida, H., Maruyama, F., Yamashita, K., and Masuda, N., PCB, PCQ concentration of blood and subcutaneous tissue in patients with PCB poisoning (Yusho). Fukuoka Acta Med., *78*: 337–342, 1987 (in Japanese).

14. Ikeda, M., Kuratsune, M., Nakamura, Y., and Hirohata, T. A cohort study on mortality of Yusho patients—A preliminary report. Fukuoka Acta Med., *78*: 297–300, 1986.

15. Kimura, H. and Baba, T. Neoplastic change in the rat liver induced by polychlorinated biphenyls. Gann, *64*: 105–108, 1973.

16. Ito, N., Nagasaki, H. J., Makiura, S., and Arai, M. Histopathological studies on liver tumorigenesis in rats treated with polychlorinated biphenyls. Gann, *65*: 545–549, 1974.

UNUSUAL OCCURRENCES AS CLUES TO CANCER ETIOLOGY, R.W. MILLER ET AL. (EDS.),
JAPAN SCI. SOC. PRESS, TOKYO/TAYLOR & FRANCIS, LTD., PP. 67–75, 1988

The Effects in the Human of Diethylstilbestrol (DES) Use during Pregnancy

Arthur L. Herbst

Department of Obstetrics and Gynecology, University of Chicago, Chicago, Illinois 60637, U.S.A.

Abstract: Intrauterine diethylstilbestrol (DES) exposure is associated with an increased risk for the development of clear cell adenocarcinoma (CCA) of the vagina and cervix. The age of the patients at diagnosis has varied from 7–35 years with the highest frequency from 14–22 years. The risk among the exposed, however, is small and is of the order of 1 per 1,000. Almost all of the cases occur in postmenarchal females. Other factors that may increase the risk are maternal history of prior miscarriage, exposure to DES in early gestation, a fall season of birth and prematurity. The occurrence of CCA has paralleled the sales of DES for pregnancy support in the U.S. Both vaginal adenosis (benign glands in the vagina) and CCA are more frequent among those whose mothers began DES in early pregnancy. An increased risk of squamous cell neoplasia has been hypothesized but not proven. The changes that occur in the female genital tract of the DES exposed appear to result from alterations in the development of the mullerian ducts. Currently there is no definitive evidence for an elevated risk of cancer among DES mothers or DES sons but studies have suggested a possible increase of breast cancer in the former group and testicular cancer in the latter group; a valid association has not been established in either.

Between 1966 and 1969 8 young women ranging in age from 15–22 years were treated in the Boston area for an extremely rare tumor, clear cell adenocarcinoma (CCA) of the vagina (in older literature referred to as a "mesonephroma"). These eight cases exceeded the number of such cases known to have occurred in young women prior to that time (*1*).

The unusual clustering of these cases led to a search for a cause. The initial clue came from the mother of one of the patients treated by Dr. Howard Ulfelder who told of her concern regarding her treatment during pregnancy with diethylstilbestrol (DES). This led to the development of a case-control retrospective study to evaluate the possible role of host, maternal and paternal roles, and environmental factors (*2*). Four control females were selected for each cancer case from the hospital in which the patient had been born. Questionnaires were completed by personal interview with the mother of each subject. During these interviews another mother of a cancer patient volunteered her positive DES history which she implicated in her daughter's disease.

Most of the factors did not differ significantly between the groups. Interestingly 7 of the 8 mothers of the cancer patients smoked at least 1/2 pack of cigarettes per day, but 21 of the 32 control mothers also had such a smoking history; not a significant difference. In addition, 7 of the mothers whose daughters developed cancer had experienced high risk pregnancy for which they had been treated during gestation with DES. Five of the 32 control mothers also had pregnancy complications but none received DES. The results of the DES association were confirmed in a subsequent study (3). The mother of one of the eight daughters with cancer did not have a high risk pregnancy nor was there any evidence of DES ingestion during her pregnancy. As already noted, these cancers occurred spontaneously albeit exceedingly rarely during the pre-DES era, and another speculative possibility is the ingestion of residues of DES from the food supply.

Current Epidemiologic Information/Registry Studies

In 1971 a Registry was formed to centralize clinico-pathologic and epidemiologic data about CCA of the genital tract. Cases occurring in young women born after 1940 were sought, whether or not there was a maternal DES history. As of July, 1987 there were 535 cases accessioned from the U.S., Canada, Australia, France, Great Britain, Mexico, Belgium, Holland, Czechoslovakia, Switzerland, Italy, West Germany, and the Ivory Coast of Africa. Among those cases with an available maternal history 60% were exposed to DES, dienestrol, or similar non-steroidal synthetic estrogens. In approximately 17% there was exposure to another hormone or an unidentified medication. In 23% of the cases there was no evidence of maternal medication. In some only fragmentary information was available so it is possible that a few of the "negative" cases may have actually been exposed. Steroidal estrogens have been prescribed during pregnancy but there is no statistically valid information currently available to relate steroidal estrogens or progestins to DES-type changes.

The years of diagnosis of DES patients with CCA of the vagina or cervix is shown in Fig. 1 (4). The highest frequencies are seen in the 1970's. Due to the passive reporting system upon which the Registry depends, there is often a delay in case accessions and thus the registration of cases for 1983 and later is probably incomplete. Currently approximately 6 DES associated CCA's treated in the U.S. are being reported to the Registry annually.

The age at diagnosis of DES patients who have developed CCA has ranged from 7 to 34 years. However 91% of the cases have been diagnosed in those between the ages of 15–27 years. The age incidence curve for 262 white female residents of the U.S. is shown in Fig. 2. The cancer has occurred in only 6 DES-exposed black females in the U.S. since few blacks received DES for pregnancy support. The cancer is rare even among the DES exposed and current estimates are 1 per 1,000 through age 34 years. The age incidence curve is unusual insofar as the disease is rare prior to the age of 14, then there is a rapid rise to reach its peak at approximately 19 years and after age 22 the rates decline sharply. Estimates for those in their mid 20's and

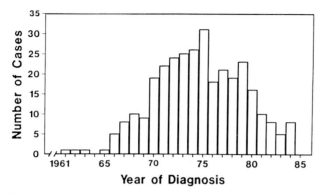

FIG. 1.   Number of DES-positive cases of clear cell adenocarcinoma according to year of diagnosis (4).

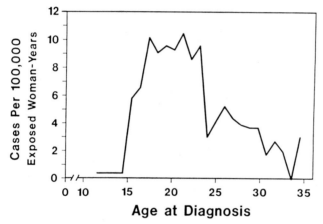

FIG. 2.   Incidence rates of clear cell adenocarcinoma, according to age, among white female residents of the United States who were prenatally exposed to DES (4).

older are imprecise because of the small number of cases. Its rate of occurrence among those over 40 is currently not known since the at risk population is currently less than 40, but CCA of the vagina and cervix was predominantly a disease of older women in the pre-DES era.

In order to compare the occurrence of CCA in the U.S. with DES usage for pregnancy support, the number of 25 mgm tablets sold yearly by one drug company for the years 1942–1961 were evaluated. Hundreds of companies manufactured the drug, but the sales of this manufacturer were sufficiently large to be representative of the usage of DES in the U.S. It was assumed that DES sold in one year would affect those born in the following year. The number of tablets sold in a 3 year period (1950–1952) was arbitrarily set to a relative value of 1 to be compared to the incidence of DES-cancer in cases born in 1951–1953, which was also set to a relative value of 1 (4, 5) (Table 1). As can be seen the occurrence of the cancer cases parallels very closely the sale of DES for pregnancy support for each 3 year cohort.

Recently a retrospective case control study was performed to evaluate factors other than DES that may contribute to the risk of development of CCA (6). One

TABLE 1. Exposure to DES and the Risk of CCA According to Birth Cohort

Year of sales of DES	Relative index of exposure[a]	Birth years	Percentage exposed[b]	Relative index of risk[a]
1947–1949	0.40	1948–1950	0.61	0.41
1950–1952	1.00	1951–1953	1.54	1.00
1953–1955	0.89	1954–1956	1.37	0.83
1956–1958	0.69	1957–1959	1.06	0.63
1959–1961	0.48	1960–1962	0.74[c]	0.33

[a] Sales years 1950–1952 and birth years 1951–1953 were assigned a value of 1.00 for comparison with other years. [b] Based on published estimates of DES exposure for birth years 1959–1965 (ref. Heinonen, O.P., 1973). [c] Partly estimated (Reprinted from Melnick et al.: N. Engl. J. Med., 316: 515–516, 1987)

TABLE 2. Variables Compared in Cases and Controls

Daughters
Birth year, birth month
Region, state of birth
Race
Birth weight
Age at menarche
Diethylstilbestrol exposure *in utero*
Day diethylstilbestrol began
Duration of diethylstilbestrol exposure
Total dosage of exposure
Progesterone in addition to DES
Mothers
Age
Prior number of pregnancies
Prior spontaneous abortions
Prior stillbirths
Prior infant deaths

(Reprinted from Herbst et al.: Am. J. Obstet. Gynecol., 154: 814, 1986)

hundred fifty-six cancer patients born in the U.S. were identified in the Registry who had written documentation of DES exposure. These were compared to 1848 DES-exposed women of similar age without cancer who were record-review participants in the National Cooperative Diethylstilbestrol Adenosis Project (DESAD), a multicenter DES evaluation project in the U.S. Table 2 displays factors in each group that were similarly recorded and could be compared. All multivariate analyses were adjusted for the difference between groups in region and years of birth. Most of the variables tested did not attain statistical significance. The relative risk for developing CCA was significantly higher among those whose mother began DES in early pregnancy (prior to the 12th week) and for those born in the fall (winter conception). In addition a maternal history of at least one prior spontaneous abortion elevated the risk. Prematurity (birth weight <2,500 g) also was a risk factor but there were an insufficient number of cases with birth weight information to allow that variable to be included in the final multiple logistic model. In this analysis many of the records had precise documentation of the time in pregnancy DES was begun, but in most there was not accurate information either on the dosage or the duration of DES treatment precluding any conclusions regarding the effect of these variables in CCA development. It should be emphasized that the elevated risk for development of CCA among those whose mothers began DES prior to the 12th week may have been mediated *via* the development of vaginal adenosis, a benign growth of glands in the vagina which also occurs with increased frequency in those whose mothers began DES in early pregnancy (see below). The elevated risk found with spontaneous abortion suggests genetic factors play a role. However it is important to emphasize that the difference in the time of exposure to DES remains statistically significant even after adjustment of the data for the maternal history of spontaneous abortion. The higher frequency of prematurity as well as a fall season of birth (winter conception) raises the speculative possibility of a role for viral infection in the development of CCA but no further data exist to support such a hypothesis (6).

Tumor Behavior

Three predominant histologic patterns of CCA have been described as clear cell (solid), papillary and tubulocystic. The 5-year survival of patients with CCA correlates closely with the stage of the tumor (I 87%) (II 76%) (III 37%) (IV—no survivors). It has also been found that those over age 19 years have an improved 5 year survival (83%) in comparison to those under age 15 years (71%) ($p<0.05$). Moreover, patients with a predominant tubulocystic pattern have a markedly better survival (88%) compared to approximately 73% for those with other tumor patterns. Detailed analyses showed that the patients over age 19 years also have a tumor with a predominant tubulocystic pattern which provides an explanation for the improved survival among the older patients.

Adenosis—Characteristics and Appearance

Vaginal adenosis (glandular epithelium or its mucinous products in the vagina) occurs in about 1/3 of DES exposed females. Two histologic variants (tuboendometrial and mucinous) are usually seen, the former lined by cells resembling tubal and endometrial epithelia and the latter resembling endocervical epithelium (7). A number of variables have been identified which influence the frequency of adenosis. Early initiation of DES in pregnancy as well as higher dosages ingested by the mother (8) increase the frequency. On the other hand adenosis appears to heal by a process of squamous metaplasia and older patients have lower frequencies (9). Furthermore one type of adenosis, namely that with a tuboendometrial histologic pattern is found topographically associated with CCA (7), and this type of adenosis appears to be associated with CCA development. However, spontaneous conversion of adenosis to CCA has only been infrequently reported and was noted in ten patients with documented adenosis followed for 1–8 years (10). Complete healing of adenosis with development of fully mature glycogenated squamous epithelium has been frequently observed (9, 11).

Due to the large areas of squamous metaplasia in the vagina and on the cervix of the DES exposed (transformation zone) there has been speculation that there will be an increased frequency of squamous cell neoplasia. An initial case-control comparison of exposed and unexposed from the DESAD study showed no evidence for a heightened risk. In a follow-up study of the same groups over a period of 7 years (12) a higher rate of dysplasia and CIS (15.7 vs. 7.9 cases per 1,000 years of follow-up) were noted among the DES exposed. Factors such as papillomaviral infection were not thoroughly evaluated in this study due to the fact that the period of evaluation began in 1974, prior to the current intensive interest in the role of papillomavirus in squamous neoplasia. Although there is a possibility that DES women may have an elevated risk for squamous neoplasia, a definite increase in risk has not been documented.

Cervicovaginal and Uterine Malformations

Concentric ridges that partially or completely encircle the cervix, and other similar anatomic abnormalities have been observed in about 20% of the DES exposed. These have been termed "hoods", "collars", "pseudopolyps" or more generally cervicovaginal ridges. Over a period of years some become less prominent or disappear (11). In addition deformities of the uterine cavity have been demonstrated by hysterosalpingogram including irregularities of the endometrial cavity, "T" shaped uteri, as well as a decrease in the size of the endometrial cavity. These changes occur in about 1/2 of the DES exposed who were record-review participants (13). These latter anatomic changes are believed to be related to the increased frequency of adverse pregnancy outcome experienced by the DES exposed including premature birth, ectopic pregnancy and midtrimester pregnancy loss (13, 14). Overall about 82% of DES exposed females who become pregnant have a viable newborn.

Histogenesis of DES Changes

The embryologic development of the human vagina is not definitely established, but it is generally believed to evolve primarily from the mullerian ducts which fuse in the midline followed by development of a solid core of squamous epithelium (vaginal plate) which extends up from the urogenital sinus. The core canalizes forming the vaginal lumen.

In utero exposure to DES in humans affects this developmental process. Mullerian-type cells resembling those of the endocervix, endometrium, and fallopian tube comprise the glandular epithelium of adenosis that is found in abnormal locations throughout the vagina in the DES-exposed. This is presumably a consequence of the nonsteroidal estrogen, DES, crossing the placenta early during intrauterine life (primarily before the 20th week). The hormone could then adhere to estrogen receptors that are present in the developing female genital tract which would lead to the observed epithelial and structural abnormalities (9). Both light microscopic and ultrastructural studies (15) suggest that CCA is of mullerian origin. Moreover both endometrium and tubal epithelium are also of mullerian origin but thus far endometrial carcinoma and fallopian tube carcinoma have not been associated with DES exposure, although a single case of endometrial cancer has been reported (16).

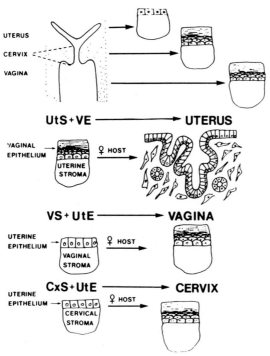

UtS+VE ⟶ UTERUS

VS+UtE ⟶ VAGINA

CxS+UtE ⟶ CERVIX

Fig. 3. A summary of recombination experiments between epithelium and stroma from uterus, cervix, and vagina from neonatal mice (1–5 days old). The upper portion of the figure depicts the morphologic organization of the epithelium in these organs; uterine epithelium is a simple columnar glandular epithelium, whereas vaginal and cervical epithelium is stratified squamous. Uterine stroma (UtS) induces uterine morphogenesis and cytodifferentiation from the vaginal epithelium (VE). In the reciprocal recombination composed of vaginal stroma (VS) plus uterine epithelium (UtE), the normally simple columnar epithelium is induced to differentiate as a vaginal epithelium. Similarly, cervical stroma (CxS) induces the development of a stratified cervical epithelium from the UtE. (ref. 9)

There is animal evidence to support these theories of histogenesis particularly from the experiments of Forsberg (17) who produced lesions similar to vaginal adenosis by administering estrogens to newborn mice who have immature vaginas at birth and are similar developmentally to the human in intrauterine life. Estrogens such as estradiol or DES given to neonatal mice appear to arrest the squamous transformation of columnar epithelium, resulting in the persistence of mullerian type epithelium in the upper vagina and cervix. Additional information on the possible mechanisms in this abnormal development come from the experiments of Cunha et al. (9) who have shown that the stroma from different parts of the embryonic female genital tract have an inductive effect on the overlying epithelium causing it to differentiate to the epithelium normally associated with that stroma (Fig. 3) i.e., combining cervical stroma and uterine epithelium leads to cerival epithelial development. Thus a stromal action of DES on the intrauterine development of the female genital tract could account for both the epithelial and structural abnormalities. The development of carcinoma requires other factors in addition to DES exposure as already noted.

DES Exposed Sons and Mothers

Conflicting data exist regarding the effects, if any, on the males exposed to DES *in utero* as well as to the mothers who ingested DES for pregnancy support. Because many DES mothers ingested high doses of DES, there has been concern that estrogen sensitive tumors such as endometrial or breast cancer could be developing with increasing frequency in this group. Bibbo *et al.* (*18*) studied DES exposed and unexposed mothers who participated in 1951–1952 in a double-blind evaluation of DES usage during pregnancy. Twenty-five years later the health status of the exposed and unexposed was ascertained. There was an increased frequency of breast cancer among the 693 exposed (32 cases) in comparison to the 668 unexposed (21 cases). The differences were not statistically significant and the greatest difference in breast cancer exposure was in the younger patients who were premenopausal and less than 20 years after DES expsoure. No other differences in cancer experience between the groups were noted. Four years later additional follow-up revealed 34 breast cancer cases among the exposed and 28 among the unexposed *i.e.*, a more comparable breast cancer experience between the groups (*9*). Subsequently Greenberg *et al.* (*19*) studied 3,033 DES exposed and 3,033 unexposed mothers and found 118 breast cancers among the exposed and only 80 among the unexposed. This difference was statistically significant and the relative risk (RR) was approximately 2.0. However, the predominant difference in this study occurred in the postmenopausal group who were more than 30 years after DES exposure, a different finding than the results of the Bibbo study. Further follow-up studies are needed to ascertain if there is an increased cancer risk to DES mothers.

Cryptorchidism, a risk factor for testicular cancer, is reported to have an increased frequency among males whose mothers used primarily hormone pregnancy tests (*20*). In a case-control study from the Mayo Clinic (*21*) no increase in testicular cancer was noted among 265 DES exposed males compared to 274 controls nor was an increase in maldescent of the testes among the DES-exposed observed.

REFERENCES

1. Herbst, A. L. and Scully, R. E. Adenocarcinoma of the vagina in adolescence: A report of 7 cases including 6 clear cell carcinomas (so-called mesonephromas). Cancer, *25*: 745–757, 1970.
2. Herbst, A. L., Ulfelder, H., and Poskanzer, D. C. Adenocarcinoma of the vagina: Association of maternal stilbestrol therapy with tumor appearance in young women. N. Engl. J. Med., *284*: 878–881, 1971.
3. Greenwald, P., Barlow, J. J., Nasca, P. C., and Burnett, W. S. Vaginal cancer after maternal treatment with synthetic estrogens. N. Engl. J. Med., *285*: 390, 1971.
4. Melnick, S., Cole, P., Anderson, D., and Herbst, A. L. Rates and risks of diethylstilbestrol-related clear cell adenocarcinoma of the vagina and cervix. An Update. N. Engl. J. Med., *316*: 514–516, 1987.
5. Herbst, A. L., Cole, P., Norusis, M. J., Welch, W. R., and Scully, R. E. Epidemiologic aspects and factors related to survival of 384 cases of clear cell adenocarcinoma of the vagina and cervix. Am. J. Obstet. Gynecol., *135*: 876, 1979.
6. Herbst, A. L., Anderson, S., Hubby, M., Haenszel, W. M., Kaufman, R. H., and

Noller, K. L. Risk factors for the development of diethylstilbestrol-associated clear cell adenocarcinoma: A case-control study. Am. J. Obstet. Gynecol., *154*: 814, 1986.

7. Robboy, S. J., Young, R. H., Welch, W. R., Truslow, G. Y., Prat, J., Herbst, A. L., and Scully, R. E. Atypical vaginal adenosis and cervical ectropion: Association with clear cell adenocarcinoma in diethylstilbestrol exposed offspring. Cancer, *54*: 869, 1984.

8. O'Brien, P. C., Noller, K. L., Robboy, S. J., Barnes, A. B., Kaufman, R. H., Tilley, B. C., and Townsend, D. E. Vaginal epithelial changes in young women enrolled in the National Cooperative Diethylstilbestrol Adenosis (DESAD) Project. Obstet. Gynecol., *53*: 300–309, 1979.

9. Herbst, A. L. and Bern, H. A. Developmental Effects of Diethylstilbestrol (DES) in Pregnancy, Thieme-Stratton, New York, 1981.

10. Sander, R., Nuss, R. C., and Rhatigan, R. M. Diethylstilbestrol-associated vaginal adenosis followed by clear cell adenocarcinoma. Int. J. Gyn. Path., *5*: 362–370, 1986.

11. Antonioli, D. A., Burke, L., and Friedman, E. A. Natural history of diethylstilbestrol-associated genital tract lesions: cervical ectopy and cervicovaginal hood. Am. J. Obstet. Gynecol., *137*: 847, 1980.

12. Robboy, S. J., Noller, K. L., O'Brien, P., Kaufman, R. H., Townsend, D., Barnes, A. B., Gundersen, J., Lawrence, W. D., Bergstrahl, E., McGorray, S., Tilley, B., Anton, J., and Chazen, G. Increased incidence of cervical and vaginal dysplasia in 3,980 diethylstilbestrol-exposed young women. JAMA, *252*: 2979–2989, 1984.

13. Kaufman, R. H., Noller, K., Adam, E., Irwin, J., Gray, M., Jeffries, J. A., and Hilton, J. Upper genital tract abnormalities and pregnancy outcome in diethylstilbestrol-exposed progeny. Am. J. Obstet. Gynecol., *148*: 973–984, 1984.

14. Herbst, A. L., Hubby, M. M., Blough, R. R., and Azizi, F. A comparison of pregnancy experience in DES-exposed and DES-unexposed daughters. J. Reprod. Med., *24*: 62, 1980.

15. Silverberg, S. G. and DeGiorgi, L. S. Clear cell adenocarcinoma of the vagina. Cancer, *29*: 1680, 1972.

16. Barter, J. F., Austin, J. M., and Shingleton, H. M. Endometrial adenocarcinoma after *in utero* diethylstilbestrol exposure. Obstet. Gynecol., *67*: 845, 1986.

17. Forsberg, J.-G. Cervicovaginal epithelium: Its origin and development. Am. J. Obstet. Gynecol., *115*: 1025, 1973.

18. Bibbo, M., Haenszel, W. M., Wied, G. L., Hubby, M., and Herbst, A. L. A twenty-five year follow-up study of women exposed to diethylstilbestrol during pregnancy. N. Engl. J. Med., *298*: 763, 1978.

19. Greenberg, E. R., Barnes, A. B., Resseguie, L., Barett, J. A., Burnside, S., Lanza, L. L., Neff, R. K., Stevens, M., Young, R. H., and Colton, T. Breast cancer in mothers given diethylstilbestrol in pregnancy. N. Engl. J. Med., *311*: 1393, 1984.

20. Depue, R. H., Pike, M. C., and Henderson, B. E. Estrogen exposure during gestation and risk of testicular cancer. J. Natl. Cancer Inst., *71*: 1151–1155, 1983.

21. Leary, F. J., Resseguie, L. J., Kurland, L. T., O'Brien, P. C., Enslander, R. F., and Noller, K. L. Males exposed *in utero* to diethylstilbestrol. JAMA, *252*: 2984–2989, 1984.

UNUSUAL OCCURRENCES AS CLUES TO CANCER ETIOLOGY, R.W. MILLER ET AL. (EDS.),
JAPAN SCI. SOC. PRESS, TOKYO/TAYLOR & FRANCIS, LTD., PP. 77–86, 1988

Development of Adenocarcinoma and Acquired Cystic Disease of the Kidney in Hemodialysis Patients

Isao Ishikawa

Division of Nephrology, Department of Internal Medicine, Kanazawa Medical University, Uchinada, Ishikawa 920-02, Japan

Abstract: Ninety-six hemodialysis patients were examined using computed tomography (CT) scan. Multiple cysts were found in 43.5% of those on hemodialysis for less than 3 years and in 79.3% of those who had been on dialysis for more than 3 years. Four patients had adenocarcinoma of the kidney; all 4 were in their 3rd and 4th decade and had been on hemodialysis for more than 5 years. Histologically, renal cell carcinomas were clear cell, or clear and granular cell carcinomas. All cancer patients had acquired cysts, intracystic epithelial hyperplasia (atypical cysts) and cysts or solid adenoma in the same kidney. Such findings are similar to those of experimental cancer of the kidney with respect to multifocal and bilateral lesions.

Of the 1,103 total reported dialysis patients in Japan and abroad, 47.1% had acquired cystic disease and 1.5% renal cell cancer. In a nationwide survey, a total of 119 patients (96 males and 23 females) with adenocarcinomas were found. Their mean age was 49.5±12.1 years. The mean duration of dialysis was 70.8±44.4 months. Twenty-five of them had metastases. Since the total number of hemodialysis patients in Japan is 66,310 (December, 1985), many adenocarcinomas may not have been discovered. Acquired cystic disease regresses rapidly after successful renal transplantation. This lends credence to the uremic metabolite accumulation hypothesis to explain the development of acquired cysts and tumors of the kidney in dialysis patients.

In conclusion, renal cell carcinoma in dialysis patients is closely related to the acquired cystic disease of the kidney. The frequency of renal cell cancer in long-term dialysis patients is increasing because of the higher incidence of acquired cysts with longer dialysis administration.

The existence of cysts in end-stage kidney was described by Frerichs (*1*) in 1851. However, little attention was paid to the contracted kidney in long-term hemodialysis patients until 1977 when Dunnill and his associates (*2*) reported acquired cystic disease of the kidney in 14 of 30 patients who had been on hemodialysis; tumors had developed in 6 of the 14 patients, with general metastasis developing in one patient. The number of hemodialysis patients is growing rapidly and had reached 73,537 in

Japan at the end of 1986 (*3*). This number is 604 per million population and 9,735 of these individuals have been on dialysis for more than 10 years (*3*). Accompanying this longer survival, new diseases unknown before the introduction of dialysis have come to light. These include acquired cystic disease and adenocarcinoma of the kidney in addition to β_2-microglobulin-derived dialysis amyloidosis and dialysis dimentia. Herein I discuss tumor formation and acquired cysts of the kidney in dialysis patients with the main focus on my own data. This is clinically important in predicting the patient's prognosis and also appears to be noteworthy because it provides important clues to solving the mechanism by which acquired cyst or tumor of the kidney develops.

The First Case in Japan of Acquired Cysts and Renal Cell Carcinoma in a Dialysis Patient

A 24-year-old male patient who had been on hemodialysis for 7 years was hospitalized for high fever and hematuria in December, 1978. He was referred to this hospital as requiring nephrectomy due to unresponsiveness to antibiotics given for "an infected autosomal dominant polycystic kidney disease." The kidneys removed in an emergency operation revealed multiple cysts and a hematoma 7 cm in diameter in the right kidney. The pathological report revealed the association of the hematoma with the autosomal dominant polycystic kidney disease. However, a detailed check of the patient's medical history revealed that a renal biopsy specimen, taken 9 years before, showed rapidly progressive glomerulonephritis, with normal sized kidneys as determined *via* intravenous pyelography. This indicated a discrepancy between the pathological report on nephrectomy and the progress of the glomerulonephritis. At this point, I recalled what I had learned in the United States, that all end-stage kidneys develop cyst formation. A search for similar reports in the literature yielded a paper by Dunnill *et al.* (*2*), published in 1977 in which it was reported that 6 out of 14 patients with acquired cysts were complicated with tumor formation, one patient showing disseminated metastasis. Our pathologist was then asked to carefully check the specimen. This check revealed the presence of renal cell carcinoma, consisting of clear and granular cells, on the wall of the hematoma. Thus was the first case detected in Japan of acquired cyst and cancer formation in the diseased kidney of a dialysis patient (*4*).

Computed Tomography to Detect Acquired Cysts and Tumor

Renal computed tomography (CT) was performed in 96 patients undergoing hemodialysis for chronic glomerulonephritis at the beginning of 1979 to measure kidney size and to detect the presence of cysts or tumors (*5*). As shown in Fig. 1, the incidence of cyst formation was surprisingly high. Multiple cysts were found in 43.5% of the patients on hemodialysis for less than 3 years and in 79.3% of those who had been on dialysis for more than 3 years (*5*). In addition, enlargement of the contracted kidney due to the presence of cysts was recognized 3 years after the induction of hemodialysis. Furthermore, 3 patients with renal cell carcinoma were found. The second case (28 years old, male, hemodialysis for 5 years 8 months) showed a carci-

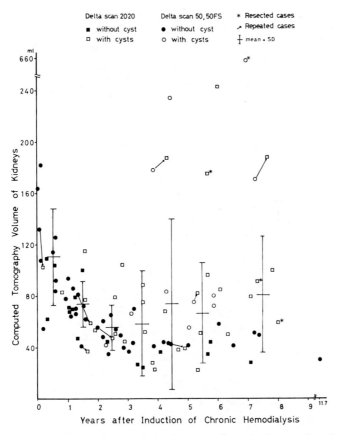

Fig. 1. Kidney volume and development of acquired cysts after the start of chronic hemodialysis. Kidney volume decreases gradually up to 3 years of dialysis. After 4 years kidney volume increases in some cases due to acquired cysts. Almost all enlarged kidneys have multiple cysts. (Cited from ref. 5).

noma in the left kidney composed of clear cells (Fig. 2a) which were seen as a tumor (2 cm in diameter) with calcified margin. In the third case (28 years old, female, hemodialysis for 8 years) normal X-ray density by CT scan showed a carcinoma of the left kidney with granular and clear cells which were a tumor formation (2.3 cm in diameter). The fourth case (31 years old, male, hemodialysis for 7 years 8 months) was one which was difficult to diagnose even by CT scan but it was later found to be a renal cell carcinoma of granular and clear cells (Fig. 2b) forming a tumor (2.5 cm in diameter) sandwiched between cysts.

Characteristics of Acquired Cysts and Tumor in Dialysis Patients

Acquired cysts predominate in the cortex and to some extent occur in the medulla (2). Most cysts are lined by flat or cuboidal epithelium. In some cysts, hyperplastic columnar cells with clear or granular cytoplasm predominate (2, 6). A scanning electron micrograph in acquired cystic disease revealed adenomatous polyps

TABLE 1.   Uremic Acquired Cystic Disease of the Kidney

	Cases	Uremic acquired cystic disease of the kidney	Renal tumor	Renal cell carcinoma
15 references (reported from outside Japan)	583	266 (45.6%)	37 (6.3%)	7 (1.2%)
autopsy 9				
CT 3				
US 3				
10 references (reported from Japan)	520	254 (48.8%)	16 (3.1%)	10 (1.9%)
autopsy 1				
CT 7				
US 1				
CT+autopsy 1				
Total	1,103	520 (47.1%)	53 (4.8%)	17 (1.5%)

US, ultrasound.

TABLE 2.   Renal Cell Carcinoma in Patients Treated with Hemodialysis

	1982[a]	1984	1986	Total
No. of patients with renal cell carcinoma	34	37	48	119
Male	25	31	40	96 (80.7%)
Female	9	6	8	23 (19.3%)
Mean age (years old)	47.9	49.6	50.5	49.5
Mean duration of dialysis (months)	49.4	73.6	83.9	70.8
No. of patients with metastasis	7	8	10	25 (21%)

[a] year of questionnaire study

I collected information on renal cell carcinomas in dialysis patients, including our own cases, by conducting a nationwide questionnaire survey (13–15). The dialysis population of Japan was 66,310 at the end of 1985. Among these, 119 adenocarcinomas of the kidney have been found; 80% of them were associated with acquired cystic disease. Thirty-four cases were found in 1982 (14), 37 in 1984 (13), and 48 in 1986 (15). The mean age of the 119 patients was 49.5 ± 12.1 years, the mean duration of hemodialysis was 70.8 ± 44.4 months, and the percentage of males was 80.7%, 4 times higher than that of females (Table 2). The male preponderance of renal adenocarcinomas may reflect the male preponderance of acquired cystic disease of the kidney in dialysis patients, as discussed later on. As shown in Table 2, 25 of the 119 patients (21.0%) had metastasis. Renal cell carcinoma associated with dialysis cannot be regarded as benign. The smallest renal cell carcinoma with metastasis was 1.2 cm in diameter (15).

Natural History and Pathogenesis of Acquired Cysts and Tumor

A prolonged duration of dialysis increases the incidence and extent of acquired cysts (*16*). The incidence of acquired cysts in non-dialysis patients is 12% (*17*). Furthermore, the development of cyst formation was observed in continuous ambulatory peritoneal dialysis patients (*18*) with almost the same incidence as in hemodialysis patients. These findings exclude the possibility that the cysts arise with specific consequence of the hemodialysis procedure. It is very impressive that after successful renal transplantation, almost all cysts have regressed and the kidney size has markedly decreased (*19–21*). There is a sex difference in acquired cysts (*16*). Males were found to have more and larger cysts and a higher rate of enlargement of the kidney. However, no age-related difference has been found in the incidence of acquired cystic disease (*5*).

Cyst fluid chemical composition was analyzed to study the pathogenesis of acquired cysts. Cyst fluid to serum ratio of sodium was 1.07 in acquired cysts (*22*). On the other hand, the cyst fluid to serum ratio of creatinine was 6.3 in acquired cysts, 1.0 in simple cysts and 0.8 in autosomal dominant polycystic kidney disease (Table 3) (*22*). Cyst fluid to serum ratio of β_2-microglobulin was very low compared to the respective serum levels (Table 3) (*23*). Therefore, an acquired cyst is a focal dilatation of the functioning proximal tubule including an altered hyperplastic epithelium.

Lectin-peroxidase conjugate reactivity (*24*) was examined in the acquired cysts. Two lectins were used; one was tetragonolobus lotus with high sensitivity for proximal tubules and the other was peanut with high sensitivity for distal tubules and collecting ducts. Positive tetragonolobus and negative peanut reaction seemed to be an indication of proximal tubule origin. Positive tetragonolobus and negative peanut reaction were observed in single-layered epithels of acquired cyst, hyperplastic epithels of atypical cysts and renal cell carcinoma. These findings suggest that renal cell carcinoma in dialysis patients is derived from the proximal tubules.

Figure 4 summarizes the results obtained together with schematic illustrations of

TABLE 3. Cyst Fluid/Serum Ratio of Sodium, Creatinine and β_2-Microglobulin

| | Case | Cyst fluid/serum ratio | | |
		Sodium	Creatinine	β_2-Microglobulin
	1	1.096 ± 0.036[a] (7)[b]	7.058 ± 1.311 (7)	0.053 ± 0.057 (7)
ACDK	2	1.087 ± 0.027 (10)	5.363 ± 1.396 (10)	0.060 ± 0.022 (8)
	3	1.038 ± 0.012 (9)	6.855 ± 1.465 (9)	0.004 ± 0.008 (7)
	Mean	1.072 ± 0.036 (26)	6.332 ± 1.581 (26)	0.040 ± 0.008 (22)
	4	1.075	0.867	
Simple cysts	5	1.077	1.000	1.864
	6	1.109	1.375	0.846
	Mean	1.087 ± 0.019 (3)	1.081 ± 0.263 (3)	1.355 (2)
PCKD	7	1.007	0.843	—

ACDK, acquired cystic disease of the kidney; PCKD, autosomal dominant polycystic kidney disease.   [a] mean $\pm$SD.   [b] numbers of cysts examined.

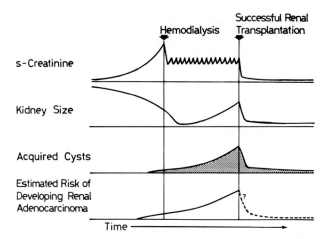

Fig. 4.   Schematic illustrations of the kidney size, number of cysts and risk factor for the development of renal cell carcinoma (see text). (Cited from ref. *8*).

the kidney size, number of cysts and the risk factor for the development of renal cell carcinoma (*8*). After 3 years or more of hemodialysis, enlargement of the kidney due to cyst formation occurs and, therefore, the risk of renal cell carcinoma becomes higher. However, if renal transplantation is successful, the cysts regress and the kidney shrinks. Furthermore a reduction in the risk of renal cell carcinoma is suspected, although this has not yet been proven. In the post transplant period, development of renal cell carcinoma in the original kidney is rare (*25*), and this appears to support the above consideration (*8*).

As to the several factors which may be involved in the etiology of renal cell carcinoma in a hemodialysis patient, impairment of immune surveillance, participation of carcinogens and involvement of local factors should be considered (*26*). Although there are several possible factors either endogenous or exogenous which may relate to carcinogens, their involvement has not been proved. I personally feel that some kind of uremic metabolite, which is a non-dialyzable and sex-related endogenous growth factor, plays a role in the pathogenesis of acquired cystic disease and renal cell carcinoma (*8*).

REFERENCES

1. Frerichs, F. T. Die Bright'sche Nierenkrankheit, p. 38, F. Vieweg, Braunschweig, 1851. (Cited from ref. *17*).
2. Dunnill, M. S., Millard, P. R., and Oliver, D. Acquired cystic disease of the kidneys: a hazard of long-term intermittent maintenance haemodialysis. J. Clin. Path., *30*: 868–877, 1977.
3. Present status of chronic dialysis therapy in Japan (1987) (Japanese). J. Jpn. Soc. Dial. Ther., *21*: 1–39, 1988.
4. Kitada, H., Kurihara, S., Suzuki, S., Onouchi, Z., Yuri, T., Ishikawa, I., Shinoda, A., Yamakawa, Y., Tsugawa, R., Konishi, F., and Kibe, Y. A case of "acquired cystic disease of the kidney" with renal cell carcinoma (Japanese). Jpn. J. Nephrol., *21*: 1145–1155, 1979.

5. Ishikawa, I., Saito, Y., Onouchi, Z., Kitada, H., Suzuki, S., Kurihara, S., Yuri, T., and Shinoda, A. Development of acquired cystic disease and adenocarcinoma of the kidney in glomerulonephritic chronic hemodialysis patients. Clin. Nephrol., *14*: 1–6, 1980.

6. Hughson, M. D., Hennigar, G. R., and McManus, J.F.A. Atypical cysts, acquired renal cystic disease, and renal cell tumors in end stage dialysis kidneys. Lab. Invest., *42*: 475–480, 1980.

7. Grantham, J. J. and Levine, E. Acquired cystic disease: Replacing one kidney disease with another. Kidney Int., *28*: 99–105, 1985.

8. Ishikawa, I. Uremic acquired cystic disease of kidney. Urology, *26*: 101–108, 1985.

9. Gardner, K. D., Jr. Acquired renal cystic disease and renal adenocarcinoma in patients on long-term hemodialysis. N. Engl. J. Med., *310*: 390, 1984.

10. Bretan, P. N., Jr., Busch, M. P., Hricak, H., and Williams, R. D. Chronic renal failure: A significant risk factor in the development of acquired renal cysts and renal cell carcinoma. Cancer, *57*: 1871–1879, 1986.

11. Hughson, M. D., Buchwald, D., and Fox, M. Renal neoplasia and acquired cystic kidney disease in patients receiving long-term dialysis. Arch. Pathol. Lab. Med., *110*: 592–601, 1986.

12. Bennington, J. L. Renal adenoma. World J. Urol., *5*: 66–70, 1987.

13. Ishikawa, I. Adenocarcinoma of the kidney in chronic hemodialysis patients in Japan —Nationwide questionnaire study and review of case reports. Jpn. J. Nephrol., *28*: 1299–1303, 1986.

14. Ishikawa, I. and Shinoda, A. Renal adenocarcinoma with or without acquired cysts in chronic hemodialysis patients. Clin. Nephrol., *20*: 321–322, 1983.

15. Ishikawa, I. Adenocarcinoma of the kidney in chronic hemodialysis patients. Int. J. Artif. Organs., *11*: 61–62, 1988.

16. Ishikawa, I., Onouchi, Z., Saito, Y., Tateishi, K., Shinoda, A., Suzuki, S., Kitada, H., Sugishita, N., and Fukuda, Y. Sex differences in acquired cystic disease of the kidney on long-term dialysis. Nephron, *39*: 336–340, 1985.

17. Mickisch, O., Bommer, J., Bachmann, S., Waldherr, R., Mann, J.F.E., Ritz, E. Multicystic transformation of kidneys in chronic renal failure. Nephron, *38*: 93–99, 1984.

18. Ishikawa, I., Moncrief, J. W., Aguirre, F., Brindley, B. W., and Mott, C. L. Acquired cystic kidney disease in continuous ambulatory peritoneal dialysis patients. *In;* M. Maekawa, K. D. Nolph, T. Kishimoto, and J. W. Moncrief (eds.), Machine Free Dialysis for Patient Convenience, pp. 131–133, ISAO Press, Cleveland, 1984.

19. Ishikawa, I., Yuri, T., Kitada, H., and Shinoda, A. Regression of acquired cystic disease of the kidney after successful renal transplantation. Am. J. Nephrol., *3*: 310–314, 1983.

20. Vaziri, N. D., Darwish, R., Martin, D. C., and Hostetler, J. Acquired renal cystic disease in renal transplant recipients. Nephron, *37*: 203–205, 1984.

21. Thompson, B. J., Jenkins, D.A.S., Allan, P. L., Winney, R. J., Dick, J.C.B., Wild, S. R., Anderton, J. L., and Chisholm, G. D. Acquired cystic disease of the kidney: an indication of renal transplantation? Br. Med. J., *293*: 1209–1210, 1986.

22. Ishikawa, I. Unusual composition of cyst fluid in acquired cystic disease of the end-stage kidney. Nephron, *41*: 373–374, 1985.

23. Ishikawa, I. β_2-Microglobulin level of cyst fluid in uremic acquired cystic disease of the kidney. Nephron, *44*: 381, 1986.

24. Faraggiana, T., Bernstein, J., Strauss, L., and Churg, J. Use of lectins in the study of histogenesis of renal cysts. Lab. Invest., *53*: 575–579, 1985.

25. Penn, I. Malignancies associated with immunosuppressive or cytotoxic therapy. Surgery, *83*: 492–502, 1978.
26. Davin, T., Cosio, F., and Kjellstrand, C. M. Association of cancer with primary renal disease and/or uremia. *In;* R. E. Rieselbach and M. B. Garnick (eds.), Cancer and the Kidney, pp. 857–868, Lea & Febiger, Philadelphia, 1982.

UNUSUAL OCCURRENCES AS CLUES TO CANCER ETIOLOGY, R.W. MILLER ET AL. (EDS.),
JAPAN SCI. SOC. PRESS, TOKYO/TAYLOR & FRANCIS, LTD., PP. 87-94, 1988

Environment and Malignancies of the Lymphatic System

Bracha RAMOT* and Isaac BEN-BASSAT

Department of Hematology, The Chaim Sheba Medical Center, Tel-Hashomer and Sackler School of Medicine, Tel-Aviv University, Israel

Abstract: The possible effects of environmental factors on childhood lymphatic leukemia and intestinal lymphoma are reviewed. It is suggested that the subtype of childhood acute leukemia is determined by a spontaneous mutation in the proliferating lymphoid pool. The latter is affected by environmental factors such as the type of infections in the pediatric population. The changing leukemia subtype pattern in the Gaza Strip and the fact that intestinal lymphoma with malabsorption has practically disappeared from Israel strongly suggest that environmental factors do play a role in lymphatic malignancies.

Marked differences in the incidence of childhood malignant diseases between developed and developing countries have been clearly documented. In the United States, leukemias, lymphomas, and tumors of the central nervous system account for 75% of the deaths from cancer of white children below the age of 15. The picture is very similar in other Western countries as well as in Israel. In Africa, however, B-cell lymphomas constitute the major form of childhood malignancy, although only partial incidence and mortality data are available.

The effect of carcinogens such as industrial pollutants, tar, cigarettes, and so on are well documented environmental factors causing malignancies in organs such as lung, bladder, and skin, but will not be dealt with in this review. In addition, however, there are less defined environmental factors such as socioeconomic status, nutrition and infections in infancy that in the proper genetic background can play a role in the multistep carcinogenic process.

We review here several hematologic malignancies in which such environmental factors may be of importance in determining the likelihood of the development of the neoplasm. Data based on our experience in Israel are discussed.

---

* Incumbent of the Gregorio and Dora Shapiro Chair of Hematologic Malignancies at The Tel-Aviv University.

Childhood Acute Lymphoblastic Leukemia (ALL)

Childhood ALL is the most common childhood cancer in developed countries, with an annual incidence around 2–3 per 10^5 for age-matched populations in Europe and the United States (*1*). Despite the major advances made in the treatment of this disease, the etiology of acute leukemia remains an enigma.

ALL is phenotypically heterogeneous. The most common phenotype in developed countries is common ALL (cALL), which is HLADR+, CD10+ CD19+; it accounts for 60–70% of ALL cases. Following in frequency in descending order are pre B-ALL, T-ALL, and B-ALL. T-ALL accounts for 10–25% of the acute childhood leukemias in the Western world (*2*); it has a constant incidence rate during childhood, a male predilection, and an older age at presentation than non-T-cell leukemias.

Epidemiologic studies from developed countries revealed a peak incidence of ALL between the ages 2 and 5 (identified by mortality statistics) (*3*). This age-related peak incidence, which is known to be due to the predilection of cALL for this age group, was interpreted by some observers to be related to socioeconomic development (*3, 4*), but others have proposed alternative explanations (*5*).

We have reported an increase in the number of cases of childhood ALL from 1967 to 1981 in the Arab population of the Gaza Strip, a region administered by Israel since 1967 (*6*). Even more striking was the high proportion of T-ALL, accounting for as much as 50% of these patients (*7*). The minimal incidence rate of ALL in the Gaza Strip did not differ significantly from that observed in the Jewish population of Israel (*7*) during the same period, where it accounted for about 30% of the immunophenotyped patients.

Of interest are the findings since 1982. While the total number of cases of acute leukemia in the Gaza Strip did not decline, the T-ALL/non-T-ALL ratio changed (Table 1). The number of T-cell cases remained constant, while the number of patients with cALL steadily increased. Figure 1 gives the age distribution of the T- and non-T-ALL in the Gaza Strip from 1982 to 1986.

Whether the changing pattern of leukemia subtypes is real or a random event attributed to the small sample size remains to be determined. Since these findings are not due to a change in cell marker techniques, this trend—if it persists—will be the first direct proof that leukemia subtypes are influenced by environmental factors, a hypothesis previously suggested by us (*4, 8*). Recent data from Egypt and from India

TABLE 1.   Subtypes of Childhood Acute Leukemia in the Gaza Strip

Year	Subtypes	
	T	Non-T
1982	8	1
1983	3	6
1984	4	3
1985	2	5
1986	4	11
Total	21	26

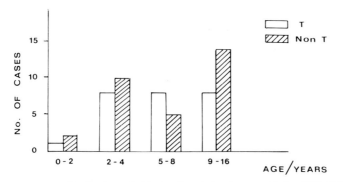

F<small>IG</small>. 1. Age distribution of childhood ALL in the Gaza Strip (1982–1987).

indicate a T/non-T-ALL ratio close to 1 (Ian Magrath, personal communication), a figure that supports our observations in the Gaza Strip.

Marked socioeconomic changes have occurred in the Gaza Strip in the past years, as evidenced by a continuous decline in infant mortality and a rise in the per capita income (4). To cite one small change, only 3% of Gaza Strip households had refrigerators prior to 1967, while over 80% have them today.

While the phenotype distribution appears to be changing, it is important to stress that a high proportion of non-T-ALL patients present with high WBC counts and are slightly older (Fig. 1), placing them in the high risk category, similar to the pattern observed in developing countries (9, 10). It is not clear whether this indicates a late diagnosis, a commonly offered explanation, or if it is a biologically different disease, possibly related to genetic and environmental factors. In this respect it is of interest that we observed two intermarried families in the Gaza Strip, in one of which two siblings had common ALL, and in the other, three siblings had T-cell lymphoma and T-ALL. From all the foregoing it is clear that genetics and environment may both be factors in determining disease type and clinical behaviour.

Changing clinical patterns of acute leukemia over the past 20 years have also been reported in American blacks by Bowman *et al.* (*11*). Their results support the view that ALL in general, and its subtypes in particular, are indeed associated with socio-economic changes. If differences in leukemia incidences are related to socio-economic factors, this observation might provide a lead in the search for leukemogenic agents, similar to those observed in Burkitt's lymphoma in Africa and T-cell leukemia in Japan.

Two hypotheses have been put forth to explain the differences between developed and developing countries. Stewart and Kneale (5) assume that death in early childhood from endemic infectious diseases obscures the true incidence rate of leukemia in countries with less developed diagnostic and medical facilities. Thus, the common ALL subtype is underdiagnosed, while the older children with T-ALL are less affected by it.

The second hypothesis, proposed by us, suggests that there is a higher proportion of T-cell leukemia in developing countries due to an absolute deficit of cALL, and environmental factors such as the type of infections in infancy—viral or bacterial—influence the incidence of the leukemia subtypes (9). Our data from the Gaza Strip support this hypothesis, where an absolute increase in the incidence of cALL occurs concurrent with improving socioeconomic circumstances. It is unlikely that this picture is due to underdiagnosis of cALL in earlier years, since the number of cases among Gaza Strip Arabs and Israeli Jews remained approximately equal. The picture does suggest that during the period of relatively poor socioeconomic conditions, there was a higher incidence of T-cell ALL. The relative decrease in T-cell ALL over time appears to be associated with a progressive increase in cALL, resulting in a roughly constant overall incidence of leukemia. We recognize, of course, that this interpretation requires verification on a larger number of cases, or data from other regions of the world undergoing similar socioeconomic development.

An international collaborative study initiated in 1982 by Greaves *et al.* (*10*) confirmed the previous observations that cALL is under-represented in developing countries, irrespective of ethnic type or geographic region. This was interpreted as supporting Stewart's hypothesis (*5*). These results could however, also be explained on the basis of a truly lower incidence of cALL rather than selective underdiagnosis of this phenotypic subgroup.

An inter-regional epidemiologic study was performed recently in Great Britain on 234 children with leukemia and lymphoma and 468 controls, matched for age and sex (*12*). The authors concluded that prenatal factors may be less important than postnatal factors or genetic makeup in the development of leukemia or lymphoma in children. None of these observations prove or deny either of the two hypotheses, since none of the data relate to leukemia incidence.

The importance of genetic factors in pediatric malignancies is well substantiated. ALL occurs at a higher frequency in children with ataxia-telangiectasia, Bloom and Down syndromes (*13*). However, these conditions account for a very small fraction of the total number of childhood ALL in any given population.

Extensive data on the genetic aspects of leukemia were summarized by Zuelzer and Cox (*14*). They could not, however, draw clear conclusions concerning genetic predisposing factors, except for a higher familial incidence in chronic lymphocytic leukemia (CLL). Controversial results were reported on the association between ALL and HLA types (*15, 16*). Our own retrospective data suggest that there is a correlation between HLA phenotypes in ALL and prognosis. The presence of HLA A11 was associated with significantly shorter survival (*17*). This finding, like other prognostic factors, may, of course, be abolished by newer and more aggressive treatment protocols.

Recently, Greaves and Chan (*18*) suggested that cALL results from a spontaneous mutation in the proliferating pre-B-cell progenitor population and that this mutation occurs at a similar frequency throughout the world. Moreover, they postulated that environmental factors have no pathogenetic role. During the fetal, neonatal, and infancy periods, clonal diversification during ontogeny occurs as a result of molecular changes on the DNA level associated with recombinational events, deletions and somatic mutations to produce functional immunoglobulins. These events may predispose the cells to a higher frequency of chromosomal breaks at the rearranging receptor gene loci, and could well be relevant to the occurrence of spontaneous mutations. The authors used the kinetic data for B-cell turnover in young mice provided by Osmond (*19*) for the calculation of relative frequencies of such mutations. They have no explanation, however, for the age-related peak of common ALL. Since spontaneous mutations should occur at a relatively constant rate (*i.e.*, the number of mutations per million cells), we feel that this could explain the constant low incidence of T-ALL in developed countries, and the higher rate in developing countries. The T-cell pool expands in response to severe viral infections, and the cell population at risk for a spontaneous mutation would depend on the proliferating lymphoid population at a given time. Thus, while we agree that spontaneous mutations ultimately account for the development of ALL, we feel that environmental factors do alter the incidence of leukemia by affecting the size of the target cell population at risk, which determines the leukemic phenotype. This challenging hypothesis awaits proof, of course, and until then the importance of environmental factors in the rate of childhood ALL and its subtypes remains an open question. If the trend observed in the population of the Gaza Strip during the last several years continues, it will challenge Stewart's hypothesis (*5*). At present, however, we require more extensive epidemiologic data.

Intestinal Lymphoma in Developing Countries

High grade and diffuse type lymphomas constitute about 80–90% of cases in developing countries, while in developed countries 30–50% of the lymphomas are nodular (*9*). In addition, there are regional and ethnic differences in incidence and phenotype. The best examples are Burkitt's lymphoma in Africa, small intestinal lymphoma around the Mediterranean basin, and adult T-cell leukemia/lymphoma in Japan. Intestinal lymphoma will be discussed here since it exhibits a regional distribution in developing countries.

Intestinal lymphoma has a high incidence in Iran, Lebanon, Algiers, Morocco, and the coloured population of South Africa. Sporadic cases have also been reported from other parts of the world. It appears to be the most common form of extranodal disease in the Middle East, accounting in some series for about 50% of extranodal and 75% of gastrointestinal lymphoma in adults (*20*). In Israel the disease affected Arabs and North African Jews (*21*).

A variant of intestinal lymphoma, called small intestinal lymphoma with malabsorption, was described by us in 1965 (*22*). This disease affected mainly young adults of both sexes and was characterized by a malabsorption syndrome for months to several years preceding the diagnosis of lymphoma.

In 1968 Seligmann *et al.* described the association between small intestinal infiltration by plasma cells and alpha heavy chain in the serum and urine, and called it alpha heavy chain disease (*23*). About 25–60% of cases of small intestinal lymphoma display alpha heavy chain in the serum (*21, 24*). Although a number of cases of nonsecreting alpha heavy chain disease have been reported (*25*), the actual prevalence of this protein abnormality in gastrointestinal lymphomas in developing countries remains unknown. This should be studied, since it is important in order to understand the evolution of this disease.

The pathology of this condition has been well described (*26–28*). Histologically, there appear to be two stages: a premalignant phase characterized by marked plasma cell infiltration called IPSID (immunoproliferative small intestinal disease) (*27*), considered to be reversible, and a malignant phase, an immunoblastic lymphoma, where alpha heavy chains were found to be expressed on the cell surface (*29, 30*). This is a disease of the Third World (*31*), and is probably one of the best human models for lymphoma pathogenesis. Gastrointestinal infections or other stimuli to the intestinal B-cells result in a clonal plasma cell response. Additional hits or hits to the proliferating pool result in a malignant transformation. It remains to be clarified whether this malignant transformation is associated with an additional oncogenic event such as a chromosomal translocation, similar to Epstein-Barr virus-associated Burkitt's lymphoma in the immunocompromised hosts. Unfortunately, no molecular studies have been reported on this disease. It is possible that the expression of an oncogene is altered because of a genetic change involving the IgA locus. This could be similar to the mechanism occurring in Burkitt's lymphoma where altered regulation of *c-myc* is a consequence of a chromosomal translocation, which probably stems from a faulty genetic recombination during the process of VDJ or VJ joining or heavy chain switching of immunoglobulin genes.

The fact that this condition has practically disappeared in Israel, and in the Gaza Strip, concomitant with a rise in living standards indicates that socioeconomic factors play a major role in the evolution of small intestinal lymphoma in developing countries.

REFERENCES

1. Breslow, N. E. and Langholz, B. Childhood cancer incidence. Geographical and temporal variations. Int. J. Cancer, *32*: 703–716, 1983.
2. Greaves, F. M. Subtypes of acute lymphoblastic leukaemia: Implications for the pathogenesis and epidemiology of leukaemia. *In;* I. Magrath, G. T. O'Conor, and B. Ramot (eds.), Environmental Influences in the Pathogenesis of Leukemias and Lymphomas, Vol. 27, pp. 129–139, Raven Press, New York, 1984.
3. Court Brown, W. M. and Doll, R. Leukemia in childhood and young adult life. Trends in mortality in relation to aetiology. Br. Med. J., *26*: 981–988, 1961.
4. Ramot, B. and Magrath, I. Hypothesis: The environment is a major determinant of the immunological sub-type of lymphoma and acute lymphoblastic leukemia in children. Br. J. Haematol., *50*: 183–189, 1982.
5. Stewart, A. and Kneale, G. W. Role of local infections in the recognition of haematopoietic neoplasms. Nature, *233*: 741–742, 1969.
6. Ramot, B., Ben-Bassat, I., Many, A., Kende, G., Neumann, Y., Brok-Simoni, F., Rosenthal, E., and Orgad, S. Acute lymphoblastic leukemia subtypes in Israel: The Sheba Medical Center experience. Leuk. Res., *6*: 679–683, 1982.
7. Ramot, B., Ben-Bassat, I., Brecher, A., Zaizov, R., and Modan, M. The epidemiology of childhood acute lymphoblastic leukemia and non-Hodgkin's lymphoma in Israel between 1976 and 1981. Leuk. Res., *8*: 691–699, 1984.
8. Ben-Bassat, I., Biniaminov, M., Rosenthal, E., and Ramot, B. T-cell acute lymphoblastic leukemia in Israel: Clinical and laboratory features. Leuk. Res., *11*: 1313–1318, 1986.
9. Magrath, I. T., O'Conor, G. T., and Ramot, B. Pathogenesis of Leukemias and Lymphomas: Environmental Influences. Raven Press, New York, 1984.
10. Greaves, M. F., Pegram, S., and Chan, L. C. Collaborative group study of the epidemiology of acute lymphoblastic leukemia subtypes: Background and first report.

Leuk. Res., *9*: 715–733, 1985.

11. Bowman, W. P., Presbury, G., Melvin, S. L., George, S. L., and Simone, J. V. A comparative analysis of acute lymphocytic leukemia in white and black children: Presenting clinical features and immunologic markers. *In;* I. T. Magrath, G. T. O'Conor, and B. Ramot (eds.), Pathogenesis of Leukemias and Lymphomas: Environmental Influences, pp. 169–177, Raven Press, New York, 1984.

12. McKinney, P. A., Cartwright, R. A., Saiu, J.M.T., Mann, J. R., Stiller, C. A., Draper, G. J., Hartley, A. L., Hopton, P. A., Birch, J. M., and others. The inter-regional epidemiological study of childhood cancer (IRESCC): A case control study of aetiological factors in leukemia and lymphoma. Arch. Dis. Childhood, *62*: 279–287, 1987.

13. German, J. Patterns of neoplasia associated with the chromosome breakage syndromes. *In;* J. German (ed.), Chromosome Mutation and Neoplasia, pp. 97–134, Alan R. Liss, New York, 1983.

14. Zuelzer, W. W. and Cox, D. E. Genetic aspects of leukemia. Sem. Hematol., *6*: 228–249, 1969.

15. Von Fliender, V. E., SultanKhan, Z., and Jeannet, M. HLADRw antigens associated with acute leukaemia. Tissue Antigens, *16*: 399–404, 1980.

16. Warren, R. P., Storb, R., Nguyen, D. D., and Thomas, E. D. Association between leucocyte group-5a antigen and acute lymphoblastic leukaemia. Lancet, *i*: 509–510, 1977.

17. Orgad, S., Cohen, I. J., Neumann, Y., Vogel, R., Kende, G., Zaizov, R., Ramot, B., and Gazit, E. Poor prognosis in childhood ALL is associated with HLA-All. Histocompatibility Immunogenetics Conference, November, 1987, New York.

18. Greaves, M. F. and Chan, Li. C. Is spontaneous mutation the major 'cause' for childhood acute lymphoblastic leukaemia? The paucity of evidence for environmental and genetic factors in acute lymphoblastic leukaemia. Annotation. Br. J. Haematol., *64*: 1–13, 1986.

19. Osmond, D. G. Population dynamics of bone marrow B lymphocytes. Immunol. Rev., *93*: 103–124, 1986.

20. Ramot, B. and Many, A. Primary intestinal lymphoma: clinical manifestations and possible effect of environmental factors. Recent Results Cancer Res., *39*: 193–199, 1972.

21. Salem, P., El-Hashimi, L., Anaissie, E., Geha, S., and others. Primary small intestinal lymphoma in adults. A comparative study of IPSID *versus* non-IPSID in the Middle East. Cancer, *59*: 1670–1676, 1987.

22. Ramot, B., Shahin, N., and Bubis, J. J. Malabsorption syndrome in lymphoma of small intestine: A study of 13 cases. Israel J. Med. Sci., *1*: 221–226, 1965.

23. Seligmann, M., Danon, F., Huerez, D., Mihaesco, E., and Preud'homme, J. Alpha chain disease: A new immunoglobulin abnormality. Science, *162*: 1396–1397, 1968.

24. Ramot, B. and Hulu, N. Primary intestinal lymphoma and its relation to alpha heavy chain disease. Br. J. Cancer, *31*: 343–349, 1975.

25. Rambaud, J. C., Modigliani, R., and Nguyen Phuoc, B. K. Nonsecretory alpha chain disease in intestinal lymphoma. N. Engl. J. Med., *303*: 353, 1980.

26. Rappaport, H., Ramot, B., Hulu, N., and Park, L. K. The pathology of so-called Mediterranean abdominal lymphoma with malabsorption. Cancer, *29*: 1502, 1972.

27. Nassar, V., Salem, P., Shahid, M., and others. "Mediterranean Abdominal Lymphoma" or immunoproliferative small intestinal lymphoma: Pathological aspects. Cancer, *4*: 1340–1354, 1978.

28. Haghighi, P. and Wolf, P. L. Alpha-heavy chain disease. Clin. Lab. Med., *6*: 477–489, 1986.

29. Moroz, Ch., Lahat, N., Biniaminov, M., and Ramot, B. Ferritin on the surface of lymphocytes of Hodgkin's disease patients a possible blocking substance removed by levamisole. J. Clin. Exp. Immunol., *29*: 30–36, 1977.

30. Brouet, J. C., Mason, D. Y., Danon, F., and others. Alpha chain disease: Evidence for a common clonal origin of intestinal immunoblastic lymphoma and plasmocytic proliferation. Lancet, *i*: 861, 1977.

31. Khojasteh, A., Haghshenass, M., and Haghighi, P. Immunoproliferative small intestinal disease: A "Third-World lesion". N. Engl. J. Med., *308*: 1401–1405, 1983.

UNUSUAL OCCURRENCES AS CLUES TO CANCER ETIOLOGY, R.W. MILLER ET AL. (EDS.),
JAPAN SCI. SOC. PRESS, TOKYO/TAYLOR & FRANCIS, LTD., PP. 95–101, 1988

Epidemiological Studies of Lung Cancer in Japanese Mustard Gas Workers

Yukio Nishimoto, Michio Yamakido, Shinichi Ishioka, Takuso Shigenobu,
and Masato Yukutake

Second Department of Internal Medicine, Hiroshima University School of Medicine, Hiroshima 734, Japan

Abstract: Until the end of the Second World War, a poison gas manufacturing plant
was operating on Okunojima, an island in the Seto Inland Sea. Of the gases produced
there, mustard gas and Lewisite were found to be associated with various malignant
tumors including lung cancer. The mortality rate for lung cancer in workers directly
or indirectly involved in the production of poison gas was significantly higher than
that of workers not involved in the production there. Lung cancer caused by poison
gas was characterized by the following features: it was found as a central pulmonary
carcinoma and was distributed from the upper airway to the hilar region. Squamous
cell carcinoma and undifferentiated carcinoma predominated, whereas adenocarcinoma and other types were rare. Retired workers who had been engaged in the manufacture of mustard gas were found to have depressed immunological competence. We
therefore started to enhance immunological competence with the use of *Nocardia rubra*
cell wall skeleton (N-CWS) in order to prevent carcinogenesis. To date, no conclusion has been reached on its effectiveness in preventing carcinogenesis, however, we
do expect it to be effective.

The defunct Japanese Army operated a poison gas factory from 1927 to 1945 on
Okunojima, an island off the coast of Tadanoumi-cho, Takehara City, Hiroshima
Prefecture. Production reached its peak in 1937. After the war the factory was closed
and the remaining poison gases were disposed of in the sea. Table 1 shows the chemical properties of these poison gases. Mustard gas (Yperite) and Lewisite are erosive
gases with high toxicity, diphenly-chlorarsine is a sneezing gas, hydrocyanic gas and
phosgene are suffocating gases, and phenacylchloride is a tear gas.

The former poison gas workers were divided into three groups according to their
type of work in the factory. As shown in Table 2, Group A consisted of workers engaged
directly in the production of poison gases such as mustard gas and Lewisite. Group
B consisted of workers who had come in contact with these gases. Group C consisted
of those engaged in the production of other gases or who were working in medical
and/or administrative work.

TABLE 1. Gases Produced at the Poison Gas Factory on Okunojima Island

Name of gas	Chemical structure	Character
β,β'-Dichlordiethylsulfide (Mustard gas, Yperite)	$(ClCH_2 \ CH_2)_2S$	Erosive
Chlorvinylarsine (Lewisite)	$CHCl: CHAsCl_2$ $(CHCl: CH)_2AsCl$ $(CHCl: CH)_3As$	Erosive
Diphenylcyanarsine	$(C_6H_5)_2AsCN$	Sneezing
Hydrocyanic acid	HCN	Asphyxiating
Chloracetophenone	$C_6H_5COCH_2Cl$	Tear gas
Phosgene	$COCl_2$	Asphyxiating

TABLE 2. Group and Type of Work[a]

Group	Type of work
A	Yperite (mustard gas) production, Yperite and Lewisite production, Lewisite production
B	Laboratory, repair, inspection, incineration
C	Tear gas, sneezing gas and other gas production, desk work, medical doctor, guard

[a] Poison gas workers were classified into Groups A, B, and C according to their type of work in the factory.

Since 1952, we have been conducting clinical and pathological studies on lung cancer among these former workers of the Okunojima Poison Gas Factory (*1*). Wada *et al.* (*2*) reported a high incidence of respiratory neoplasia among former poison gas workers in 1968. This present report describes the results of epidemiological and pathological studies on subjects who developed cancer between 1952 and 1986, and the measures taken for the prevention of carcinogenesis.

Standardized Mortality Ratios of Malignant Tumors in Former Poison Gas Workers Compared with That of Japanese Males Overall

The subjects of our study were 1,632 regular male workers of the factory. In 1981, the standardized mortality ratio (SMR) was determined based on the number of subjects who had developed cancer between 1952 and 1980 among this population and the number of expected cases based on person-years, and a comparison was made between the occurrence of cancer in the former poison gas workers and data on Japanese males overall.

Table 3 shows that the SMRs for malignant tumors of the respiratory organs such as lung cancer and laryngeal cancer, and the SMR for all malignant tumors combined were significantly elevated. The results indicated that the former poison gas workers are a high-risk group for malignant tumors of the respiratory organs.

SMRs for the workers according to their type of work were also obtained. SMRs for malignant tumors of the respiratory organs in workers belonging to Groups A and B were significantly elevated to 4.6 and 4.9, respectively (Fig. 1a). On the other hand, the SMR for Group C was 1.4, showing no significant difference.

A similar study was conducted concerning the duration of work in the factory (Fig. 1b). The SMR for cancer of the respiratory organs among former workers who had worked for 5 or more years was 7.17. The SMR for workers whose duration of

TABLE 3. Standardized Mortality Ratio (SMR)[a] for Malignant Tumor in Poison Gas Workers as Compared with That of Japanese Males Overall

	Total number of malignant tumors	Cancer of respiratory tract	Cancer of gastrointestinal tract	Other malignant tumors
Person years		41,368		
Observed cases[b]	173	70	59	44
Expected cases	141.96	17.81	64.54	59.46
SMR[a]	1.2**	3.9***	0.92	0.74

** $p < 0.01$. *** $p < 0.001$.

[a] $SMR = \dfrac{\text{Number of observed cases}}{\text{Number of expected cases}}$.   [b] Clinical observations were conducted from 1952 to 1980.

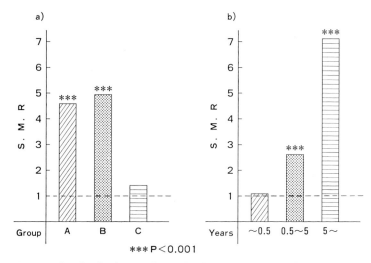

FIG. 1. Standardized mortality ratio of lung cancer in poison gas workers as compared with that of Japanese males overall. a: poison gas workers were divided into Groups A, B and C according to type of work done in the factory. b: These workers were divided into three groups according to duration of work in the factory.

work at the factory was 7 or more months was also significantly elevated. Thus former workers who had engaged in the production of mustard gas and Lewisite or related work for a period of 6 or more months are a high-risk group for respiratory tract cancer.

Table 4 shows that deaths due to cancer of the respiratory organs was significantly elevated in the fifth decade, the SMR being 10.3. With age the expected number of cases tended to increase and the SMRs tended to decrease, but in the eighth decade there was still a significantly high value of 2.5. This indicates that influence of exposure to mustard gas and Lewisite for a given period adds to the effect of aging.

Figure 2 shows the duration from starting work until death due to lung cancer. The period was 37.4±5.9 years for workers who were exposed at less than 19 years of age, 32.3±7.6 years for those who were first exposed at 20–29 years, and 30.7±

TABLE 4. Distribution of Age at Death Due to Malignant Tumors

		30–39 yrs	40–49 yrs	50–59 yrs	60–69 yrs	70–79 yrs	80– yrs
Number of total malignant tumors	Observed cases	0	11	39	63	49	11
	Expected cases	1.59	9.89	34.25	54.52	36.79	6.58
	S.M.R.	0	1.1	1.1	1.2	1.3*	1.7
Cancer of respiratory tract	Observed cases	0	8	15	31	15	1
	Expected cases	0.31	0.78	3.83	7.07	5.94	0.89
	S.M.R.	0	10.3***	3.9***	4.4***	2.5**	1.1
Cancer of gastrointestinal tract	Observed cases	0	2	15	18	21	3
	Expected cases	0.75	5.17	16.14	24.55	15.36	2.57
	S.M.R	0	0.4*	0.9	0.7	1.4	1.2

* $p < 0.05$.　** $p < 0.01$.　*** $p < 0.001$.

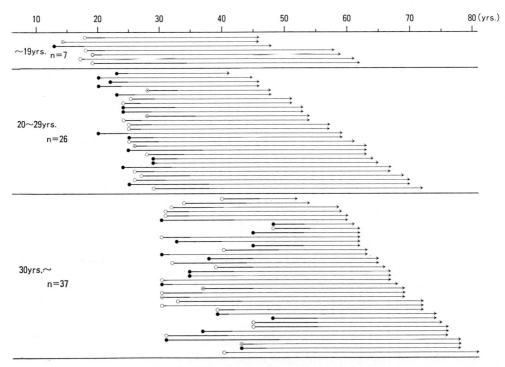

FIG. 2. The duration from starting work until death due to lung cancer. All cases were divided into three groups depending on age at time of starting work: less than 19 years of age, 20 to 29 years, and 30 years or more. ● Group A; ○ Group B; ⊙ Group C; ■ duration of work.

8.5 years for those first exposed at 30 years or more. There was no significant difference among the three age-groups.

Characteristics of Malignant Tumors of the Respiratory Tract among Poison Gas Workers

As shown in Table 5, the total number of patients who developed malignant tumors between 1952 and 1986 was 336 (20.6%) with the rate for malignant tumors of

TABLE 5.   Number of Malignant Neoplasms from 1952 to 1986

Group	A	B	C	Total
Number of survivors[a] in 1952	674	598	360	1,632
Number of malignant neoplasms from 1952 to 1986	161 (23.9)[c]	119 (19.9)	56 (15.6)	336 (20.6)
Respiratory system	74 (11.0)	49 (8.2)	14 (3.9)	137 (8.4)
Tongue		1		1
Paranasal Sinus	1	2		3
Pharynx	3	5	1	9
Larynx	11	8	1	20
Trachea	1	1		2
Lung	53	30	10	93
Pleura			1	1
Mediastinum	1		1	2
Lung (character unknown)	4	2		6
Gastrointestinal tract and liver	91 (13.5)	57 (9.5)	36 (10.0)	184 (11.3)
Others	7 (1.0)	16 (2.7)	7 (1.9)	30 (1.8)

[a] Clinical observations were started in 1952.   [b] Data include dead and living cases.   [c] Percent in parenthesis.

TABLE 6.   Histological Types of Lung Cancer by Group (1952–1986)

Group	Cases	Squamous cell ca.	Undifferentiated cell ca. Large	Undifferentiated cell ca. Small	Adenoca.	Combined sq. and ad.
A	31	16[a]	4	6[a]	4	1
B	14	9	2	3	0	0
C	7	1	0	2	2	2
Total	52	26[a]	6	11[a]	6	3
			17[a]			

[a] Includes a case with two separate cancers.

the respiratory tract being 8.4%. At the site of development of lung cancer, there was a predominance of the central type in the pulmonary hilus. An increase was also seen for cancers of the larynx, pharynx, and lung, which are considered to be directly exposed to the poison gases. Of these cases, there were 19 cases of multiple cancers including 14 cases of lung cancer and 2 cases of laryngeal cancer associated with malignant tumors of other organs.

The histological type (Table 6) could be confirmed by autopsy or biopsy in 52 cases of lung cancer. Squamous cell carcinoma was found in 26 cases (50%), undifferentiated carcinoma in 17 cases (33%) and there were a few cases with adenocarcinoma.

Attempt to Prevent the Development of Cancer by N-CWS

In April 1984, to prevent carcinogenesis, 175 patients were intradermally administered once a month with 200 μg of *Nocardia rubra* cell wall skeleton (N-CWS).

TABLE 7.   Number of Malignant Tumors in N-CWS and Control Groups from April 1984 to October 1987

	Malignant (+) tumor	Malignant (−) tumor	Total
N-CWS group	7 (1)[a]	168	175
Control group	14 (4)	161	175
Total	21 (5)	329	350

$\chi_c^2 = 1.824$ $(p < 0.1)$
[a] Number of respiratory tract cancers in parenthesis.

The incidence of cancer was then compared with that of a control group matched by age, type and duration of work. During the 3-year and 6-month follow-up from April 1984 to October 1987, 7 cases of malignant tumor developed in the group administered N-CWS and 14 cases in the control group (Table 7). By the chi square test, this difference was not significant $(p < 0.1)$.

There was one case of malignant tumor of the respiratory tract in the N-CWS administered group and 4 cases in the control group.

DISCUSSION

Animal experiments have demonstrated that mustard gas is carcinogenic (3, 4). A high incidence of cancer of the respiratory tract was reported among the Allied troops exposed to this during the First World War (5).

The poison gas workers of our study are regarded to be a group which inhaled a small amount of the gas over an extended period. The 1,632 workers who were employed in the factory were found to be a high-risk group for cancer of the respiratory tract. The standardized mortality ratio was significantly elevated in Groups A and B who had inhaled mustard gas for a period of more than 7 months. The results indicate that cancer of the respiratory tract is induced by mustard gas.

The development of lung cancer in these cases occurred 30 years after exposure. Cancer of the respiratory tract in these workers was regarded as an occupational cancer that developed even after cessation of exposure to poison gas. The cancer in these workers developed from the upper respiratory tract including the paranasal sinus and the pulmonary hilus. Histologically, squamous cell carcinoma and undifferentiated carcinoma were the predominant types, whereas adenocarcinoma was rare. According to a histological study of 4,931 cases of lung cancer in Japan by Yoshimura and Yamashita (6), squamous cell carcinoma accounted for 40.4%, adenocarcinoma for 37.6%, and undifferentiated carcinoma for 18.4%.

Because early clinical detection of cancer is important, these workers have been examined regularly in an attempt to develop useful tumor markers (7). In addition, we have attempted to prevent carcinogenesis by immunological means.

N-CWS was developed by Azuma et al. (8), and the animal experiments conducted by Hirao et al. (9) have shown that it prevents carcinogenesis. Immunological abnormalities, such as depressed mitogen response and T-cell subset abnormalities have been reported in poison gas workers (10, 11). It was also reported that N-CWS is capable of normalizing depressed immunocompetence in poison gas workers (12).

Our results showed that the incidence of cancer was slightly lower in the group administered N-CWS than in the control group.

Further studies are needed to clarify the usefulness of N-CWS in the prevention of carcinogenesis.

REFERENCES

1. Wada, S., Nishimoto, Y., Miyanishi, M., Katsuta, S., Nishiki, M., Yamada, A., Tokuoka, S., Umisa, H., and Nagai, M. Review of Okunojima poison gas factory regarding occupational environment. Hiroshima J. Med. Sci., *11*: 75–80, 1962.
2. Wada, S., Miyanishi, M., Nishimoto, Y., Kanbe, S., and Miller, R. W. Mustard gas as a cause of respiratory neoplasia in man. Lancet, *i*: 1161–1163, 1968.
3. Boyland, H. and Horning, E. S. The induction of tumors with nitrogen mustards. Br. J. Cancer, *3*: 118–123, 1948.
4. Griffin, A. C., Brandt, E. L., and Tatum, E. L. Nitrogen mustards as cancer inducing agents. JAMA, *144*: 571, 1950.
5. Beebe, G. W. Lung cancer in World War I veterans: Possible relation to mustard gas injury and 1918 influenza epidemic. J. Natl. Cancer Inst., *25*: 1231–1253, 1960.
6. Yoshimura, K. and Yamashita, N. Clinical statistical observation of 4,931 cases with lung cancer by histological types. Results of field study in Japan. Lung Cancer, *22*: 1–17, 1982 (in Japanese).
7. Maruishi, J., Yamakido, M., Onari, K., Kamitsuna, A., Inamizu, T., Ishioka, S., Mukoda, K., Akiyama, M., Goriki, K., Fujita, M., and Nishimoto, Y. Clinical significance of pregnancy associated α_2-glycoprotein (α_2-PAG) in lung cancer. Lung Cancer, *24*: 273–283, 1984 (in Japanese).
8. Azuma, I., Yamawaki, M., Yasumoto, K., and Yamamura, Y. Antitumor activity of *Nocardia rubra* cell-wall skeleton preparations in transplantable tumors in syngeneic mice and patients with malignant pleurisy. Cancer Immunol. Immunother., *4*: 95–100, 1978.
9. Hirao, F., Sakatani, M., Nishikawa, H., Yoshimoto, T., Namba, M., Ogura, T., Azuma, I., and Yamamura, Y. Effect of *Nocardia rubra* cell-wall skeleton on the induction of lung cancer and amyloidosis by 3-methylcholanthrene in rabbits. Gann, *71*: 398–401, 1980.
10. Yamakido, M., Yanagida, J., Ishioka, S., Matsuzaka, S., Hozawa, S., Takaishi, M., Inamizu, T., Akiyama, M., and Nishimoto, Y. Immune functions of former poison gas workers. I. Mitogenic response of lymphocytes and serum factors. Hiroshima J. Med. Sci., *35*: 117–126, 1986.
11. Yamakido, M., Yanagida, J., Ishioka, S., Matsuzaka, S., Hozawa, S., Takaishi, M., Inamizu, T., Akiyama, M., and Nishimoto, Y. Immune functions of former poison gas workers. II. Lymphocyte subsets and interleukin 2 production. Hiroshima J. Med. Sci., *35*: 127–134, 1986.
12. Yamakido, M., Ishioka, S., Onari, K., Matsuzaka, S., Yanagida, J., and Nishimoto, Y. Changes in natural killer cell, antibody-dependent cell mediated cytotoxicity and interferon activities with administration of *Nocardia rubra* cell wall skeleton to subjects with high risk of lung cancer. Gann, *74*: 896–901, 1983.

Etiology of Lung Cancer at the Gejiu Tin Mine, China

Sun SHIQUAN

Institute for Radiation Protection, Ministry of Nuclear Industry, Taiyuan, Shanxi Province, China

Abstract: There were 1,724 lung cancer cases registered at the Yunnan Tin Corporation in the period 1954–1986, of which 90% had a history of working underground. Previous exposure to radon, and radon daughters and arsenic is considered to be responsible for the high incidence of lung cancer in these miners. Arsenic may come from inhalation of arsenic-containing ore dust or other environmental arsenic pollution. It appears that radon exposure accounts to a greater extent than arsenic for the increase of lung cancer in these miners. Pathological study was made of 100 surgically resected lung cancer specimens. In this way the distribution and composition of dust retention was determined in relation to peripheral lung cancer.

Most of the reports of occupational lung cancer in miners are concerned with underground (UG) exposure to radon and its daughters (*1–4*). The problem of radon accumulation and lung cancer in uranium and non-uranium mines, and the concerns over environmental radon in the development of lung cancer in the general population (*5*) have evoked wide attention. Dust exposure and pneumoconiosis are other agents implicated in the etiology of lung cancer in miners (*6*) and merit further investigation.

The situation at the Gejiu tin mine in Yunnan province is somewhat different from the mines in the United States and Europe (*7–10*), not only in its seriousness but also for the complexity of etiology. The mine in China involves radon and dust, UG and surface, mining and smelting, occupational and environmental, and makes analysis complicated. Studies of the etiology of lung cancer there started 15 years ago. Investigations have been made of the role of radon daughters, ore dust, arsenic, ferric oxide and the combined effect of smoking, and environmental pollution (*11–17*). The authorities involved are paying a great deal of attention to the problem by improving UG protection, medical treatment, mass screening, prophylactic treatment, and related research work. This paper will present our point of view on the etiology of lung cancer based on data available up to now.

General Description of the Mine and Lung Cancer

The Gejiu tin mine in Yunnan province, China, has a history of more than a thousand years. Extensive exploitation started from the 1920–1930's. After the foundation of the Peoples's Republic of China (1949), the unified Yunnan Tin Corporation was established. It is now an important non-ferrous metal integrated complex including mining, dressing, and smelting operations. The number of active miners working underground (WUG) has fluctuated between 6,000 and 7,000 and the total number of persons with histories of WUG for more than one year has ranged from 11,000 to 14,000 in the past 20 years.

The high incidence of lung cancer attracted attention beginning in the 1960s. Then it increased year after year, with a total of 1,724 lung cancer cases registered and 1,571 deaths by the end of 1986 (Fig. 1). About 90% were miners and had histories of WUG at Gejiu, a majority of whom had worked in narrow and deep crude tunnels without mechanical ventilation before 1949.

Our investigation of lung cancer in Gejiu miners started in 1973. On the basis of data available, previous exposure to radon daughters and arsenic was considered to be responsible for the high rate of lung cancer; arsenic may come from inhalation of arsenic-containing ore dust or from environmental arsenic pollution (Fig. 2).

The ores mined at Gejiu are mainly soil-like reddish oxides, containing tin, lead, and copper; arsenic is present at a concentration of about 1–3%. Arsenic trioxide, lead, and copper are important by-products of the tin smeltery operated nearby. The iron content (ferric oxide) is about 50%, while nickel, cobalt, chromium, cadmium, and uranium are present in negligible amounts. The free silica (SiO_2) content is less than 5%. The possible effect of these various components of ore dust in the initiation and promotion of lung cancer in miners cannot yet be ruled out. The concentration of UG air dust has been monitored since the middle of the 1950s; radon since 1972. There was high exposure to dust and radon in tunnels before the 1960–1970s. The proportion of smokers with different degrees in the mines was generally similar to that of surface workers. The frequency of lung cancer in smoking miners was about

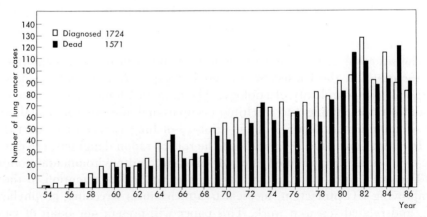

FIG. 1.   Number of lung cancers occurring among miners in Yunnan Tin Corporation. All were males, two females were excluded.

two times higher than in non-smoking miners; smoking itself cannot explain the high risk of lung cancer in miners WUG.

It is evident that to control the risk of lung cancer in Gejiu miners, systematic UG ventilation must be improved to obtain a simultaneous decrease in the air concentration of ore dust and radon. But measures used for decreasing radon and dust are not identical in every aspect, so it is important to estimate the effect of radon and dust separately in the etiology of lung cancer; this is difficult to do, however, because miners WUG were exposed to them simultaneously. To overcome this difficulty, UG exposure conditions and their relationship to lung cancer were studied in miners who worked in different mines and different jobs.

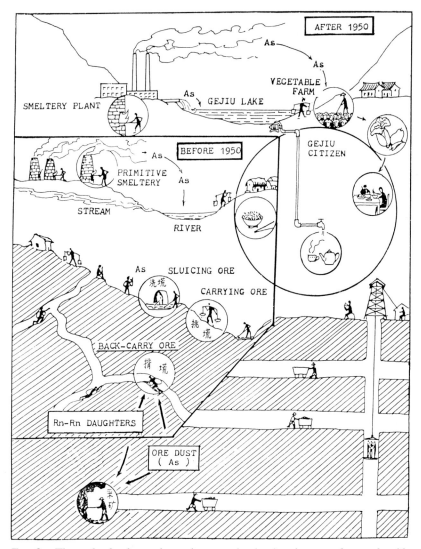

FIG. 2.   The path of radon and arsenic contamination in miners, smelters and residents before and after the foundation of PRC (1949).

Exposure to Arsenic-containing Ore Dust

Under the prior regime, mining practices were primitive and operated manually. Ore was back-carried from narrow deep tunnels to the surface. After 1950 there was extensive mechanical development of galleries and shafts through the use of pneumatic drills. UG air dust concentration reached 20–40 mg/m³ for a time, then dropped to about 6 mg/m³ on the average as a result of changing from dry to wet drilling during the 1960–1970s; now there is only 2–3 mg/m³ on the average. Generally, miners at the post of tunneling have the highest dust exposure, followed by mining and auxiliary jobs: prop setting, transport, and winching of dust, *etc.*. Mines L, M, and S which are near one another, have similar styles of working, characteristics of ores, air concentration of dust and arsenic, and historical changes. There is a much higher arsenic content in ores (oxides) than in the limestone rock encountered in tunneling. Therefore, the highest air concentration of arsenic occurs in mining, followed by tunneling and auxiliary jobs (Fig. 3).

Arsenic in pulmonary tissues taken from miners with lung cancer is 43.4 mg/kg dry weight on the average. This is 8 times higher than that of miners without cancer and 36 times higher than in lung cancer cases in the general population. Figure 3

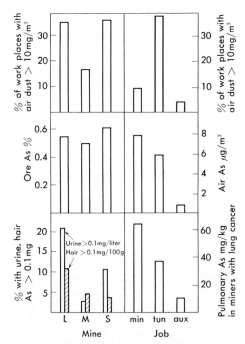

Fig. 3.   Underground air concentration of dust and arsenic, arsenic in ore (measured in 1965–1970), arsenic in urine, hair, and pulmonary tissue (in 1977–1979), in different mines (L,M,S) and different job categories (mining, tunneling, auxiliary job).

Note: urine As >0.1 mg/l in 88% and hair As >0.1 mg/100 g in 71% of Gejiu inhabitants (1968). Pulmonary As in Gejiu miners without lung cancer was 5.7 mg/kg, and that in non-miners with lung cancer at Gejiu was 1.2 mg/kg. (Data collected from the Institute of Labour Protection, Yunnan Tin Corporation).

shows that the pattern of pulmonary arsenic had a similar relationship to the air arsenic in different jobs. Arsenic in the urine and hair of miners measured after 1968 was not higher, but was actually lower than that of the Geiju non-mining population. This occurred because the mines are located in hills beyond the reach of arsenic air pollution from the smeltery located in Gejiu city. Arsenic deposited in pulmonary tissues may be transported to the urine and hair in insignificant amounts, because arsenic dust is in a less-soluble state. Drinking water was contaminated with arsenic at these mine areas before 1950, and that situation still occasionally existed at mine L even after the 1970s, which is probably the reason for higher arsenic levels in the urine and hair of L miners as compared with M and S miners.

To study the relationship between previous dust exposure and lung cancer occurrence in the three mines (L, M, S), lung cancer standard mortality ratio (SMR) (1974–1978) was calculated using the miner population data registered in 1976. The result shows that the mortality in mines L and M was apparently higher than in mine S (Fig. 4A), which seems difficult to explain by their previous exposure levels of dust or arsenic. The job categories of the miners were relatively stable in the Gejiu mine, but were not identical. To compare the lung cancer risks in different job categories, the miners with lung cancer working at different posts were compared with all miners. The result shows that the excesses were similar for mining and auxiliary jobs, both of which have apparently higher frequencies than tunneling. This means that even though tunneling was subject to the highest concentration of dust, the probability of lung cancer was the lowest; on the contrary, auxiliary workers were exposed to the lowest concentration of dust and arsenic, but their lung cancer risk was similar to that

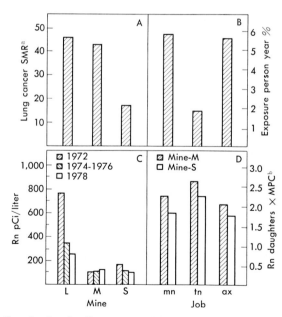

Fig. 4.   Levels of lung cancer risk in different mines and different job categories compared with levels of radon exposure. a) using lung cancer mortality of Yunnan population to calculate SMR. b) maximum permissible concentration (4×10^4 MeV/1); mn, mining; tn, tunneling; ax, auxilary job.

of miners. These findings taken together are contradictory to the concept that dust or arsenic is the main cause of Gejiu miner lung cancer.

Environmental Arsenic Pollution

It has been found that the high rate of lung cancer at Gejiu occurred not only in miners but also in people working or staying on the surface, including smeltery workers and the general population with a history of living in the districts polluted by arsenic. In early years, because of a lack of water in the mine area, people living there used to drink water which was used for, or contaminated by ore-sluicing. Most of the suffereres were dressing workers and miners. Another population exposed to previous arsenic pollution were residents living near clusters of small crude smelteries (old smeltery pollution) and farmers living near a big smeltery rebuilt in 1954 (new smeltery pollution). It is also important to study the effect of surface arsenic pollution in the development of lung cancer in Gejiu miners.

Quantitative estimation of the levels of previous arsenic pollution is nearly impossible, but this can be partially remedied by the investigation of the incidence of characteristic arsenic skin lesions, such as arsenic keratosis on palms and soles, pigmentation of skin and skin cancer, which are lifelong unchangeable signs of previous arsenic pollution.

Figure 5 shows the results of mass screening conducted in 1977 on the incidence of skin keratosis in different cohorts with different supposed levels of arsenic pollu-

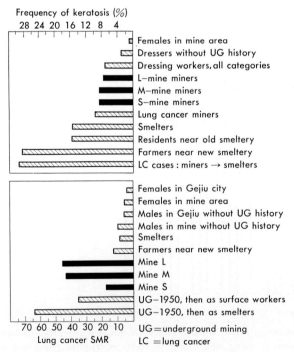

FIG. 5. Relationship between the frequency of lung cancer and arsenic-induced skin keratosis. Note: lung cancer mortality of Yunnan population (male) is used to calculate SMR.

tion, compared with their lung cancer risks. The frequency of keratosis ranked in the following order: smeltery workers and residents living in the districts polluted by smelteries>miners>women in the mine area. Miners had a high lung cancer risk without a parallel frequency of skin keratosis. The three mines (L,M,S) had similar frequencies of skin keratosis but the lung cancer risks were quite different; the frequency of keratosis in miners with lung cancer was only a little higher than that in miners without lung cancer, which was similar to that in dressing workers. Both groups had similar exposure to drinking arsenic-polluted water in the early years. All the above-mentioned facts seem to indicate that skin keratosis probably comes not from UG ore dust exposure, but mainly from previous environmental arsenic pollution.

The highest frequencies of lung cancer and keratosis were found in miners who started smeltery work after ceasing WUG in small tunnels, and they were exposed to arsenic from both polluted drinking water and the smeltery. The level of lung cancer risk in that "combined" group was higher than the sum of risks of smeltery alone and mining WUG before 1950 alone.

There were 10 cases of miners with lung cancer and skin cancer. Similar findings were also found in the general Gejiu population. The prevalence and mortality of skin cancer in the mine area was apparently higher than in the control area. Most of these skin cancers have the typical clinical and histological appearance of arsenic skin cancer (18), and provide evidence of previous environmental arsenic pollution. It presumably contributed to the development of lung cancer, but is by no means the primary occupational origin of lung cancer in miners with a history of WUG.

Radon Daughter Exposure and Its Relationship with the High Incidence of Gejiu Miner Lung Cancer

1. Estimated level of radon exposure

Underground monitoring of radon in the Gejiu tin mine started in 1972. The highest value was found in mine L: 2.9×10^4 Bq/m³ (780 pCi/l) on the average. The estimated concentration of radon daughters was 5.4 WL, and the unattached fraction of radon daughters was 0.018–0.034, depending on the existing dust concentration. Uranium content in ores (oxides) may reach 0.05–0.2% occasionally, but in most samples it is only a little higher than that in the earth crust, *i.e.*, 0.001–0.008% on the average. Radium is generally in a concentration of $1–3 \times 10^{-11}$ g/g. As a result of a comprehensive survey of ventilation and radiation protection by engineers, it is believed that radon comes from huge unsealed vacant places and rock fissures, and accumulates in the absence of effective mechanical ventilation. The following facts indicate that the value obtained in mine L in 1972 (5 WL) can be used to represent the typical exposure for Gejiu miners before the 1950s: 1) the concentration of radon at some blind ends of tunnels without mechanical ventilation reached 5.6×10^4 Bq/m³ when measured in 1978; 2) even higher concentrations, 24 WL on the average, were encountered in mine Q in 1978 (see Fig. 6), which was owned by the local community and was in a preliminary stage of exploitation without mechanical ventilation (such a situation probably existed in tunnels of mines L, M, and S 20–30 years ago); 3) concentration of radon daughters measured in 1978–1980 in some small

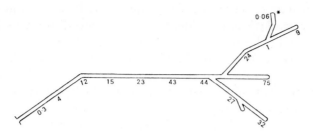

FIG. 6. Results of radon daughter monitoring in a tungsten-copper (previously tin) mine at Gejiu (mine Q), in March, 1978. One opening blind-end tunnel, 200 meters long, without mechanical ventilation. Figures denote radon daughter concentration in WL. *Pneumatic drill was running, radon daughters were diluted by the released compressed air.

crude tunnels operated manually by villagers was 2.6 WL on the average; these tunnels were generally similar to those operated before 1950 but with some improvement of working conditions.

Most miners with lung cancer worked UG for more than 10–20 years before the 1950s and may have accumulated 600–1,200 WLM ($1 WL = 1.3 \times 10^5$ MeV/1 or 2.08×10^{-5} J/m³; 1 WLM = 170 WL.hr or 3.5×10^{-3} J.hr/m³). Pb-210 in ribs measured from 25 miners with lung cancer was 1.25 pCi/g wet weight on the average *(13)*. After correction for the time between last mining and analysis based on the occupational records, the calculated cumulative exposure was only about 400 WLM on the average, which is much smaller than the value mentioned above, the value calculated from the occupational histories and from data on monitoring by individuals themselves (716 WLM on the average). In fact, UG concentration of radon dropped significantly after the 1970s. If the time correction in the calculation of Pb-210 *(19)* is based on the time "high exposures were gotten rid of" instead of "leaving the tunnel" (there may be a lag of 5–10 years), the obtained WLM will be 2–3 times higher, and similar to the value obtained from the estimated radon concentration.

2. Radon exposure and lung cancer frequency in different job categories

Because radon comes from unsealed vacant places and from a lack of effective UG ventilation systems, there were no regular differences of radon concentration in different job categories (Fig. 4D). The level of radon exposure in auxiliary jobs was similar to mining; that might explain the similar lung cancer risk levels. But tunnel workers who would have been exposed to similar radon concentration had a much lower lung cancer risk. There are two possible explanations: 1) tunneling was often accompanied by high dust exposure (Fig. 3), so it would have the lowest fraction of unattached radon daughters, and their deposition on the bronchial surface and alpha dose contribution will be decreased *(20)*. This may be related to a similar finding noticed in an early report of lung cancer in Jachymov *(21)*: most of the lung cancers were in miners who worked at places with low dust exposure, *e.g.*, carpenters and pumpers. The second explanation is that as the pneumatic drill was used more often in tunneling, the released compressed air may have diluted the concentration of radon in the driller's respiratory zone; that would not be reflected in the routine monitoring which had to be at a distance from the running drills (Fig. 6).

3.   Different radon exposures in different mines

The proportion of miners transferring between mines L, M, and S was less than 7%, before 1975 in those over 40 years of age. So, the lung cancer frequency in different mines can be compared with respect to previous exposure levels. Figure 4C shows that radon exposure can be used to explain the high risk in mine L and low risk in mine S, but cannot explain the high risk in mine M. This discrepancy arose possibly from mismatching of the date of data available, *i.e.*, the lack of radon monitoring data in the early years, especially before the 1960s.

In the absence of effective mechanical ventilation, UG concentration of radon depends mainly on natural ventilation, due to man-made openings and geological conditions. So, a rough estimation of the relative levels of previous radon concentration in different mines can be obtained from the analysis of historical information. The following impressions were obtained concerning mines L, M, and S: mine L had fewer openings and small altitude variation, and its natural ventilation would have been poor in both early and recent years; mine M was similar to mine L in early years, but it might have improved after the development of openings and the collapse of the surface on evacuated tunnels after the 1960s; the expelled air arising from the collapsed surface fissures contained radon in a concentration of about 2×10^3 Bq/m³. Mine S was developed along a steep hill with a large number of openings and great altitude variations, and its natural ventilation would have been better in both early and recent years, which is consistent with the fact that lung cancer risk in mine S was lower than that in mines L and M in recent years. If so, the lung cancer incidence should be decreased in miners who started WUG after the middle of the 1950s in mine M; *i.e.*, their UG experience began mainly after the natural ventilation had been improved. The preliminary study of miners starting WUG after 1954 shows that similar to the sequence of radon concentration monitored in the 1970s, the lung cancer excess in both mine M and mine S was lower than that in mine L. But the number of lung cancer cases was too small to be statistically significant; and a longer follow-up is needed to determine the truth of the above explanation.

Patho-histogenesis of Lung Cancer in Miners: Etiological Contributions of Radon and Dust Exposure

One hundred specimens of surgically resected lung cancers were examined, in the hope of finding a basis to evaluate the relative importance of radon and dust in the etiology of lung cancer among Gejiu miners. According to the site of origin, 56 were central, arising from large bronchi (higher than segmental) and 44 were peripheral. As a result of annual screening, 27 (48.2%) of the central lung cancers were detected in early stages, the original lesions were limited to well defined areas. Thus, the local histologic environment can be examined for its influence on carcinogenesis. The histologic distribution was epidermoid 73, small cell 8, adenocarcinoma 18, and unclassified 1.

There is prominent dust retention in pulmonary tissue. The brown dust particles are iron positive and may be mixed with nucleated or slender "ferruginous bodies" (Fig. 7). Energy-wavelength dispersive microanalysis (EDX-WDX) shows that the brown dust particles contain iron in about 60% and arsenic in about 2% of the

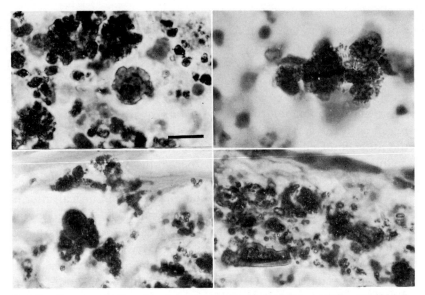

FIG. 7. Dust particles in pulmonary tissue: brown dust particles and dissociated brown granules making conglomerates (upper left), or attached to black axis (upper right) and black core (lower left) making ferruginous bodies. There is hyperplasia of alveolar epithelial cells above these particles and bodies (lower right). HE stain, bar=10 μm.

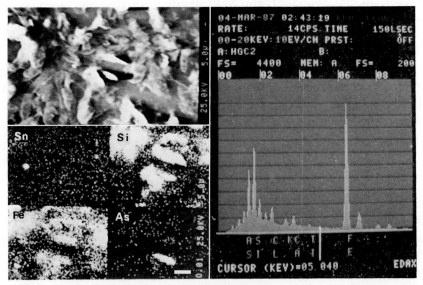

FIG. 8. Dust particles in back scattered image of scanning electron microscope (upper left), X-ray mapping of the same area shows the distribution of Sn, Si, Fe, and As (lower left), EDX microanalysis of a dust particle shows the elements detected (right). Bar=5 μm.

detectable elements (Fig. 8), the same amount as in Gejiu ores. The free brown granules and the brown capsule of ferruginous bodies contain plenty of iron and a trace of arsenic. They may represent iron dissociated from deposited ore dust and conjugated with protein. In Gejiu ores arsenic generally exists in combination with

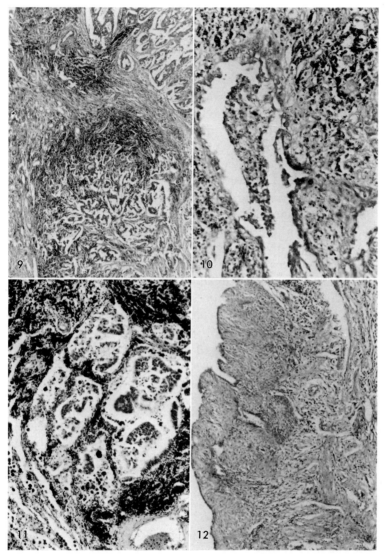

FIG. 9.   Scar cancer: dust retention, fibrosis, and malignant change of alveolar epithelial cells; alveolar cell carcinoma (upper right). HE stain, ×30.

FIG. 10.   Dust retention and malignant change of bronchiolar epithelial cells. HE stain, ×156.

FIG. 11.   Dust related malignant change in an early peripheral alveolar cell carcinoma. HE stain, ×78.

FIG. 12.   Carcinoma *in situ* of segmental bronchus with early infiltration. There is no dust retention in submucosa. HE stain, ×78.

iron. Dissociation of iron from less-soluble ore dust would be accompanied by local release of arsenic, which may explain how arsenic induces lung cancer in Gejiu miners.

Eleven of the 44 peripheral lung cancers appeared to be dust related malignant change of bronchiolar and alvolar epithelial cells; 9 of them met the criteria for "scar cancer" (Figs. 9 and 10). In the case of central lung cancer with the highest amount of pulmonary arsenic (109.4 mg As/dry weight), a small early alveolar carcinoma 3 mm in diameter was accidentally found in an area of heavy dust retention (Fig. 11). This may be regarded as evidence for dust (arsenic) carcinogenesis. It is worth noting that never was dust found in the submucosa of large bronchi (Fig. 12). It may be concluded that ore dust has little chance for continuous contact with stem cells in the large bronchi. So, dust retention cannot be invoked to explain the development of central lung cancer arising from large bronchi.

The possibility of a quantitative approach to the etiology of these lung cancers based on histologic observations arises from the following: only two occupational carcinogens are recognized, *i.e.*, radon and dust; arsenic is the only acceptable carcinogen in the ore dust; local release of arsenic from deposited ore dust next to the target tissue is the basis for its carcinogenic effect; and there is no distinctive histological type for lung cancer induced by radon or arsenic. Thus, arsenic may be a cause when dust retention exists at the site of origin of lung cancer; if it is not, radon is the only occupational carcinogen which can be considered.

It is evident that the reasoning described above is mainly based on relative differences which are insufficient for a definite quantitative evaluation of the carcinogenic effects of radon, dust, and arsenic separately. But it seems to be enough to support the following conclusion: arsenic contamination, including exposure to UG arsenic, contained in ore dust or free in the environment, is an important etiological agent in the high incidence of Gejiu miner lung cancer. The principal etiological agent involved in WUG, however, is radon and radon daughters.

ACKNOWLEDGMENTS

We thank Zhang Fuming, Xiang Shouxian, Zhao Guifen, and Tan Shong Yin for providing data of underground monitoring, chemical analyses, epidemiological surveys and pathological examinations; also, Meng Xiangyu, Liu Shengen, Jiang Hong, Luo Yingliang, and You Zhanyun for technical assistance.

REFERENCES

1. Whittemore, A. S. and McMillan, A. Lung cancer mortality among U.S. uranium miners: A reappraisal. J. Natl. Cancer Inst., *71*: 489–499, 1983.
2. Sevc, J., Kunz, E., and Placek, V. Lung cancer in uranium miners and long term exposure to radon daughter products. Health Phys., *30*: 433–437, 1976.
3. Morrison, H. I., Semenciw, R. M., Mao, Y., Corkill, D. A., Dory, A. B., deVilliers, A. J., Stocker, H., and Wigle, D. T. Lung cancer mortality and radiation exposure among the Newfoundland fluorspar miners. *In;* H. Stocker (ed.), Occupational Radiation Safety in Mining, Vol. 1, pp. 365–368, Canadian Nuclear Association, Toronto, 1985.
4. Radford, E. R. and St. Clair Renard, K. G. Lung cancer in Swedish iron miners exposed to low doses of radon daughters. N. Engl. J. Med., *310*: 1485–1494, 1984.
5. Evans, R. D., Harley, J. H., Jacobi, W., McLean, A. S., Mills, W. A., and Stewart, C. G. Estimate of risk from environmental exposure to radon-222 and its decay products. Nature, *290*: 98–100, 1981.
6. Yasuda, S., Koroku, T., and Sasaki, Y. Lung cancer associated with pneumoconiosis in coal and metal miners. Lung Cancer, *25*: 179–185, 1985 (in Japanese).

7. Rostoski, O., Saupe, E., and Schmorl, G. Die Bergkrankheit der Erzbergleute in Schneeberg in Sachsen ("Schneeberg Lungenkrebs"). Z. Krebsforsch., *23*: 360–384, 1926.

8. Teleky, L. Occupational cancer of the lung. J. Indust. Hyg. Toxicol., *19*: 73–85, 1837.

9. Seltser, R. Lung cancer and uranium mining. Arch. Environ. Health, *10*: 923–936, 1965.

10. Buechley, R. W. Epidemiological consequences of an arsenic-lung cancer theory. Am. J. Pub. Health, *53*: 1229–1232, 1963.

11. Sun, S. Q., Meng, X. Y., Yuan, L. Y., You, Z. Y., Liu, S. E., Yang, X. O., Yang, L., and Chen, H. Y. Etiological analysis of lung cancer among miners at Gejiu Yunnan province. Radiat. Prot., *1*(2): 1–8, 1981 (in Chinese).

12. Mao, B. L. An etiological approach to the lung cancer in tin miners. Tumor, *2*(2): 1–5, 1982 (in Chinese).

13. Wang, X. H., Huang, X. H., Huang, S. L., Zhang, X. Q., Zhang, J. Y., Zhang, F. M., Mao, B. L., Yang, S. W., and Pan, Z. M. Radon and lung cancer in miners. Chin. J. Radiol. Med. Prot., *4*(3): 10–14, 1984 (in Chinese).

14. Zhang, F. M. The analysis of ridge regression about occupational factors of the lung cancer of Yunnan tin miners. Chin. J. Prev. Med., *20*: 151–153, 1986 (in Chinese).

15. Sun, S. Q. and You, Z. Y. Discussion on etiology of miner lung cancer in Gejiu tin mine, Yunnan province, China. Chin. J. Radiol. Med. Prot., *7*: 225–229, 1987 (in Chinese).

16. Liu, Y. T., Chen, Z., and Wang, A. T. Problems of the etiology of Yunnan tin miner lung cancer. Chin. J. Indust. Hyg. Occup. Dis., *5*: 20–21, 1987 (in Chinese).

17. Zhao, G. F., Sun, L. H., Ji, X. M., Xuan, Q. F., Liu, C. L., and Li, J. X. Experimental study on lung cancer induced by exposure of mine dust and radon daughters. Radiat. Prot., *7*: 203–209, 1987 (in Chinese).

18. Yeh, Y., How, S. W., and Lin, C. S. Arsenic cancer of skin: histologic study with special reference to Bowen's disease. Cancer, *21*: 312–339, 1968.

19. Black, S. C., Archer, V. E., and Dixon, W. C. Correlation of radiation exposure and lead-210 in uranium miners. Health Phys., *14*: 81–93, 1968.

20. Jacobi, W. Relation between the inhaled potential α energy of Rn-222 and Rn-222 daughters and the absorbed α energy in the bronchial and pulmonary region. Health Phys., *23*: 3–11, 1972.

21. Pirchan, A. and Sikl, H. Cancer of the lung in the miners of Jachymov (Joachimsthal). Am. J. Cancer, *16*: 681–722, 1932.

22. Sun, S. Q., You, Z. Y., Tan, S. Y., and Zhao, G. F. Patho-histogenetic approach to the etiology of Yunnan tin miner lung cancer (unpublished).

Radiation-induced Cancer and Its Modifying Factor among A-bomb Survivors

Hiroo KATO

Department of Epidemiology, Radiation Effects Research Foundation, Hiroshima 732, Japan

Abstract: The Atomic Bomb Casualty Commission (ABCC) and its successor, the Radiation Effects Research Foundation, have conducted a long-term follow-up study of a cohort of 120,000 atomic bomb (A-bomb) survivors and non-exposed controls since 1950. The most recent findings regarding cancer mortality and incidence in this cohort can be briefly summarized as follows:

1) An increase in leukemia mortality among A-bomb survivors peaked 5–6 years after the bombing and has decreased with time thereafter. In addition to leukemia, the incidence of cancer of the lung, breast, esophagus, stomach, colon, thyroid, ovary, urinary tract, and multiple myeloma increases with dose. At present, there is no indication of an increase in cancer of the rectum or uterus among A-bomb survivors. In general, radiation-induced solid cancers begin to appear after the age at which they are normally prone to develop, and have continued to increase with time in proportion to the natural increase in mortality of the control group. 2) There are factors which modify the effects of radiation, such as age at the time of bombing (ATB) and sex. Sensitivity to radiation, in terms of cancer induction, is higher for persons who were young ATB in general, than for those who were older ATB. 3) There was no increase in childhood cancer among those exposed while *in utero*, but there is a recent indication of an increase in cancer incidence among these persons as they age. 4) There seems to be no interaction in a multiplicative way between radiation and smoking and lung cancer induction.

The basis of the epidemiological studies being carried out by the Radiation Effects Research Foundation (RERF) (formerly the Atomic Bomb Casualty Commission in collaboration with the Japanese National Institute of Health) is a cohort of 109,000 atomic bomb (A-bomb) survivors and their controls, the so-called Life Span Study sample. Recently this cohort was expanded to 120,000 by inclusion of 11,000 distally exposed subjects in Nagasaki (LSS-E85) (*1*). Follow-up includes mortality surveillance, which is practically complete at the death certificate level, periodical medical examinations of members of a large clinical subsample, the so-called

Adult Health Study sample, and record linkage with tissue and tumor registries in Hiroshima and Nagasaki. In addition, a cohort consisting of 2,600 *in-utero* exposed children and another of 72,000 children of A-bomb survivors are also under follow-up observation.

The existence of a radiation-related excess cancer risk in the A-bomb exposed population has been well established, but its clarification in terms of cancer site and dose-response remains as a major task of the RERF program. The influences modifying the excess risk of such host factors as age, sex, hormonal or other physical status at the time of exposure, and of environmental factors subsequent to exposure such as smoking and diet, are highly relevant to models of carcinogenesis in general and radiation carcinogenesis in particular.

Before reaching this stage, increasingly more complex studies had to be made beginning with the first indications that radiation is oncogenic, and gradually improving knowledge about the exposures and the effects. Topics of this paper will be concentrated on the temporal pattern of radiation-induced cancer and its modifying factors such as age at time of exposure.

Cancer Incidence by Site

Analyses of mortality based on the Life Span Study sample, 1950–1985, using the recently revised radiation dose (DS-86 dose) (2) have shown a significant excess in mortality from malignant tumors, but the excess in terms of relative risk at 1 Gy

TABLE 1. Summary Measures of Radiation Dose-response for Mortality from Malignant Neoplasms, 1950–1985

Site	No. of cases	Statistical test (P)[a]	Relative risk at 1 Gy	Excess risk per 10^4 PYGy	Attributable risk (%)
All malignant neoplasms	5,936	0.000	1.39 (1.32, 1.47)	10.1 (8.43, 11.9)	10.4 (8.67, 12.2)
Leukemia	202	0.000	4.97 (3.89, 6.39)	2.30 (1.88, 2.73)	56.6 (46.3, 67.1)
All cancer except leukemia	5,734	0.000	1.30 (1.23, 1.37)	7.49 (5.90, 9.15)	8.04 (6.33, 9.82)
Esophagus	176	0.02	1.43 (1.09, 1.92)	0.34 (0.08, 0.67)	12.8 (2.95, 25.0)
Stomach	2,007	0.000	1.23 (1.13, 1.34)	2.09 (1.20, 3.06)	6.41 (3.68, 9.38)
Colon	232	0.000	1.56 (1.25, 1.99)	0.56 (0.26, 0.91)	15.2 (7.05, 24.9)
Rectum	216	0.66	0.92 (, 1.27)	−0.08 (−0.17, 0.25)	−2.20 (−4.79, 7.08)
Liver	77	0.57	1.12 (0.87, 1.71)	0.05 (−0.05, 0.25)	4.03 (−4.47, 21.0)
Gallbladder	149	0.10	0.40 (1.00, 1.99)	0.24 (0.0002, 0.54)	8.78 (0.01, 19.9)
Pancreas	191	0.54	0.88 (, 1.24)	−0.11 (, 0.20)	−3.37 (, 6.42)
Lung	638	0.000	1.46 (1.25, 1.72)	1.26 (0.70, 1.89)	11.6 (6.48, 17.4)
Breast	156	0.000	2.02 (1.48, 2.76)	1.04 (0.53, 1.61)	22.4 (11.5, 35.0)
Uterus	382	0.07	1.22 (1.02, 1.50)	0.61 (0.04, 1.30)	5.49 (0.40, 11.8)
Ovary	82	0.03	1.80 (1.14, 2.85)	0.45 (0.09, 0.89)	18.6 (3.62, 37.1)
Prostate	52	0.84	1.05 (, 1.73)	0.03 (, 0.40)	1.95 (, 24.9)
Urinary tract	133	0.000	2.06 (1.46, 2.90)	0.56 (0.27, 0.90)	23.4 (11.2, 37.4)
Malignant lymphoma	110	1.00	0.99 (, 1.44)	−0.004 (, 0.20)	−0.28 (, 15.2)
Multiple myeloma	36	0.002	2.89 (1.56, 5.45)	0.22 (0.08, 0.39)	32.9 (11.5, 59.8)

[a] Statistical test for linear increase with radiation dose. ( ): 90% confidence interval. (From ref. 2)

(100 rad), excess death and attributable risk for various malignant tumors, vary considerably by site (Table 1). A significant increase is evident for leukemia, for cancers of the lung, breast, stomach, colon, esophagus, urinary tract, and ovary, and for multiple myeloma. When the observation is extended to include cancer incidence data, the relative risk is also significant for thyroid cancer (3). No increase is yet evident for mortality from cancer of the pancreas, rectum or uterus. Other studies on the same fixed population have shown no increase in chronic lymphatic leukemia (4), liver cancer (4), intracranial tumors (4) or osteosarcoma (4). As the risk can be expected to increase in the future as the cohort ages, careful follow-up will be necessary before any conclusion regarding differences in the risk of carcinogenesis by site can be drawn.

Temporal Patterns and Latent Period of Radiation Induced Cancer

In man, cancers do not appear immediately after exposure to ionizing radiation, but only after some latent period. Since the A-bomb survivors were exposed to relatively large amounts of radiation almost instantly, they should provide an exceptional cohort in which to investigate the temporal patterns of appearance of radiation induced cancer, when compared with occupational groups (exposed to radiation continuously but usually to rather small doses) or patients exposed to diagnostic or therapeutic, often fractionated radiation.

The temporal pattern does differ between leukemia and other solid tumors. An increase in leukemia incidence began to appear in both cities about 3 years after exposure to the A-bombs and reached a peak around 1951–1952 (5). Since then, the leukemia rates in the exposed persons have declined steadily. The rate in the Nagasaki exposed survivors has not exceeded that of the control population since the early 1970s, but in Hiroshima there is still evidence of continuation of a slightly higher leukemia rate in the exposed even in the most recent period of observation from 1981 to 1985 (6).

It has been demonstrated that the younger the age at the time of bombing (ATB), the greater was the risk of leukemia during the early period, and the more rapid was the decline thereafter. Moreover, the length of the latency period seems to decrease with dose (5).

Malignancies other than leukemia such as cancers of the lung, stomach, and other organs exhibit a different latency pattern over time. Radiation-induced cancers begin to appear after the age is attained at which the cancer is normally prone to develop (so-called cancer age). Even for those individuals who had already reached cancer age ATB, the shortest latency period is 10–15 years with no evident shortening of the latency period in the high-dose group.

For leukemia, the first and second mutational steps necessary for radiation to cause transformation in cells may occur simultaneously or very nearly so. Therefore, the greater the exposure dose, the earlier was the development of leukemia irrespective of age ATB. For solid tumors such as lung cancer, however, probably only the first mutational step is the result of exposure to radiation and the second and possibly another step occurs only when some other factor acts as a promoter. Cell transformation and proliferation then occur, leading to the development of cancer. In this case, the time when the promoter acts to initiate the second step may be unrelated to the

TABLE 2. Relative Risk at 1 Gy and Absolute Risk (Excess Death per 10^4 PYGy) by Age ATB and Age at Death for All Cancer Except Leukemia, 1950–85

A: Relative risk (at 1 Gy)

Age ATB	Age at death						
	<20	20–29	30–39	40–49	50–59	60–69	70+
<10	70.07	5.89	1.96	1.86			
10–19		0.82	1.66	1.59	1.68		
20–29			1.38	2.09	1.74	1.37	
30–39				1.12	1.11	1.23	1.48
40–49					1.12	1.13	1.33
50+						0.95	1.15

B: Absolute risk (excess deaths per 10^4 PYGy)

Age ATB	Age at death						
	<20	20–29	30–39	40–49	50–59	60–69	70+
<10	0.43	1.32	2.85	5.16			
10–19		−0.12	2.00	5.84	13.91		
20–29			1.39	9.40	15.71	14.33	
30–39				1.33	3.16	11.00	41.01
40–49					3.37	7.31	37.30
50+						−2.88	17.21

(From ref. 6)

radiation dose, the initiator of the process. Hence, the latent period is unrelated to radiation dose, and cancer develops only when the age at which it is normally prone to develop is attained. Thus, the two different latency patterns can be explained by a two- (multi-) step mutational theory (7, 8).

At least one animal experiment (9, 10) has been designed to test this thesis directly. These experimental findings indicate that radiation acts as the initiator and prolactin as the promoter in the induction of breast cancer in the rat and are generally supported by the present analysis of the epidemiological survey.

There are two different models (relative risk and absolute risk models) that have been employed to project the risk of death due to radiation-induced solid cancer during life (11). The absolute risk model assumes that the excess deaths are constant by age at death throughout one's life, while the relative risk model assumes that the relative risk is constant by age at death throughout life, though excess deaths increase with age at death in proportion to age-specific mortality rates of the control group.

The absolute risk (excess deaths per 10,000 person-years-Gray) and relative risk at 1 Gray of "all cancers except leukemia" were observed and classified by seven decades of age at death for six specific age ATB cohorts for the period 1950–1985 (Table 2) (6). The excess deaths increase with age at death for the same age ATB cohort in proportion to the age-specific death rate from cancer in the control population, whereas the relative risk at 1 Gray shows a constant value by age at death for the same age ATB cohort in general. Thus, the present data more strongly support the relative risk model projection.

Effects of Age ATB and Sex

It should be mentioned, however, that the relative risk of the cohort of the youngest age, *i.e.*, under age 10 ATB, was extremely high at the youngest attained age *i.e.*, under 30 years of age as compared with later attained age (Table 2) (*6*). This may imply that the latent period for solid cancer induction was shortened in this youngest cohort ATB. To demonstrate this, cumulative mortality rates were calculated using life-table methods for the 1.00+ Gy group, the 0.50–0.99 Gy group, and the 0–0.09 Gy group (as a comparison) and contrasted (Fig. 1a). In the 1.00+ Gy dose group, the cumulative cancer death rate over the entire study period is four times higher than the rate in the 0–0.09 Gy group. Moreover, cancers develop earlier than in the 0–0.09 Gy group, with the first death from stomach cancer, a boy of age 9 ATB, occurring 13 years after exposure. The 0.50–0.99 Gy group exhibits an intermediate pattern, a higher cumulative cancer death rate than that seen in the 0–0.09 Gy group. Though the number of cancer deaths is small, the distribution by site in the high-dose group is not conspicuously different from that in the general population. The very high relative risk in the early period (which results from the shortening of the latent period) for the age 0–9 ATB survivors may reflect the existence of persons who are highly sensitive to radiation in the population (*7, 12*).

Because radiation-induced cancer begins to appear after attaining the age when the cancer is normally prone to develop, it is necessary to investigate the effect of age ATB on the estimation of the risk of radiation-induced cancers either adjusted or specific for age at death. For age-at-death specific groups the relative risk as well as absolute risk for all cancers except leukemia is higher the younger the age ATB (Table 2) (*6*).

The same tendency was also observed for other sites of solid tumors such as cancers of the lung, breast and stomach (*1, 6*). Thus, the effect of age ATB and the at-

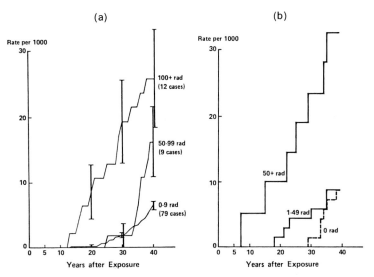

FIG. 1.   a: Cumulative mortality rate for all cancer except leukemia—those exposed at under 10 years of age. b: Cumulative incidence rates for all cancer—those exposed while *in utero*.

tained age has to be considered in estimating the risk of induction of cancer by radiation in man. However, it is difficult at present to estimate accurately the magnitude of the risk during one's lifetime from the magnitude of the risk observed in A-bomb survivors. Survivors exposed at younger ages will have to be followed for some time into the future to evaluate their cancer experience.

The risk of cancer induction does not differ by sex in general, but does differ for some sites of cancer. The relative risk of cancer of the thyroid and lung is higher for women than for men. For lung cancer, since their absolute risks do not differ, the lower relative risk for males is probably a reflection of their higher background lung cancer mortality rate. The recent mortality analysis discloses the difference in relative risk of lung cancer by sex to be smaller and no longer statistically significant when differences in smoking habits are taken into account (6). Similar results were obtained in a study of lung cancer incidence in the years 1950–1981 on the same cohort (13).

Cancer Incidence among In-utero Exposed Children

There are some reports which suggest an increase in incidence of childhood cancers among children born to mothers who received medical X-ray during pregnancy (14, 15).

According to the data from A-bomb survivors, cancer deaths have been reported among *in-utero* exposed children till 1976, but no increase with dose was observed (16). Recently the observation was updated to 1984 and the cancer incidence based on the data of the tumor registries of Hiroshima and Nagasaki were used in order to increase the number of cancer cases. A total of 18 cancer cases including two leukemia cases were observed during the period 1950–1984 among 1,627 children exposed *in utero* (in preparation). The relative risk increased with dose, and the linear increasing trend with dose is statistically significant at 5% level. As shown in Fig. 1b, cumulative incidence rates by years after bombing indicate that the latent period in the high dose group seems to be shorter (the earliest cancer occurred at the age of 6 years) as compared with that of the control group. There was no difference in cancer induction by sites of cancer and trimester of mother at exposure.

Thus, although there was no increase in childhood cancer, as the subjects have approached the cancer age, the incidence of cancer seems to increase with dose. As it is expected that the number of cancer cases will increase as they age, careful follow-up of those *in-utero* exposed children should be made.

Relationship between Radiation and Other Carcinogenic Factors

Both cohort type (6, 13) and case-control type studies (17) suggest that atomic radiation and smoking combine in an additive manner to increase lung cancer risk. This is in contrast to the multiplicative synergism between alpha-radiation from radon and smoking reported among uranium miners (18), though another study indicates no interaction between radon and smoking in lung cancer induction (19).

In this connection, the attributable risk of radiation in cancer mortality during 1950–1985 among those exposed to 1 rad and over (average exposure dose was 29.5

rad) (*2*) were 56.6%, 8.04%, 6.41%, 11.6%, and 22.4% for leukemia, all cancers except leukemia, and cancers of stomach, lung, and breast (Table 1).

REFERENCES

1. Preston, D. L., Kato, H., Kopecky, K. J., and Fujita, S. Studies of the mortality of A-bomb survivors. Report 8. Cancer mortality, 1950–82. Radiat. Res., *111*: 151–178, 1987.
2. Shimizu, Y., Kato, H., Schull, W. J., Preston, D. L., Fujita, S., and Pierce, D. A. Life Span Study Report 11. Part 1. Comparison of risk coefficients for site-specific cancer mortality based on the DS86 and T65DR shield kerma and organ dose. Radiation Effects Research Foundation Technical Report (RERF TR), 12–87, 1987.
3. Wakabayashi, T., Kato, H., Ikeda, T., and Schull, W. J. Studies of the mortality of A-bomb survivors, Report 7. Part III. Incidence of cancer in 1959–1978, based on the tumor registry, Nagasaki. Radiat. Res., *93*: 112–146, 1983.
4. Kato, H. Cancer mortality. GANN Monograph on Cancer Res., *32*: 53–74, 1986.
5. Ichimaru, M., Ishimaru, T., and Belsky, J. L. Incidence of leukemia in atomic bomb survivors, Hiroshima and Nagasaki 1959–71 by radiation dose, years after exposure, age and type of leukemia. J. Radiat. Res., *19*: 262–282, 1978.
6. Shimizu, Y., Kato, H., and Schull, W. J. Cancer mortality in the years 1950–85 based on the recently revised dose (DS86). Life Span Study Report 11, Part II, RERF TR, in preparation.
7. Kato, H. and Schull, W. J. Studies of the mortality of A-bomb survivors. Report 7. Mortality 1950–78: Part 1. Cancer mortality. Radiat. Res., *90*: 395–432, 1982.
8. Land, C. E. and Norman, J. E. Latent periods of radiogenic cancers occurring among Japanese A-bomb survivors. *In;* Late Biological Effects of Ionizing Radiation, vol. 1, pp. 29–47, International Atomic Energy Agency, Vienna, 1978 [ST1/PUB/489].
9. Yokoro, K., Nakano, M., Ito, A., Nagano, K., Kodama, Y., and Hamada, K. Role of prolactin in rat mammary carcinogenesis: detection of carcinogenicity of low-dose carcinogens and persisting dormant cancer cell. J. Natl. Cancer Inst., *58*: 1777–1783, 1977.
10. Kamiya, K., Inoh, A., Fujii, Y., Kanda, K., Kobayashi, T., and Yokoro, Y. High mammary carcinogenicity of neutron irradiation in rats and its promotion by prolactin. Jpn. J. Cancer Res. (Gann), *65*: 449–456, 1985.
11. National Research Council, Committee on the Biological Effects of Ionizing Radiation. Effects on Populations of Exposure to Low Levels of Ionizing Radiation (BEIR-III). National Academy of Sciences—National Research Council, National Academy Press, Washington, DC, 1980.
12. United Nations Scientific Committee on the Effects of Atomic Radiation. 1986 Report. Annex A: Genetic Effects of Radiation. III. Genes, Chromosomes and Cancer, pp. 54–62, and Annex B: Dose-response relationships for radiation-induced cancer, F. Population heterogeneity and susceptibility to cancer induction, pp. 182–183, United Nations, New York, 1986.
13. Kopecky, K. J., Nakashima, E., Yamamoto, T., and Kato, H. Lung cancer, radiation and smoking among A-bomb survivors. RERF TR, 13–86, 1986.
14. Bithell, J. F. and Stewart, A. M. Pre-natal irradiation and childhood malignancy: a review of British data from the Oxford Survey. Br. J. Cancer, *35*: 271–287, 1975.
15. Harvey, E. B., Boice, J. D., Jr., Honeyman, M., and Flannery, J. T. Prenatal x-ray exposure and childhood cancer in twins. N. Engl. J. Med., *312*: 541–577, 1985.

16. Kato, H. Mortality of *in-utero* children exposed to the A-bomb and of offspring of A-bomb survivors. IAEA-SM-224, *603*: 49–60, 1978.
17. Blot, W. J., Akiba, S., and Kato, H. Ionizing radiation and lung cancer; a review including preliminary results from a case-control study among A-bomb survivors. *In;* R. L. Prentice and D. J. Thompson (eds.), Atomic Bomb Survivor Data: Utilization and Analysis. SIAM, Philadelphia, 1984.
18. Whittemore, A. S. and McMillan, A. Lung cancer mortality among US uranium miners: a reappraisal. J. Natl. Cancer Inst., *71*: 489–499, 1983.
19. Radford, E. P. Radiogenic cancer in underground miners. *In;* J. Boice and J. Fraumeni (eds.), Radiation Carcinogenesis: Epidemiology and Biological Significance, pp. 225–230, Raven Press, New York, 1984.

UNUSUAL OCCURRENCES AS CLUES TO CANCER ETIOLOGY, R. W. MILLER ET AL. (EDS.),
JAPAN SCI. SOC. PRESS, TOKYO/TAYLOR & FRANCIS, LTD., PP. 125–134, 1988

Chromosome Aberrations and Transforming Genes in Leukemic and Non-leukemic Patients with a History of Atomic Bomb Exposure

Nanao KAMADA,*[1] Kimio TANAKA,*[1] and Akira KASEGAWA*[2]

Research Institute for Nuclear Medicine and Biology, Hiroshima University, Hiroshima 734, Japan[1] *and
Fundamental Research Laboratory, Toa Nenryo Kogyo Co. Ltd, Saitama 345, Japan*[2]

Abstract: To investigate leukemogenesis in atomic bomb (A-bomb) survivors, chromosome aberrations in bone marrow cells, and T- and B-lymphocytes from 135 healthy persons who had been exposed within 1,000 m of the hypocenter of the Hiroshima A-bomb were sequentially examined. Leukemic marrow cells from 468 patients with acute or chronic type of leukemias, including 25 acute leukemias exposed to 1 rad or more of radiation were also studied cytogenetically. Analysis of breakpoints observed in T-lymphocytes with stable types of abnormalities revealed a nonrandom distribution, and clustering in specific regions of chromosomes such as 22q1, 14q3, and 5q3. Statistical analysis revealed a higher incidence of translocations in 50 bands, including those containing cellular oncogenes such as 8q22, 8q24, and 9q34. Of these 50 bands, 20 were matched with bands specific for leukemia and cancer and 14 with constitutive fragile sites. In leukemic marrow, all 10 patients who had been exposed to radiation of more than 200 rad and then developed acute non-lymphocytic leukemia had chromosome aberrations. Their aberrations were more complex than those in patients exposed to less than 200 rad (33 patients) and in the non-exposed patients (134 patients). DNA samples extracted from bone marrow cells of 13 survivors, including 4 healthy survivors with more than 30% chromosome abnormalities in the bone marrow and 9 leukemia patients were used for *in vivo* selection assay of transforming genes. Tumor formation in nude mice was observed in 3 of the 4 healthy survivors and 9 leukemia patients. All of the transfectants were shown to contain Alu sequences. The transforming N-ras gene was detected for the first time in the bone marrow cells from 3 heavily exposed survivors and from 7 leukemia patients with a history of radiation exposure.

Atomic bomb (A-bomb) survivors are a unique population that experienced whole-body exposure to large and mixed doses of gamma rays and neutrons. Among the exposed individuals, radiation-induced leukemia has been well documented (*1, 2*). A significant increase of malignant tumors such as cancer of the thyroid, breast, lung and, more recently, of multiple myeloma has also been observed among A-bomb survivors, especially those who were exposed within 1 km of the hypocenter (3–5). They have a high frequency of chromosome aberrations in their bone marrow cells and T- or B-lymphocytes more than 35 years after the exposure (6–8). However, the biological significance of these chromosome abnormalities remains unclear, especially in relation to possible leukemia or malignant tumor development.

So far, more than 40 human proto-oncogenes and their respective chromosomal localizations have been determined. Interestingly, most of the proto-oncogenes have been mapped to breakpoints on or near breakpoints involving specific chromosome translocations in leukemia. The translocations at the chromosomal sites containing cellular oncogenes seem to be associated with the development and progress of leukemia. We report here the characteristics of chromosome aberrations in A-bomb survivors including evidence of significantly higher frequencies of translocations on chromosomal sites containing human proto-oncogenes, and the presence of the activated transforming N-ras gene in DNA extracted from bone marrow cells of non-leukemic patients in the exposed group. The possible leukemic process is discussed based on observations of chromosome aberrations and transforming N-ras gene among A-bomb survivors.

Chromosome Aberrations in Bone Marrow Cells and Lymphocytes of Physically Normal Atomic Bomb Survivors

A-bomb survivors who were exposed within 1 km from the hypocenter and who were apparently in good health had a 10–40% frequency of chromosome aberrations in their bone marrow cells and peripheral lymphocytes. Table 1 shows the chromosome aberration frequencies in bone marrow cells of 105 survivors exposed within 3 km of the hypocenter in Hiroshima. Eighteen of the 20 survivors (90%) exposed within 0.5 km had chromosome aberrations; the average aberration frequency was 23.2%. Eleven of the 21 survivors (52.4%) exposed within a radius of 0.5–1.0 km had chromosome aberrations. Abnormal clone formation in the bone marrow was found in 14 survivors exposed within 1 km (heavily exposed group). Serial observations of 6 heavily exposed survivors also demonstrated that the percentage of abnormal clones changed annually and some were replaced by a new abnormal clone.

Examination of 3,136 metaphases obtained from 39 healthy survivors by means of banding techniques revealed 627 cells with structural aberrations. The frequency of cells containing chromosome aberrations was 20.8%. Of the 651 observed abnormal

TABLE 1.　Bone Marrow Chromosome Aberrations in A-bomb Survivors

Distance (km)	No. of cases	Cells observed	Chromosome aberrations		
			No. of cells (%)	Subjects (%)	Clone
0–0.5	20	1,127	262 (23.2)	18 (90)	7
0.5–1	21	789	101 (12.8)	11 (52.4)	7
1–1.5	18	556	1 (0.2)	1 (5.6)	0
1.5–2.0	23	728	0	0	0
2.0–3.0	23	737	3 (0.4)	1 (4.3)	0
Controls	17	624	0	0	0

cells, 627 (96.3%) contained stable type aberrations such as translocations and inversions. Only 24 cells (3.7%) contained unstable aberrations such as dicentric and ring chromosomes. Reciprocal translocations among the stable type of aberrations were the most frequent abnormality (53.6%) followed by complex aberrations involving two or more translocations and inversions, (17.2%), deletions (10.3%), and inversions (5.1%). Most of the observed cells (82.8%) were balanced type chromosome exchanges without any loss of chromosome segments.

The distribution of 1,414 breakpoints in the 627 cells with chromosome aberrations from the 39 survivors was in all chromosomes, but some chromosomes such as Nos. 8, 15, 18 and 22 had a significantly higher incidence ($p<0.05$). Furthermore, the site of breakpoints within a chromsome was nonrandom, indicated by the high frequency of breaks in 12 regions: 5q3, 4q3, 14q3, 15p1 ($p<0.001$), 22q1, 18p1, 13q3, 21q2 ($p<0.01$), 18q2, 7q3, 16q1 and 11q2 ($p<0.05$). Bands having a significantly higher frequency of breaks were also identified. In calculations, it was postulated that the 322 bands on the haploid set of the chromosomes are of the same size. On the assumption that the development of breaks in these bands would show a Poisson distribution, Poission analysis was made for statistical differences of breaks in various bands. Fifty bands had a significantly higher frequency of breaks (1p36, 1p31, 1q22, 1q32, 2p25, 2q21, 3p25, 3q21, 3q27, 4p16, 4q31, 4q35, 5q22, 5q31, 5q34, 6q21, 6q25, 7q32, 8p23, 8q13, 8q22, 8q24, 9q22, 9q34, 10q24, 10q26, 11q22, 11q23, 12q24, 13q14, 13q22, 13q34, 14p11, 14q23, 14q24, 14q32, 15p11, 15q22, 15q24, 16q13, 16q24, 17p11, 17q23, 18p11, 18q21, 19q14, 20q11, 21q12, 22q11, 22q13). Our preliminary study of 296 chromosome breakpoints on bone marrow cells in 13 healthy survivors revealed that these cells also have similar clusters of breakpoints.

To investigate the relationship between chromosome aberrations and malignant transformation, we compared the breakpoints among 50 bands that had a significantly higher frequency of breaks in heavily exposed survivors with those relating to neoplasms and fragile sites. Mitelman found 61 breakpoints involving 54 specific chromosome changes observed in human cancer and leukemia (9). Yunis and Soreng identified 51 constitutive fragile (c-fra) sites that were prone to chromsomal breakage and rearrangement under conditions of folic acid deficiency (10). Interestingly, 20 of the 50 bands with a high incidence of breaks in A-bomb survivors were consistent with the 61 breakpoints in 54 specific chromosome changes for neoplasms and 16 of them were consistent with 51 c-fra sites. Furthermore, 6 of 50 bands in A-bomb survivors, 5q31, 6q25, 8q22, 8q24, 11q23 and 17q23, are completely common to the breakpoints in 54 specific aberrations for neoplasms and in the 51 c-fra sites. Strikingly, all locations of the 6 sites were correlated with the localization of proto-oncogenes of fms, myb, mos, myc, ets, and erb-A, respectively (11–15).

A significantly higher frequency of breakpoints in lymphocytes and bone marrow cells from A-bomb survivors was observed at 8q22 ($p<0.01$), 8q24 ($p<0.01$), and 9q34 ($p<0.05$), which are the sites containing c-mos, c-myc and c-abl. The site of translocation to which chromosome material moved was investigated, especially in chromosomal sites involving proto-oncogenes such as 8q22, 8q24, and 9q34. No identical combinations of 8;21, 8;14 and 9;22 translocations, which are common to leukemic cells, could be found. However, a very small percentage of karyotypes similar to those in leukemias were observed. For example, 12 aberrant cells with deletion of

TABLE 2.   Chromosome Aberration Frequencies and Complexity in Acute Leukemia Patients among A-bomb Survivors

	No. of cases	No. of cases with abnormal clone (%)	Average of aberrant chromosomes per stem line
A-bomb exposed patients			
200 rad<	10	10 (100)	3.00
1–200 rad	15	8 (53.3)	1.07
<1 rad	18	10 (55.6)	0.89
Non-exposed patients	134	83 (61.9)	1.24

chromosome 22 (22q-) resembling Ph¹ chromosomes were found in both lymphocytes and bone marrow cells from 52 A-bomb survivors; they accounted for 0.2% of all aberrant cells. However, no true 9;22 translocation was found (*16*).

Chromosome Aberrations in Leukemia Patients among A-Bomb Survivors

Cytogenetic analysis was performed on 25 acute leukemia patients who were exposed to more than one rad of A-bomb irradiation. All of 10 acute leukemia patients with a history of exposure to more than 200 rads of radiation showed cytogenetically abnormal clones and the frequency of forming abnormal clones was much higher than that of the patients exposed to less than 200 rads (53.3–61.9%) (Table 2). The heavily exposed leukemia patients had a tendency to show abnormalities in chromosomes 5 and 8. Furthermore, chromosome aberrations in the heavily exposed leukemia patients were observed to be of a more complex nature. The average number of aberrant chromosomes per abnormal clone of leukemia cells (stem line) was 3.0 in survivors exposed to more than 200 rads and 0.89–1.07 in those exposed to less than 200 rads.

Detection of Transforming Gene in DNA Extracted from Bone Marrow Cells

To clarify the relation of chromosome abnormalities and leukemic development, transforming activity of DNA extracted from bone marrow cells of A-bomb survivors was examined by means of the *in vivo* selection assay method (*17*). DNA from patients and the plasmid pSV2Neo gene DNA were co-transfected into NIH3T3 cells and the transfected cells were selected with the antibiotic, neomycin, and then injected into subcutaneous sites of nude mice. Tumors appeared 4–8 weeks after inoculation of transfected cells. Tumor formation in nude mice was observed in 3 of 4 healthy survivors, with 2 to 4 tumors arising from 4 inoculated sites, and in all 9 leukemic patients with different frequencies of tumor formation in nude mice. DNA extracted from the tumors had an Alu sequence specific for human DNA in all cases (Fig. 1). However, the N-ras transforming gene was detected in 7 out of 9 leukemic patients and 3 of the 4 heavily exposed survivors with a chromosome aberration frequency of 30–40% (Table 3). As a control, 5 DNA samples extracted from bone marrow cells of healthy students in medical school were tested in the same way and no positive

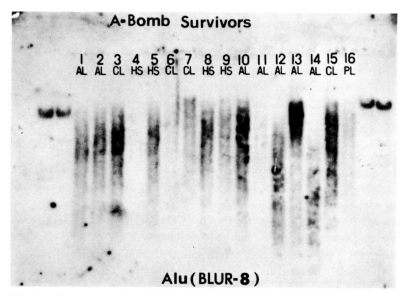

Fig. 1. Alu sequences in DNAs extracted from tumors derived from DNAs of A-bomb survivors. AL: acute leukemia. CL: chronic myelocytic leukemia. HS: healthy survivors.

TABLE 3.   Detection of Transforming Gene in A-bomb Survivors

Case	Distance from hypo-center (km)	Esti-mated dose (rad)	Clinical Dx	Karyotype	Alu sequence in tumor arisen in nude mice	N-ras gene in tumor cell
Healthy survivors						
1	0.3	600	—	48.3%⎫	+	+
2	0.3	661	—	35.7%⎪ of non-clonal chromosome		
3	0.4	565	—	30.7%⎬ abnormalities in bone marrow cells	+	+
4	0.5	667	—	37.5%⎭	+	—
Leukemic patients						
5	0.8	—	ALL (L2)	46, XX, −3, +der (3) t(3; ?)(q12; ?), −3, +der (3) t(3; ?)(q12; ?)del (3) (p23), −13, −14, −17, +der (17) t(3; 17)(q21; q21), +2mar	+	—
6	1.0	200	AML (M4)	46, XY, del (11)(q13)	+	—
7	1.0	185	CML-bc	46, XY, t(9; 22)(q34; q11)	+	+
8	1.2	—	AML (M1)	46, XY	+	+
9	1.8	<20	AML (M2)	46, XY, t(9; 22)(q34; q11)	+	+
10	1.8	<20	AML (M3)		+	+
11	2.0	<10	CML-bc	46, XX, t(9; 22)(q34; q11)	+	+
12	2.0	<10	CML-bc	47, XY, t(9; 22)(q34; q11), −12, +der (12), t(3; 12)(p12; p12), +Ph[1]	+	+
13	2.0	<10	AML (M5)	46, XY	+	+

ALL: acute lymphocytic leukemia. AML: acute myelocytic leukemia. CML: chronic myelocytic leukemia.

results were obtained. The point mutation sites within the N-ras gene which showed activation are now under investigation.

Significance of Chromosomal Aberrations in A-Bomb Survivors with Relation to Malignant Transformation

It has been well documented that severely exposed A-bomb survivors have a significantly high incidence of chromosome abnormalities in bone marrow cells and lymphocytes. Furthermore, the site of breakpoints in the chromosomes was nonrandom with a high incidence of breaks at regions specific for breakpoints in leukemia cells. Our recent study revealed that 20 of the 50 bands with a high frequency of breaks in A-bomb survivors are consistent with the 61 breakpoints in 54 specific chromosome changes for neoplasia, and that 6 breakpoints common to A-bomb survivors, neoplasia, and c-fra sites were related to the sites known to be the location of some proto-oncogenes.

Strikingly, 20 of the c-fra sites and 6 of the heritable fragile (h-fra) sites were correlated with breakpoints that have been localized at or near the breakpoints of human malignancy (*10, 18*). The chromosomal rearrangements of malignancy coincided with the c-fra sites and h-fra sites in lymphocytes. Cancer patients with chromosomal rearrangements also carried fragile sites. For example, patients with small cell lymphoma with t(12;14) (q13;q32) or with acute myelomonocytic leukemia with inv (16) (p13q22) or del (16) (q22) showed a fragile site at 12q13 or 16q22 in lymphocyte chromosomes, respectively (*19, 20*). Fragile site 3p14 has been described as a breakpoint in the deletion of 3p14-3p23 in small cell carcinoma of the lung (*21*) and fragile site 7q31 was involved in a terminal deletion of 7q in 5 patients with acute non-lymphocytic leukemia (ANLL) with a history of exposure to radiation, alkylating agents, or pesticides (*22*). These findings are of interest, indicating that fragile sites act as predisposing factors for certain chromosome rearrangements in human malignancies. Therefore, the sites with a high frequency of breaks in A-bomb survivors may also play a similar role in radiation-induced leukemia. However, at present, it is not clear whether there is a correlation between c-fra and proto-oncogenes.

The hypothesis that a normal proto-oncogene could be activated by translocation is also of interest, considering that most of the observed chromosome aberrations in the heavily exposed survivors were translocations and that a significantly higher frequency of translocation was observed at 8q22, 8q24, and 9q34 where proto-oncogenes of c-mos, c-myc and c-abl are located. It is necessary to determine whether or not any of these proto-oncogenes are expressed or are altered in the A-bomb survivors.

Cytogenetic study of leukemia patients among A-bomb survivors revealed that patients who had been exposed to more than 200 rads tended to have significantly higher aberration rates than less exposed and unexposed patients. Furthermore, chromosome aberrations in survivors were seen to be more complex, and chromosomes 5 and 8 were involved in the aberrations in several cases. These observations suggest that the leukemic cells of the patients with a history of heavy exposure to atomic radiation could have developed from an abnormal cell with complex types of chromosome abnormalities induced by the radiation. There are two stages (initiation and promotion) in the development of animal cancer. At least two oncogenes are necessary to convert normal cells to neoplastic cells in some experiments. Thus, c-myc and c-H-ras-1 have been shown to transform primary rat embryo fibroblasts to a neoplastic

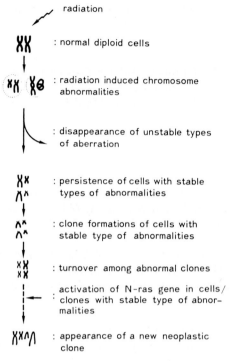

radiation

: normal diploid cells

: radiation induced chromosome
  abnormalities

: disappearance of unstable types
  of aberration

: persistence of cells with stable
  types of abnormalities

: clone formations of cells with
  stable type of abnormalities

: turnover among abnormal clones

: activation of N-ras gene in cells/
  clones with stable type of abnormalities

: appearance of a new neoplastic
  clone

FIG. 2.   A possible mechanism of leukemogenesis.

cell line, whereas either one of these alone cannot affect cell growth. From our cytogenetic findings, leukemia development after irradiation seems to involve many
stages such as: appearance of the cells with breakpoints at hot spots, disappearance of
cells with unstable-type aberrations, clone formation of cells with abnormal karyotypes,
turnover by newly developed abnormal clones, and the ultimate appearance of more
malignant clones (Fig. 2). Heavily exposed survivors had abnormal cells with breakpoints at the site of proto-oncogenes, the site involving the chromosome aberrations
in human cancer, and fragile sites 35 years after exposure. It remains to be clarified
how these cells ultimately are transformed to malignant cells after the action of some
triggering factor. Recently cellular oncogenes belonging to the ras family have been
identified in a wide variety of human tumors either by DNA transfection assay (23–
25) or by the application of synthetic oligonucleotide hybridization probes to detect
the single base changes associated with acquisition of oncogenicity (26). These substitutions are known to occur at codons 12, 13 or around codon 61 and result in a
single amino acid change in the 21 KD (p21) ras oncogene product. In human leukemias, a number of examples of activated ras oncogenes have been reported (27–32).

In our study, 7 out of 9 radiation induced leukemia cases were found to have activated N-ras genes. For leukemia development, activation of the N-ras gene seems to
play some important role as a triggering factor. Recently, Bos et al. (26) and Forrester et al. (33) independently reported evidence for K-ras mutational activation in
pre-malignant colon tissue. Our results of N-ras activation in heavily exposed survivors who have a 30–40% frequency of chromosome aberrations in the bone marrow

cells provide further evidence for the association of ras activation in the early stage of human leukemogenesis (Fig. 2).

ACKNOWLEDGMENTS
This work was supported in part by Grants-in-Aid for Cancer Research from the Ministry of Education, Science and Culture of Japan and grants from the Japan Medical Association (1986) and from the Japanese Foundation for Multi-Disciplinary Treatment of Cancer (1987).

REFERENCES

1. Ichimaru, M., Ohkita, T., and Ishimaru, T. Leukemia, multiple myeloma, and malignant lymphoma. *In;* Shigematsu, I. and Kagan, A. (eds.), Cancer in Atomic Bomb Survivors, Gann Monograph on Cancer Research No. 32, Japan Sci. Soc. Press, Tokyo, 1986.
2. Kato, H. and Schull, W. J. Studies of the mortality of A-bomb survivors. 7. Mortality, 1950–1978: Part 1. Cancer Mortality. Radiat. Res., *90*: 395–432, 1982.
3. Kato, H. Cancer Mortality. *In;* Shigematsu, I. and Kagan, A. (eds.), Cancer in Atomic Bomb Survivors, Gann Monograph on Cancer Research No. 32, Japan Sci. Soc. Press, Tokyo, 1986.
4. Miller, R. W. and Boice, J. D. Radiogenic cancer after prenatal or childhood exposure. *In;* Upton, A., Albert, R. E., Burns, F. J., and Shore, R. E. (eds.), Radiation Carcinogenesis, Elsevier, New York, 1986.
5. Ichimaru, M., Ishimaru, T., Mikami, M., and Matsunaga, M. Multiple myeloma among atomic bomb survivors in Hiroshima and Nagasaki 1950–76: Relationship to radiation dose absorbed by marrow. J. Natl. Cancer Inst., *69*: 323–328, 1982.
6. Awa, A. A., Neriishi, S., Honda, T., Yoshida, M. C., Sofuni, T., and Matsui, T. Chromosome-aberration frequency in cultured blood cells in relation to radiation dose of A-bomb survivors. Lancet, *ii*: 903–905, 1971.
7. Kamada, N. Chromosome aberrations induced by radiation with special reference to possible relation between chromosome aberrations and carcinogenesis. Cancer Chemother., *7* (Suppl.): 140–149, 1980.
8. Kamada, N., Kuramoto, A., Katsuki, T., and Hinuma, Y. Chromosome aberrations in B lymphocytes of atomic bomb survivors. Blood, *53*: 1140–1147, 1979.
9. Mitelman, F. Restricted number of chromosomal regions implicated in aetiology of human cancer and leukaemia. Nature, *310*: 325–327, 1984.
10. Yunis, J. J. and Soreng, A. L. Constitutive fragile sites and cancer. Science, *226*: 1199–1204, 1984.
11. Groffen, J., Heisterkamp, N., Spurr, N., Dana, S., Wasmuth, J. J., and Stephenson, J. R. Chromosomal localization of the human c-fms oncogene. Nucleic Acids Res., *11*: 6331–6339, 1983.
12. Harper, M. E., Franchini, G., Love, J., Simon, M. I., Gallo, R. C., and Wong-Staal, F. Chromosomal sublocalization of human c-myb and c-fes cellular onc genes. Nature, *304*: 169–171, 1983.
13. Neel, B. G., Jhanwar, S. C., Chaganti, R.S.K., and Hayward, W. S. Two human c-onc genes are located on the long arm of chromosome 8. Proc. Natl. Acad. Sci. U.S.A., *79*: 7842–7846, 1982.
14. de Taisne, C., Gegonne, A., Stehelin, D., Bernheim, A., and Berger, R. Chromosomal localization of the human protooncogene c-est. Nature, *310*: 581–583, 1984.

15. Dayton, A. I., Selden, J. R., Laws, G., Dorney, D. J., Finan, J., Tripputi, P., Emanuel, B. S., Rovera, G., Nowell, P. C., and Croce, C. M. A human c-erbA oncogene homologue is closely proximal to the chromosome 17 breakpoint in acute promyelocytic leukemia. Proc. Natl. Acad. Sci. U.S.A., *81*: 4495–4499, 1984.

16. Tanaka, K. and Kamada, N. Leukemogenesis and chromosome aberrations: *de novo* leukemia in humans—with special reference to atomic bomb survivors. Acta Haematol. Jpn., *48*: 1830–1842, 1985.

17. Southern, P. J. and Berg, P. Transformation of mammalian cells to antibiotic resistance with a bacterial gene under control of the SV40 early region promoter. J. Mol. Appl. Genet., *1*: 327–341, 1982.

18. Sutherland, G. R. Heritable fragile sites on human chromosomes. 1. Factors affecting expression in lymphocyte culture. Am. J. Hum. Genet., *31*: 125–135, 1979.

19. Yunis, J. J. Fragile sites and predisposition to leukemia and lymphoma. Cancer Genet. Cytogenet., *12*: 85–88, 1984.

20. LeBeau, M. M. and Rowley, J. D. Heritable fragile sites in cancer. Nature, *308*: 607–608, 1984.

21. Whang-Peng, J., Kao-Shan, C. S., Lee, E. C., Bunn, P. A., Carney, D. N., Gazdar, A. F., and Minna, J. D. Specific chromosome defect associated with human small-cell lung cancer deletion 3p (14–23). Science, *215*: 181–182, 1982.

22. Yunis, J. J. The chromosomal basis of human neoplasia. Science, *221*: 227–236, 1983.

23. Yuasa, Y., Gol. R. A., Chang, A., Chiu, I-M., Reddy, E. P., Tronick, S. R., and Aaronson, S. A. Mechanism of activation of an N-ras oncogene of SW-1271 human lung carcinoma cells. Proc. Natl. Acad. Sci. U.S.A., *81*: 3670–3674, 1984.

24. Der, C. J., Krontiris, T. G., and Cooper, G. M. Transforming genes of human bladder and lung carcinoma cell lines are homologous to the ras genes of Harvey and Kirsten sarcoma virus. Proc. Natl. Acad. Sci. U.S.A., *79*: 2637, 1982.

25. Feinberg, A. P., Vogelstein, B., Droller, M. J., Baylin, S. B., and Nelkin, B. D. Mutation affecting the 12th amino acid of the c-Ha-ras oncogene product occurs infrequently in human cancer. Science, *220*: 1175, 1983.

26. Bos, J. L., Fearon, E. R., Hamilton, S. R., de Vries, M. V., van Boom, J. H., van der Eb, A. J., and Vogelstein, B. Prevalence of ras gene mutations in human colorectal cancers. Nature, *327*: 293–297, 1987.

27. Murray, M. J., Cunningham, J. M., Parada, L. F., Dautry, F., Lebowitz, P., and Weinberg, R. A. The HL-60 transforming sequence: A ras oncogene coexisting with altered myc genes in hematopoietic tumors. Cell, *33*: 749–757, 1983.

28. Eva, A., Tronick, S. R., Gol, R. A., Pierce, J. H., and Aaronson, S. A. Transforming genes of human hematopoietic tumors: Frequent detection of ras-related oncogenes whose activation appears to be independent of tumor phenotype. Proc. Natl. Acad. Sci U.S.A., *80*: 4926–4930, 1983.

29. Gambke, C., Signer, E., and Moroni, C. Activation of N-ras gene in bone marrow cells from a patient with acute myeloblastic leukaemia. Nature, *307*: 476–477, 1984.

30. Hirai, H., Tanaka, S., Azuma, M., Anraku, Y., Kobayashi, Y., and Fujisawa, M. Transforming genes in human leukemia cells. Blood, *66*: 1371–1378, 1985.

31. Bos, J. L., Toksoz, D., Marshall, C. J., de Vries, M. V., Veeneman, G. H., van der Eb, A. J., van Boom, J. H., Janssen, J.W.G., and Steenvoorden, A.C.M. Amino-acid substitutions at codon 13 of the N-ras oncogene in human acute myeloid leukemia. Nature, *315*: 726–730, 1985.

32. Bos, J. L., de Vries, M. V., van der Eb, A. J., Janssen, J.W.G., Delwel, R., Lowenberg, B., and Colly, L. P. Mutations in N-ras predominate in acute myeloid leukemia. Blood, *69*: 1237–1241, 1987.

33. Forrester, K., Almoguera, C., Han, K., Grizzle, W. E., and Perucho, M. Detection of high incidence of K-ras oncogenes during human colon tumorigenesis. Nature, *327*: 298–303, 1987.

VIRUSES AND OTHER MICROORGANISMS

UNUSUAL OCCURRENCES AS CLUES TO CANCER ETIOLOGY, R. W. MILLER ET AL. (EDS.),
JAPAN SCI. SOC. PRESS, TOKYO/TAYLOR & FRANCIS, LTD., PP. 137–147, 1988

Malignant Lymphoma in African Children: Three Decades of Discovery

Gregory T. O'Conor

Anatomic Pathology, Loyola University Medical Center, Maywood, Illinois 60153, U.S.A.

Abstract: The recognition of Burkitt lymphoma (BL) as a clinical syndrome and a pathological entity in African children resulted from astute clinical observations (bedside epidemiology), the availability of cancer registry data and accurate pathological interpretation. Following the early studies in Africa, it soon became evident that this tumor occurred worldwide and the excess of cases in Africa was an incidence phenomenon associated with specific environmental factors. The sentinel discovery of the Epstein Barr virus (EBV) and its association with BL stimulated a wide variety of scientific investigations which have had an impact of virtually every discipline and biology. Epidemiological observations linked to modern laboratory techniques have provided etiological insights which implicate specific environmental factors and genetic events in the pathogenesis of BL and other immunoproliferative diseases. Early infection with EBV and holoendemic malaria are clearly of paramount importance in the development of endemic BL (eBL). These factors do not play a role in the majority of sporadic BL (sBL) cases, but immunosuppression and T-cell deregulation almost certainly are common denominators. The final or principle genetic event in both instances would appear to be the chromosome 8 translocation involving the *c-myc* oncogene and structural alteration. It is expected that the BL model will continue to be a useful one for identifying basic mechanisms in carcinogenesis which may be applicable as well to a variety of non-neoplastic diseases.

Africa has been referred to as the cradle of civilization and of "modern humans" (*1*). Be that as it may, it is at least fair to say that geographical pathology and/or geographical epidemiology as an approach to etiological hypothesis building, particularly in respect to cancer, was born and found fertile field on this continent. Clinical observations by astute physicians (bedside epidemiology), the establishment of cancer registries and accurate histopathological interpretation made it possible to characterize specific entities, to recognize significant variations in relative frequency and to make etiological correlations with extant environmental conditions. The Committee of Africa of the International Union against Cancer (UICC), later to become the Geographical Pathology Committee and then the Committee on Epidemiology was the principal group encouraging international communication in this area of research and provided the initiative as well as a forum for scientific exchange of data and observations. For many years Dr. Harold L. Stewart was Chairman and the driving force behind this committee which also included some of the great medical pioneers of African pathology and epidemiology; George Oettle and John Higginson in South Africa, Robert Camain in Senegal, George Eddington in Nigeria, Rafael Prates in Mozambique, and Jack Davies in Uganda. These men truly set the stage, stimulated their local colleagues and initiated the early investigations which have provided much of what we know about cancer in Africa today.

The subject of this presentation is perhaps the most outstanding example of an important entity first recognized as such in Africa and which has proven to be an invaluable model for the study of human cancer with broad implications in many areas of biomedical research.

Discovery and Definition

The initial description of what is now called Burkitt lymphoma (BL) as a "Clinical Syndrome" and a "Pathological Entity" was published in 1961 (2, 3) and its recognition as such resulted from correlations made on the basis of astute clinical observations, the availability of cancer registry data and accurate pathological interpretations; the three essential elements mentioned earlier.

Mr. Burkitt, a British Government surgeon, had observed, collected and documented a series of cases which he published as "sarcoma's of the jaw" in 1958 (4). He noted the frequency with which jaw and abdominal tumors occurred in the same patient and suggested a relationship. Quite independently and unaware of Mr. Burkitt's work a review, with Professor J.N.P. Davies in whose department I was working in 1958, of all childhood tumors from the Kampala Cancer Registry indicated that more than half were malignant lymphomas. Of these, most were extra nodal, localization in the jaw and abdominal organs was unusually frequent and all were of poorly differentiated or undifferentiated cell type. Many of the abdominal tumors had been interpreted previously as neuroblastoma, granulosa cell tumor of the ovary or simply as small cell sarcoma. This study was presented at a meeting of the East African Association of Physicians in 1958 and published in the Journal of Pediatrics in 1960 (5). It was only on Mr. Burkitt's return from home leave, that the necessary communication was established between surgeon and pathologist. An appropriate synthesis followed with the publication of the two papers in 1961 which represented the first description of a new clinical-pathological entity now generally referred to as Burkitt's Lymphoma.

Subsequently, it was realized that many observers in different parts of Africa had, in fact, recorded the occurrence of unusual jaw tumors in children as well as a high relative frequency of "small cell sarcomas" or lymphosarcomas. A summary of many such observations is shown in Table 1 (2–13).

Of particular historical interest, is the brief clinical note in the Mengo (Uganda) Hospital records in 1904 by Sir Albert Cook (6). This may be the first documentation of BL in Africa. Of even greater interest perhaps are the sculptured models found

TABLE 1.   Early Observations of Lymphoma in African Children

1904	Sir Albert Cook (6) —Uganda: first recorded clinical description of BL
1934	Smith and Elmes (7) —Nigeria: three sarcomas of jaw, ten sarcomas of orbit, one sarcoma of ovary
1953	Capponi (8) —Cameroun: lymphosarcoma frequent in children, four ovarian tumours
1954	Camain (9) —Senegal: "hematosarcoma" frequent, jaw and orbital tumours
1956	De Smet (10) —Belgian Congo: lymphosarcoma frequent, tumours of jaw, thyroid, abdomen in children
1957	Thijs (11) —Ruanda and Belgian Congo: small round cell sarcomas in jaw, thyroid, ovaries
1958	Prates (12, 13) —Mozambique: plaster models of jaw and orbital tumours in children
1958	Burkitt (4) —Uganda: sarcomas of jaw in children
1960	O'Conor and Davies (5) —Uganda: 50% childhood tumours—lymphomas, 50% present with jaw tumours
1961	Burkitt and O'Conor (2, 3)—Uganda: malignant lymphoma in African children, a clinical syndrome, a pathological entity

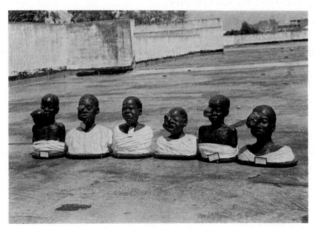

Fig. 1.   Models from Pathology Museum in Lorenzo Marques. From D. Burkitt, A lymphoma syndrome dependent on environment, Part II. Epidemiological features. In; F. C. Roulet (ed.), Symposium on Lymphoreticular Tumours in Africa, pp. 119–136, S. Karger, Basel/New York, 1964.

in the pathological museum in Lorenzo Marques (13). These were made by Professor Prates from patients he had observed over a number of years (Fig. 1).

Following these early studies in Africa, it soon became apparent that the occurrence of this tumor was not limited to Africa nor, in fact, to children (14). This, however, was not immediately accepted by all; one respected hematopathologist was quite adamant in stating that in all his years of experience, he had never seen such a tumor! Nevertheless, subsequent publications from Africa and many other countries established without any doubt that the tumor occurred world-wide and the excess of cases in Africa represented an incidence phenomenon associated with specific environmental factors (15).

Countries in sub Sahara Africa and Papua New Guinea (16) are the two areas of the world where BL is known to be highly "endemic". In the West and in all developed countries it is relatively uncommon, but yet it may represent up to 30–

40% of malignant lymphomas in children. In many developing countries outside of Africa and Papua New Guinea, although incidence data are limited, BL probably has an intermediate prevalence which may be related to socio-economic status and to a variety of environmentally induced aberrations in immune response.

The acceptance of the eponymic designation of this tumor is partly a reflection of the difficulty which existed and still exists in reaching an agreement on the classification of malignant lymphomas. Interest in this newly described African entity served as the focal point for a meeting of the International Union Against Cancer in Paris in 1963 (17). At this meeting, many of the participants did not yet recognize that the tumor occurred outside of Africa. Although it was generally agreed that it was a lymphoreticular neoplasm, a malignant lymphoma, any agreement on nomenclature was not feasible. The meeting decided, therefore, to sanction the eponym in recognition of Mr. Bukitt's contributions. Although, we now have a clearer concept in respect to cell-type there remain some semantic problems in classification and the eponym continues to enjoy universal acceptance.

The gross anatomical and microscopic characteristics of the entity as originally described by O'Conor (3) and elegantly refined by Wright (18) were the basis for a definition of BL endorsed by a World Health Organization sponsored meeting in 1964 and are still valid (19). BL is a malignant lymphoma of B cell type classified as undifferentiated (20) small noncleaved (Working Formulation (21) or lymphoblastic (Kiel) (22). The monomorphism of the cell and nucleus, the presence of multiple nucleoli, the starry sky effect, due to numerous tingible body macrophages, and the high mitotic rate are important and distinctive features readily recognized in properly fixed histological and cytological preparations. Technical artifacts as well as the growth pattern in some tissues such as breast, gonads, and intestinal wall can at times obscure the diagnostic criteria. In some tumors, particulary in non-African cases, there may be a varying degree of cellular and nuclear pleomorphism which has led to the term undifferentiated non-Burkitt. The significance and the parameters for such a separation are a matter of continuing investigation (23). The most characteristic marker for BL is the presence of one of the three specific and reciprocal chromosomal translocations. The $t(8; 14)$ translocation is most frequent and found in 75 to 80% of cases; less common are the $t(8; 22)$ in 15% and the $t(2; 8)$ in 5% of cases (24). The specificity of the cytogenetic anomaly in BL appears to be absolute. To date, there has not been any sufficiently documented case in which one of the specific translocations was absent. Conversely, however, there are some cases of malignant lymphoma of non-Burkitt type which have the $t(8; 14)$ translocation. These may represent variant types of lymphoma arising from cells of the same lineage as the classic BL, but in which one of the transforming events occurs at a slightly different stage of differentiation (25).

The priority that has been given to what is a relatively rare neoplasm and the immense literature which has accumulated over the last 25 to 30 years is quite remarkable. This attention, however, has clearly been justified by the generation of a wealth of new information which has had a resounding impact, not only in oncology but in many other fields of medicine as well. Burchenal referred to this African lymphoma in the early days as a "stalking horse" for chemotherapy (26). What was, in fact, a rapidly fatal cancer in virtually all cases is now curable at the 80 to 90% level with appropriate therapy. The model has also been a stalking horse and has provided strong stimulus for the application of a variety of new and multi-disciplinary techniques in almost every area of oncology.

Etiology and Pathogenesis

Epstein Barr virus: With the discovery, the early definition and some descriptive epidemiology of BL there quickly followed the search for environmental risk factors and relevant etiological correlations. Mr. Burkitt's famous tumor safari in Africa emphasized the relationship of tumor prevalence to altitude and rainfall and identified a so-called "tumor belt" (27). This focused attention on a possible viral etiology and the potential role of an insect vector. This in turn, stimulated vigorous and frantic attempts to isolate a putative virus and led to the truly landmark discovery of the Epstein Barr virus (EBV) (28). Infection with EBV is paradoxically not temperature or rainfall dependent. However, holoendemic malaria is and appears to be the factor of major importance along with EBV in the pathogenesis of Burkitt's tumor in those areas of highest incidence.

Following its isolation, EBV was quickly characterized as a new human herpes type virus and a number of viral or virus-induced antigens were identified. Methods for detection of these antigens in cells, and related antibodies in sera, which were applicable for field use in population studies were soon developed (29–33).

EBV was found to be ubiquitous but with differing patterns of infection in different populations: early infection being the rule in developing countries while in developed countries exposure and infection occur later; that is in puberty or early adulthood.

EBV was subsequently identified as the causative agent of infectious mononucleosis (34), but its precise role in the pathogenesis of BL remained unclear. A large prospective study in Uganda conducted by the International Agency for Research on Cancer demonstrated a significantly higher titer of antibodies to EBV in infants who later developed BL than in the normal population (35). This suggested that early infection, perhaps its intensity, and the host's ability to limit viral replication may all be factors in the genesis of the disease at is occurs in Africa. There would appear to be no etiological association with EBV in the majority of non-endemic or Western cases, 80 to 90% of which are EBV negative. Again, there are geographic areas where the EBV association with BL is intermediate.

An important characteristic of EBV most relevant to its pathogenetic role in a variety of neoplastic and non-neoplastic diseases is its mitogenic effect and functional capacity for immortalizing B lymphocytes. In the X-linked lymphoproliferative disease, described by Purtilo, EBV is associated with fatal mononucleosis and the development of lymphoid tumors including Burkitt's lymphoma (36). EBV induces lymphomas in appropriate laboratory animals (37–39) and its association with nasopharyngeal carcinoma (NPC) is also indicative of its oncogenic potential (40, 41).

Cytogenetic characteristics: BL cells synthesize both light and heavy chain immunoglobulins. The heavy chains usually of the M-type and the light chains may be difficult to detect as secreted products but this is likely a matter of quantitation since BL cells are at an early stage of maturation (42). Along with the limited spectrum of

differentiation in different tumors which may account for some morphological variations, one should expect a level of functional variation as well (25).

As already mentioned, BL cells carry one of three specific and reciprocal chromosomal translocations. In each instance the breakpoint corresponds to an immunoglobulin gene locus; in chromosome 14 it is the *mu* heavy chain, in chromosome 2
the kappa light chain, and in chromosome 22 the lambda light chain. There is then
a clear functional correlation between the type of variant translocation and the type
of immunoglobulin expressed in the tumor (43). Following closely on these observations it was shown that the cellular oncogene *c-myc* is located at or near the breakpoint
of chromosome 8 (44). Since the three types of translocation are reciprocal, the rearrangements all bring the *c-myc* in close contact or relationship with an immunoglobulin
gene which results in alteration of the oncogene expression. It should be emphasized
that although the specific translocations are not observed in EBV immortalized B-cell
lines, *c-myc* expression may be amplified at levels similar to those in tumor cell lines.
Activation of *c-myc* by EBV, therefore, probably contributes to the proliferative capacity and the immortalization of B cells but is not dependant on gene rearrangement and does not result in transformation. It appears likely that activation of other
oncogenes or transforming genes may participate in the genesis of the translocation
and in the structural alterations of *c-myc* associated with malignancy (45).

Endemic vs. sporadic BL: Although, it is now well accepted that BL occurs world
wide, there are obvious differences between the endemic BL (eBL) and the sporadic
cases as seen in the western hemisphere and in other areas where the disease is relatively uncommon (sBL) (46). These differences have obvious etiological as well as
clinical significance and, therefore, must be the focus of continuing investigation.
EBV and holoendemic malaria are believed to be the principal risk factors in eBL,
and recent experimental data strongly support the early hypotheses (47). Neither
alone, appear to be necessary or sufficient for tumorigenesis but evidence for their interaction in the pathogenesis of eBL is convincing. The very early work of McGregor
in The Gambia clearly demonstrated the effect of heavy malarial infection on immunoglobulin production in children (48). These were sentinel observations at a time
when serum immunoglobulin was perhaps the only useful parameter for measuring
reticulo-endothelial stimulation and B cell proliferation. An appropriate relationship
could also be demonstrated in the incidence and level of parasitemia with the age
distribution of BL which was consistent with an etiological association.

The role of T cells in the regulation of B cell proliferation is, of course, now well
established. Investigators in Papua New Guinea where BL is also endemic have demonstrated impaired T cell immunity in individuals from areas of holoendemic malaria (49) and in Sweden, the T helper/suppressor ratio has been reported depressed
in patients with falciparum malaria (50). It is again however, from the Medical Research Council Laboratories in The Gambia that has come a critical experiment
which, I believe, provides the strongest evidence for the role of malaria and its association with EBV in the induction of eBL. Whittle and colleagues have shown that
T cells from patients during an attack of P. falciparum malaria lose their ability to
control the growth of EBV-infected B lymphocytes in culture resulting in an abnormal
proliferation and accompanied by production of excessive amounts of immunoglobulin
and viral capsid antigen (51). Thus, malaria acts as a T cell immunosuppressor

permitting an uncontrolled and aberrant proliferation of B cells with the attendant increased risk for mutational events.

Reference has been made herein and in the abundant literature to the immortalizing capability of EBV *in vitro* and its tumorigenicity in nonhuman primates under specified conditions (*38*). The distinction between immortalizing and transforming functions, however, and the underlying mechanisms have been unclear. Recent experiments serve to identify the critical event necessary for EBV oncogenicity (*52*). Transfection of EBV infected human lymphocytes with activated *c-myc* resulted in cell transformation *in vitro*. These cells then readily grew and produced undifferentiated lymphomas in immunodeficient mice. Furthermore, the degree of malignancy was correlated with the level of *c-myc* RNA. As the authors note, this model would appear to be an in *vitro* recapitulation of key events in the pathogenesis of EBV-associated BL. In sBL, malaria is obviously not a factor and EBV association is found in only a small proportion, 10 to 15%, of cases. In sBL and in some undifferentiated lymphomas occurring in patients with AIDS as well as in patients with the X-linked lymphoproliferative syndrome (XLP), EBV does however appear to be involved in the tumorigenic process. Significant, but not necessarily discriminant, clinical and phenotypic differences between eBL and sBL are recognized (*46*). The common denominator and therefore the most objective marker is the presence of one of the three characteristic translocations which involve the *c-myc* locus on chromosome 8 and which result in alteration and/or deregulation of this oncogene. At the cytogenetic level these translocations are consistent. However, at the molecular level there are clear differences in the site of the break-point on chromosome 8 and in the type of structural alteration of *c-myc* (*53*). In eBL, the break-point is outside the *c-myc* locus, whereas in sBL the translocation truncates the gene. In both however, the same 5 prime sequences are affected by several variant mutations which are identifiable utilizing different restrictive enzymes. These observations while supporting the concept of BL as an entity provide a more firm basis for subclassification. As stated earlier it is quite logical to relate some of the clinical and functional differences between tumors of the same type or class to such genetic structural and mutational variations.

The type of undifferentiated lymphoma which is classified as small non-cleaved non-Burkitt (Working Formulation) or lymphoblastic non-Burkitt type (Kiel) deserves further comment. If indeed these tumors do represent a definable subgroup, a less cumbersome designation would seem to be Burkitt-like lymphoma (BLL). This has been a controversial matter for many years and to some extent remains so. BLL, as described, is a B cell tumor also of early lineage or stage of maturation with many morphologic features mimicking the classical BL whether it be eBL or sBL. At the same time morphometric, ultrastructural and immunophenotypic differences have been documented which may delineate a subset with clinical and/or pathogenetic significance (*23*). Since both BL and BLL outside of endemic areas are uncommon it has been difficult to obtain adequately preserved tissue on a sufficient number of cases to make a definitive comparison. Of critical importance would be the cytogenetic studies, but to my knowledge there are no data on a sufficient number of well documented BLL cases.

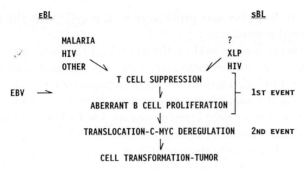

FIG. 2.   Risk factors and proposed sequence of genetic events in the pathogenesis of eBL and sBL.

DISCUSSION

In summary, one may return to a unifying theme by referring to the concept proposed by Klein for BL tumorigenesis; "a diversity of initiation followed by convergent cytogenetic evolution" (*54*). At the current state of our knowledge a major if not the final genetic event in the pathogenesis of BL and perhaps BLL is the chromosome 8 translocation involving the *c-myc* oncogene and its resultant structural alteration, activation and deregulation. Variations in the break-point site appear to relate to other genetic and/or epigenetic factors which in turn may be determinants of the subtype of BL *e.g.*, eBL or sBL. The clinical, morphological and functional variations may simply reflect the stage of B cell maturation when the final and critical genetic event takes place. If we think in terms of the two mutation model proposed for human cancer by Moolgavkar and Knudson (*55*), the first genetic event in eBL and those cases of sBL associated with EBV, may be considered as infection and immortalization of B lymphocytes by the virus. In the non-EBV associated sBL cases, the parallel event or events remain unclear (Fig. 2).

Immunosuppression with T cell deregulation resulting in an abnormal proliferation of B cells may be caused by a variety of different agents in different populations and at any age, but it is assumed that the chances for a specific non-random mutation in this expanded cell pool are then increased. In Africa holoendemic malaria is believed to be at least one of the most significant immunosuppressing factors (before AIDS) and all evidence suggests it is also a major stimulus to the B cell proliferation of EBV infected cells. Early infection with EBV and the profound effect of falciparum malaria in children readily explains the characteristic age distribution and the uniformity of the lymphoma as seen in Africa. In sBL the interplay of a variety of epigenetic as well as the genetic specific events may occur at different ages.

The thirty years since the recognition of this malignant lymphoma in African children have seen a remarkable evolution in biomedical science and in cancer research. A multidisciplinary approach to the investigation of this unique, but uncommon tumor has been an important part of this evolution. As the focus shifts to greater emphasis on molecular genetics one confidently expects that the BL model will continue to be a particularly useful one for identifying some of the basic mechanisms in carcinogenesis which may be amenable to preventive measures and applicable as well to a variety of non-neoplastic diseases.

REFERENCES

1. Lewis, R. Africa: Cradle of modern humans. Science, *237*: 1292–1295, 1970.
2. Burkitt, D. P. and O'Conor, G. T. Malignant lymphoma in African children. I. A. clinical syndrome. Cancer, *10*: 258–269, 1961.
3. O'Conor, G. T. Malignant lymphoma in African children. II. A pathological entity. Cancer, *14*: 270–283, 1961.
4. Burkitt, D. P. A sarcoma involving the jaws in African children. Br. J. Surg., *46*: 218–223, 1958.
5. O'Conor, G. T. and Davies, J.N.P. Malignant tumours in African children with special reference to malignant lymphoma. J. Pediatr., *56*: 526–535, 1960.
6. Cook, A. R. Mengo Hospital Notes. (unpublished), 1904.
7. Smith, E. C. and Elmes, B.G.T. Malignant disease in natives of Nigeria: analysis of 500 tumours. Trop. Med. Parasit, *28*: 461–476, 1934.
8. Capponi, M. Note sur le cancer au Cameroun. Bull Soc. Path. Exot., *46*: 604–611, 1953.
9. Camain, R. Apercu sur le cancer en A.O.F. Bull Soc. Path exot., *47*: 614–630, 1954.
10. De Smet, M. P. Observations cliniques de tumeurs malignes des tissus reticuloendotheliaux et des tissus hemolymphopoietiques au Congo. Ann. Soc. Belge Med. Trop., *36*: 53–70, 1956.
11. Thijs, A. Considerations sur les tumeurs malignes des indigenes du Congo Belge et du Ruanda-Urundi; a propos de 2,536 cas. Ann. Soc. Belge Med. Trop., *37*: 483–514, 1957.
12. Prates, M. D. Malignant neoplasms in Mozambique. Br. J. Cancer, *12*: 177–194, 1958.
13. Burkitt, D. A lymphoma syndrome dependent on environment. Part II. Epidemiological features. *In;* F. C. Roulet (ed.), Symposium on Lymphoreticular Tumours in Africa, pp. 119–136, S. Karger, Basel/New York, 1964.
14. O'Conor, G. T., Rappaport, H., and Smith, E. B. Childhood lymphoma resembling Burkitt tumor in the United States. Cancer, *18*: 411–417, 1965.
15. Parmin, D. M., Sohier, R., and O'Conor, G. T. Geographic distribution of Burkitt's lymphoma. *In;* G. Lenoir, G. T. O'Conor, and C.L.M. Olweny (eds.) Burkitt's Lymphoma: A Human Cancer Model, pp. 155–164, International Agency for Research on Cancer, Lyon, 1985.
16. Booth, K., Burkitt, D., Bassett, D. J., Cooke, R. A., and Buddulph, J. Burkitt lymphoma in Papua, New Guinea. Br. J. Cancer, *21*: 657–664, 1967.
17. F. C. Roulet (ed.). Symposium on Lymphoreticular Tumors in Africa. S. Karger, Basel/New York, 1964.
18. Wright, D. H. Cytology and histochemistry of the Burkitt's lymphoma. Br. J. Cancer, *17*: 50–55, 1963.
19. Berard, C. W., O'Conor, G. T., Thomas, L. B., and Torloni, H. Histopathological definition of Burkitt's tumour. Bull. WHO, *40*: 601–607, 1969.
20. Rappaport, H. Tumors of the hematopoietic system. *In;* Atlas of Tumor Pathology, Section 3, Fascicle, 8, U.S. Armed Forces Institute of Pathology, Washington, D.C., 1966.
21. National Cancer Institute Sponsored Study of Classifications of Non-Hodgkin's Lymphomas. Cancer, *49*: 2112–2135, 1982.
22. Lennert, K. Malignant Lymphomas Other Than Hodgkin's Disease. Springer-Verlag, New York/Heidelberg/Berlin, 1978.
23. Payne, C. M., Grogan, T. M., Cromey, D. W., Bjore Jr., C. G., and Kerrigan, D. P.

An ultrastructural morphometric and immunophenotypic evaluation of Burkitt's and Burkitt-like lymphomas. Lab. Invest., *57*: 200–218, 1987.

24. Berger, R. and Bernheim, A. Cytogenetics of Burkitt's lymphoma-leukemia: A review. *In;* G. Lenoir, G. O'Conor, and C.L.M. Olweny (eds.), Burkitt's Lymphoma: A Human Cancer Model, pp. 155–164, International Agency for Research on Cancer, Lyon, 1985.

25. Magrath, I. T. Lymphocytic differentiation. An essential basis for the comprehension of lymphoid neoplasia. J. Natl. Cancer Inst., *67*: 501–514, 1981.

26. Burchenal, J. H. Geographic chemotherapy-Burkitt's tumor as a stalking horse for leukemia: Presidential address. Cancer Res., *26*: 2393–2405, 1966.

27. Burkitt, D. P. A "tumour safari" in East and Central Africa. Br. J. Cancer, *16*: 379–386.

28. Epstein, M. A., Achong, B. G., and Barr, Y. M. Virus particles in cultured lymphoblasts from Burkitt's lymphoma. Lancet, *i*: 702–703, 1964.

29. Henle, G. and Henle, W. Immunofluorescence in cells derived from Burkitt's lymphoma. J. Bacteriol., *91*: 1248–1256, 1966.

30. Henle, G., Henle, W., Clifford, P., Diehl, V., Kafuko, G. W., Kirya, B. G., Klein, G., Morrow, R. H., Munube, G.M.R., Pike, M. C., Tukei, P. M., and Ziegler, J. L. Antibodies to Epstein-Barr virus in Burkitt's lymphoma and control groups. J. Natl. Cancer Inst., *43*: 1147–1157, 1969.

31. Henle, W., Henle, G., Zajac, B. A., Pearson, G., Waubke, R., and Schriba, M. Differential reactivity of human serums with early antigens induced by Epstein-Barr virus. Science, *169*: 188–190, 1970.

32. Reedman, B. M. and Klein, G. Cellular localization of an Epstein-Barr virus (EBV)-associated compliment-fixing antigen in producer and nonproducer lymphoblastoid cell lines. Int. J. Cancer, *11*: 499–520, 1973.

33. Lindahl, T., Klein, G., Reedman, B. M., Johansson, B., and Singh, S. Relationship between Epstein-Barr Virus (EBV) and the EBV-determined nuclear antigen (EBNA) in Burkitt lymphoma biopsies and other lymphoproliferative malignancies. Int. J. Cancer, *13*: 764–772, 1974.

34. Evans, A. S., Niederman, J. C., and McCollum, R. W. Seroepidemiologic studies of infectious mononucleosis with EB virus. N. Engl. J. Med., *279*: 1121–1127, 1968.

35. de-The, G., Geser, A., Day, N. E., Tukei, P. M., Williams E. H., Beir, D. P., Smith, P. G., Dean, A. G., Bornkamm, G. W., Feorino, P., and Henle, W., Epidemiological evidence for causal relationship between Epstein-Barr virus and Burkitt's lymphoma from Ugandan prospective study. Nature, *274*: 756–761, 1978.

36. Purtilo, D. T. X-linked lymphoproliferative syndrome: An immunodeficiency disorder with acquired agammaglobulinemia, fatal infectious mononucleosis, or malignant lymphoma. Arch. Pathol. Lab Med., *105*: 119–121, 1981.

37. Shope, T., Dechairo, D., and Miller, G. Malignant lymphoma in cotton-top marmosets following inoculation of Epstein-Barr virus, Proc. Natl. Acad. Sci. U.S.A., *70*: 2487–2491, 1973.

38. Miller, G. Oncogenicity of Epstein-Barr virus. J. Infect. Dis. *130*: 187–205, 1974.

39. Miller, G., Shope, T., Coope, D., Waters, L., Pagano, J., Bornkamm, G. W., and Henle, W. Lymphoma in cotton-top marmosets after innoculation with Epstein-Barr virus: Tumor incidence, histologic spectrum, antibody responses, demonstration of viral DNA, and characterization of viruses. J. Exp. Med., *145*: 948–967, 1977.

40. Nonoyama, M., Huang, C. H., Pagano, J. S., Klein, G., and Singh, S. DNA of Epstein-Barr virus detected in tissue of Burkitt's lymphoma and nasopharyngeal carcinoma. Proc. Natl. Acad. Sci. U.S.A., *70*: 3265–3268, 1973.

41. zur Hausen, H., Schulte-Holthause, H., Klein, G., Henle, W., Henle, G., Clifford, P., and Santesson, L. EB-virus DNA in biopsies of Burkitt tumors and anaplastic carcinomas of the nasopharynx. Nature, *228*: 1056–1057, 1970.

42. Benjamin, D., Magrath, I. T., Maguire, R., Janus, C., Todd, H., and Parsons, R. Immunoglobulin secretions by cell lines derived from African and American undifferentiated lymphomas of Burkitt's and non-Burkitt's type. J. Immunol., *129*: 1336–1342, 1982.

43. Lenoir, G., Preud'homme, J. L., Bernheim, A., and Berger, R. Correlation between immunoglobulin light chain expression and variant translocation in Burkitt's lymphoma. Nature, *298*: 474–476, 1982.

44. Taub, R., Kirsch, I., Morton, C., Lenoir, G., Swan, D., Tronick, S., Aaronson, S., and Leder, P. Translocation of the *c-myc* gene into the immunoglobulin heavy chain locus in human Burkitt lymphoma and murine plasmacytoma cells. Proc. Natl. Acad. Sci. U.S.A., *79*: 7837–7841, 1982.

45. Lenoir, G. M. and Bornkamm, G. W. Burkitt's lymphoma, a human cancer model for the study of the multistep development of cancer: Proposal for a new scenario. *In;* G. Klein (ed.), Advances in Viral Oncology, New York, Vol. 7, pp. 173–206, Raven Press, 1987.

46. Magrath, I. and Sariban, E. Clinical features of Burkitt's lymphoma in the U.S.A. *In;* G. Lenoir, G. O'Conor, and C.L.M. Olweny (eds.), Burkitt's Lymphoma: A Human Cancer Model, pp. 155–164, International Agency for Research on Cancer, Lyon, 1985.

47. O'Conor, G. T. Persistent immunologic stimulation as a factor in oncogenesis with special reference to Burkitt's tumor. Am. J. Med., *48*: 279–285, 1970.

48. McGregor, I. A., Gilles, H. M., Walters, J. H., and Davies, A. H. Effects of heavy and repeated malarial infections of Gambian infants and children. Br. Med. J., *2*: 686–692, 1956.

49. Moss, D. J., Burrows, S. J., Castelino, D. J., Kane, R. J., and Pope, J. H. A comparison of Epstein-Barr virus specific T-cell immunity in malaria-endemic and non-endemic regions of Papua New Guinea. Int. J. Cancer, *31*: 727–732, 1983.

50. Troye-Blomberg, M., Sjoholm, P. E., Perlmann, H., Patarroyo, M. E., and Perimann, P. Regulation of the immune response in plasmodium falciparum malaria. I. Nonspecific proliferative responses *in vitro* and characterization of lymphocytes. Clin. Exp. Immun., *53*: 335–344, 1983.

51. Whittle, H. C., Brown, J., Marsh, K., Greenwood, B. M., Seidelin, P., Tighe, H., and Wedderburn, L. T-cell control of Epstein-Barr virus infected B-cells is lost during *P. falciparum* malaria. Nature, *312*: 449–450, 1984.

52. Lombardi, L., Newcomb, E. W., and Dalla-Favera, R. Pathogenesis of Burkitt lymphoma—Expression of an activated *c-myc* oncogene causes the tumorigenic conversion of EBV-infected human B lymphoblasts. Cell, *49*: 161–170, 1987.

53. Pelicci, R., Knowles, II, D. M., Magrath, I., and Dalla-Favera, R. Chromosomal breakpoints and structural alterations of the *c-myc* locus differ in endemic and sporadic forms of Burkitt lymphoma. Proc. Natl. Acad. Sci. U.S.A., *83*: 2984–2988, 1986.

54. Klein, G. Lymphoma development in mice and humans: Diversity of initiation is followed by convergent cytogenetic evolution. Proc. Natl. Acad. Sci. U.S.A., *46*: 218–223, 1979.

55. Moolgavkar, S. H. and Knudson, A. G. Mutation and cancer: a model for human carcinogenesis. J. Natl. Cancer Inst., *66*: 1037–1052, 1981.

UNUSUAL OCCURRENCES AS CLUES TO CANCER ETIOLOGY, R.W. MILLER ET AL. (EDS.),
JAPAN SCI. SOC. PRESS, TOKYO/TAYLOR & FRANCIS, LTD., PP. 149-158, 1988

X-linked Lymphoproliferative Syndrome Provides Clues to the Pathogenesis of Epstein-Barr Virus-induced Lymphomagenesis

David T. Purtilo, Norimasa Yasuda, Helen L. Grierson, Motohiko Okano, Beda Brichacek, and Jack Davis

Departments of Pathology and Microbiology, Pediatrics, and the Eppley Institute for Research in Cancer and Allied Diseases, University of Nebraska Medical Center, Omaha, NE 68105-1065, U.S.A.

Abstract: X-linked lymphoproliferative disease (XLP) is a rare genetic syndrome that continues to serve as a useful model to understand more broadly the role of immunodeficiency and the pathogenetic mechanisms for the spectrum of Epstein-Barr virus (EBV)-induced diseases to which XLP is predisposed. Apart from XLP, EBV infection is related to the high frequency of non-Hodgkin's lymphoma in children with various primary immune deficiency diseases and in allograft recipients. More recently, EBV has been implicated in several lymphoproliferative diseases in individuals with acquired immune deficiency syndrome. Studies thus far on patients with XLP suggest that immune deficiency is a major determinant of these diseases. Additional molecular aberrations must be necessary in the pathogenesis of lymphoma to convert polyclonal to monoclonal disease.

The limited range of histopathological types of tumors which occur in immune compromised individuals—malignant lymphomas (ML), squamous cell carcinomas of skin and uterine cervix, and Kaposi's sarcomas—suggests that ubiquitous viruses can induce specific cancers in immune suppressed individuals (*1*). Such is the case for B cell malignant lymphoma in males with the X-linked lymphoproliferative syndrome (XLP), which is induced by Epstein-Barr virus (EBV). XLP is a model for studying the pathogenesis of EBV-induced diseases in patients with inherited or acquired immunodeficiency syndromes (*2*). The association of EBV with Burkitt's lymphoma (BL), infectious mononucleosis (IM), and nasopharyngeal carcinoma (NPC) was firmly established by 1975. At that time two competing hypotheses prevailed. The outcome of infections was postulated to be the result of differences in EB viral strains or immune responses to the virus.

EBV-induced Diseases in X-linked Lymphoproliferative Syndrome

Six males in the Duncan family died during the period from 1964 to 1973 with IM, acquired hypogammaglobulinemia, or ML following EBV infection (*2*). Pro-

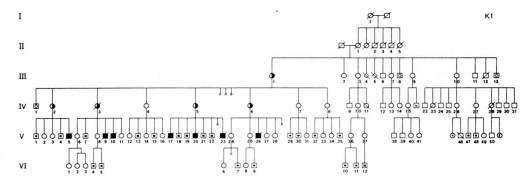

FIG. 1.   Pedigree of the Duncan kindred in 1987. Closed squares: males with XLP. Half-closed circles: carriers. Asterisk indicates seronegative individual.

TABLE 1.   Males in the Duncan Kindred Affected with X-linked Lymphoproliferative Syndrome

Pedigree #	Age (yrs.) at death†/ present age	Phenotypes	EBV serology	Serum immunoglobulin concentration	Response to bacteriophage $\phi \times 174$ challenge
V-005	9.5†	IM → hypogamma	NT	Hypo G, A, M after IM	NT
V-009	18.0†	IM → lymphoma	NT	Hypo A	NT
V-010	3.5†	Lymphoma	Defective response to EBV		NT
V-017	3.0†	Fatal IM	NT		NT
V-020	8.5†	Fatal IM	NT	Hyper M and G after IM	NT
V-023	2.0†	Fatal IM	NT	Hyper G, A, M after IM	NT
V-026	18.5†	Hypo IgA, hyper M RCA, IM, agamma	Defective response to EBV	Hypo A → hyper M → hypo G,A,M	Defective
V-047	15.0 alive	At risk	Seronegative	Hypo A, M	Borderline
V-048	13.5 alive	At risk	Seronegative	Hypo A	Normal
VI-004	13.0 alive	At risk	Seronegative	Hypo A, hyper M	Defective
VI-005	8.0 alive	At risk	Seronegative	Hypo G, A, hyper M	Defective
VI-009	2.4 alive	At risk	Seronegative	Normal	Borderline
VI-010	6.0 alive	At risk	Seronegative	Hypo A, M	Defective
VI-011	9.0 alive	At risk	Seronegative	Hypo A, M	Defective
VI-012	6.0 alive	Hypogamma	Defective response to EBV	Hypo G, A, M	Borderline

EBV=Epstein-Barr virus, IM=infectious mononucleosis, NT=not tested, G=IgG, A=IgA, M=IgM, EBNA=Epstein-Barr nuclear-associated antigen, RCA=red cell aplasia.

spective study of this family has revealed 9 additional males who may be affected (Fig. 1, Table 1). Continuing study of this family has offered an unique opportunity to prospectively explore EBV-induced diseases within a spectrum between a benign infectious disease, IM, and malignant lymphoma. Thereby, mechanisms responsible for these diseases are being discovered.

In 1976 Purtilo proposed (3) that the different diseases observed in males with XLP are due to defective T cell immune regulation of B cells following infection with EBV. For example, failure of suppressor T cells to eliminate EBV-infected B cells likely accounts for the fatal IM phenotype. Survivors of IM who manifest a gradual sustained proliferation of B cells may with time develop a malignant lymphoma. The third major phenotype, acquired hypogammaglobulinemia, would develop because of excessive suppressor T cell activity or failure of T helper cells in survivors of IM (*3*). The phenotypic variability in XLP has been attributed to faulty control of lymphoproliferation. Thus, we have called the genetic locus the "lymphoproliferative control gene(s)."

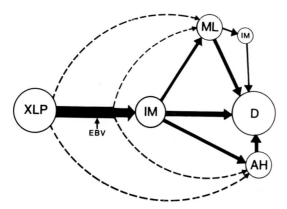

FIG. 2.   The frequency of the various phenotypes of XLP is depicted with the postulated events occurring during the natural history of patients with the defect. The size of the circles and thickness of the arrows indicate the relative frequency of the events. These events have been determined based on analysis of patients in the XLP Registry. Dotted lines indicate postulated rare events. (Published with permission of Ann. Intern. Med.)

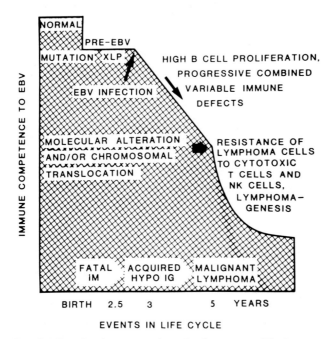

FIG. 3.   Postulated events and mechanisms responsible for EBV-induced fatal IM, acquired hypogammaglobulinemia (hypogamma) and malignant lymphoma in males with the X-linked lymphoproliferative syndrome.

In 1978, we developed the registry of XLP to test the foregoing hypotheses. Each patient referred to the registry is evaluated for established criteria diagnostic of XLP: one or more of the diseases observed in the Duncan family must occur in two or more maternally-related males (*4*). Through November 1987, 50 kindreds worldwide with 200 affected males have been registered (5, unpublished observations).

The mortality of males with XLP is 85% by 10 years of age and 100% by 40 (*5*). The phenotypes of XLP may occur concurrently or evolve with time in long-term survivors (Fig. 2). For example, recurrent lymphoma has occurred in patients at intervals of from 3 to 17 years following initial diagnosis. Fatal IM may occur years following apparent cure of malignant lymphoma (*6*). Immunopathologic studies have disclosed mechanisms partially explaining the diseases evoked by EBV (Fig. 3).

Fatal Infectious Mononucleosis

Within 32 days (median duration) following onset of infectious mononucleosis, approximately two-thirds of males with XLP who were acutely infected with EBV succumbed (*5, 7*). The signs, symptoms, laboratory findings, and lesions result from an explosive EBV-evoked polyclonal B cell proliferation. Concomitantly, a polyclonal T cell proliferative response occurs and natural killer cell activity is increased. The T cells in peripheral blood and tissues predominantly mark with CD8 antibodies, while the lymphoproliferative lesions within the hematopoietic organs (*7–9*) and liver (*10*) contain slightly more B than T cells (3 : 2 ratio). The T cells surrounding the EBV-carrying B cells almost always bear the CD8 surface antigen. Anomalous killing cytotoxic T cells and natural killer cells occur in immune competent individuals with acute infectious mononucleosis (*11*), and may account for the hematopoietic, hepatic, and other lesions in the fatal IM phenotype of XLP.

Most of the cases of XLP that we had previously considered to be hypoplastic or aplastic anemia (*4*) are more precisely diagnosed as the virus-associated hemophagocytic syndrome (VAHS) of Risdall (*12*). Other patients (non-XLP) with VAHS have defective immune responses to EBV or other viruses. Rash, high fever, hepatosplenomegaly, progressive pancytopenia and erythrophagocytosis by macrophages in bone marrow and lymph nodes are found. The diagnosis of VAHS is vital: the patients require restoration of immunity and antiviral therapy rather than cytotoxic therapy. Only rarely have we documented bona fide aplastic anemia in males with XLP (*5*).

Malignant Lymphoma

Immune deficient patients are predisposed to develop EBV-carrying malignant lymphomas (*13–16*). Infectious mononucleosis, a polyclonal lymphoproliferative disease (*11*) is a benign counterpart to endemic monoclonal EBV-carrying Burkitt's lymphoma. Approximately 20% of patients with XLP have developed ML. Among 161 patients with XLP studied in detail, we have found ML alone in 23 males, ML associated with hypogammaglobulinemia in 6, and a combination of severe IM or fatal IM, hypogammaglobulinemia, and ML in 6 patients (*5, 17*).

A careful clinicopathologic analysis of 17 of these patients with XLP and ML

TABLE 2.   Immunological Defects in X-linked Lymphoproliferative Syndrome

Findings	Publication
X-linked progressive combined variable immune deficiency is described.	1975
Pre-EBV infection IgA deficiency and borderline hypogammaglobulinemia	1978
Defective anti-EBNA response of affected males	1979
Natural killer cell activity defect post-EBV infection	1980
Inverted T4/T8 ratio and lymphocyte responses to PWM are decreased.	1982
Elevated EBV antibodies occur in carrier females.	1982
Defective memory T cell responses are identified in the regression assay.	1982
Deficient leukocyte migration inhibition responses to EBV antigens.	1982
Defective $\phi \times 174$ switching IgM $\longrightarrow$ IgG antibody response to 2° challenge	1983
Delayed onset of infectious mononucleosis with subsequent HG	1984
Evolving new phenotype — necrotizing lymphoid vasculitis	1985
Defective NK cell activity, but retention of ADCC	1986
Anti-EBNA antibody deficiency with selective IgG2 and 3 deficiency	1986
EBV-infected B cells and T cells invade thymus & epithelium is destroyed.	1986
B cell proliferation oligo and monoclonal in fatal IM	1986
T cell suppression of production of IgA and IgG by LCL *in vitro* in HG	1986
Restoration of immunity with allogeneic bone marrow transplantation	1986
Reduced frequency and CD4 and cytotoxic T cells in blood of survivors	1987
Decreased production interferon-gamma by T helper cells of survivors	1987
IgG subclass immune deficiency	1987
Anti-tetanus antibody deficiency	1987

EBV = Epstein-Barr virus, EBNA = Epstein-Barr nuclear-associated antigen, HG = hypogammaglobulinemia, ADCC = antibody dependent cellular cytotoxicity, NK = natural killer cell, IM = infectious mononucleosis, LCL = lymphoblastoid cell lines.

revealed a median age of 4.0 years (range 2–19 years) at diagnosis and median survival of 12 months (range, 1–220 months); however, 8 patients are long-term survivors (*17*). All ML occurred at extranodal sites, mostly in the ileocecal region. Localized disease (Stages I and II) predominated. All of the ML were intermediate grade or high grade diffuse malignant lymphomas similar to the general pediatric population; however, lymphoblastic lymphoma, which accounts for 30 to 50% of all pediatric lymphomas, was not observed in XLP. Morphologically, the tumors were B cell types, especially Burkitt's lymphoma. Characteristics distinguishing ML with XLP from others cases include the maternal family history, early age of onset, acquired hypogammaglobulinemia post EBV infection, ileocecal involvement, and favorable prognosis.

A recent review of the American Burkitt's Lymphoma Registry revealed that 39 of 42 cases (93%) with primary involvement of the ileum were males (*18*). Eight of the XLP cases were of the Burkitt and Burkitt-like subtype of ML and all involved the ileocecal region. Thus, young males with malignant lymphoma involving the ileocecal region ought to be evaluated for XLP.

Detection of XLP Pre-EBV Infection

Detection of affected males prior to infection with EBV is complicated, but can be achieved with a high degree of certainty by pedigree analysis (*2, 4*) (Fig. 1, Table

1), and failure of switching from IgM to IgG antibody response following a secondary challenge with bacteriophage $\phi \times 174$ (*19*). Techniques for direct detection of the defective gene are being sought. Preliminary studies by Skare *et al.* (*20*) suggest linkage of the XLP locus in the X chromosome with the gene probe DXS42 using restriction fragment length polymorphisms (RFLPs).

Second Wave of Acquired Immunological Defects Post-EBV Infection

Depicted in Fig. 3 is the progressive deterioration of immune competence occurring in males with XLP following EBV infection. Patients who survive primary infection with EBV, predominantly acquire hypogammaglobulinemia. For example, patient V-016 (Fig. 1, Table 1) acquired hypogammaglobulinemia following acute IM (*21*). His suppressor T cells became activated and B cells disappeared from his circulating blood. EBV-transformed lymphoblastoid cell lines from the patients with hypogammaglobulinemia fail to secrete normal amounts of immunoglobulin *in-vitro* when they are exposed to autologous T cells. Thus, sustained suppressor T cell activity probably prevents EBV-induced B cell proliferation, but induces hypogammaglobulinemia. This phenomenon was observed in the Duncan family and thus in the seminal report of XLP we described the entity as being a "X-linked recessive progressive combined variable immune deficiency disease" (*2*).

Multistep Mechanisms Converting Pre-malignant B Cell Proliferative Lesions to Malignant Lymphoma

For forty years, studies of the initiation/promotion model of carcinogenesis have confirmed that cancer is a multi-step process (*22*). With rare exceptions, malignancies are monoclonal (*23–25*).

A three-step hypothesis has been proposed by Klein (*26*) for endemic BL: 1) EBV evokes polyclonal B cell proliferation, 2) malarial infection causes further polyclonal B cell proliferation and suppresses T cell surveillance, and 3) a reciprocal chromosomal translocation involving breakpoints at *myc* and Ig loci endow the cell with survival advantages. Political problems prevailing in the region of Africa endemic for Burkitt's lymphoma, and the rarity of BL ($8–10$/year/10^6) in this region, preclude prospectively testing of these patients. Such studies are being done in XLP: 20% develop malignant lymphomas including BL. We propose that EBV, immune deficiency and cytogenetic and molecular alterations are involved in the multistep evolutionary process from the premalignant state to malignant lymphoma in males with XLP.

Immune deficient patients can develop a poorly controlled polyclonal B cell proliferation evoked by EBV which increases chances for a molecular or cytogenetic error to occur. Whether the genetic aberration is chromosomal and/or molecular and involves one or more proto-oncogenes is unclear. According to the multi-step carcinogenesis (*22*) scenario, several genetic mistakes should transpire during evolution to a monoclonal malignancy.

We have found clonal lymphoproliferative lesions within tissues of 10 patients who died of IM from 1 to 20 weeks following onset of illness (*27*). These findings support the hypothesis that polyclonally proliferating B cells might evolve into a monoclonal malignant B cell lymphoma. Molecular hybridization of DNA from tissues using DNA probes for EBV genome, and the human heavy chain joining region of immunoglobulin (J$_\text{H}$) in Southern blots has revealed EBV DNA in all tissues; minor differences in viral strains were observed by restriction endonuclease analyses (*27*). Rather than finding the expected polyclonal B cell proliferation possessing a large number of B cell clones (*28*), we found oligoclonal or monoclonal B cell populations by J$_\text{H}$ gene rearrangement analyses. Cleary *et al.* (*25*) have noted monoclonal EBV-induced lymphoproliferative lesions in organ-transplant recipients several months following transplantation. Furthermore, our studies demonstrated oligoclonal and monoclonal lesions associated with rearranged *myc* proto-oncogene within a few weeks of onset of IM in patients with fatal IM. In the majority of cases, the rearranged *myc* fragments were present in the same position in the gel as a rearranged J$_\text{H}$ fragment. Cloning of the DNA derived from these lesions will assist in determining whether transposition of chromosomes with breakpoints at immunoglobulin and *myc* loci occurs in the lesions (*27*). Using flow cytometry, formalin-fixed paraffin-embedded tissues of these and other cases in the Registry are being evaluated for aneuploidy, cell cycle analysis and expression of *myc* protein (*29*).

The exact mechanism of EBV-induced lymphocyte immortalization, and its relationship to malignant transformation, remains unknown. EBV-immortalized normal lymphocytes are karyotypically normal, polyclonal, and unable to form subcutaneous tumors when injected into nude mice. In contrast, BL cells have chromosomal aberrations, are monoclonal and can form subcutaneous tumors in nude mice (*26*). EBV is not likely a tumor initiator as it is not a complete carcinogen. Thus, additional events are required for progression to the full neoplastic phenotype of BL.

Prevention and Treatment

Protection of males at high risk for EBV-induced lymphoproliferative diseases is feasible by detecting males with XLP by $\phi \times 174$ challenge (*19*) and linkage of the XLP locus by RFLP analysis using DNA probes nearby DXS42. Immunoglobulin with neutralizing antibodies to EBV can then be provided to affected males prior to EBV infection (*30*). Moreover, detection of active EBV infection in organ transplant recipients by serologic or virologic means can permit withdrawal of immune suppression and some EBV-induced lymphoproliferative lesions regress (*31, 32*). Whether regression occurs with decreased immune suppression regardless of the clonality of the lesions is disputed (*33*). Modrow and Wolf (*34*) and others (*35, 36*) have suggested that genetically-altered monoclonal B cell proliferations are more resistant to cytotoxic T cells than are diploid, polyclonal populations. Anti-viral agents have been incompletely assessed such as various interferons, Acyclovir™ and its analogs for combating EBV-induced diseases in immune deficient patients (*30*).

ACKNOWLEDGMENTS

This work was supported in part by grants PHS CA30196, awarded by the National

Cancer Institute DHHS, NCI Laboratory Research Center Support Grant, CA36727, the Lymphoproliferative Research Fund, and the State of Nebraska Department of Health LB506.

The authors thank Hans Ochs, M.D., Ph.D., for performing $\phi \times 174$ assays and our Japanese collaborators Professor Yorio Hinuma, M.D., Shinji Harada, M.D., Eiji Tatsumi, M.D., Kiyoshi Sakamoto, M.D., Toyoro Osato, M.D., for their substantial contribution to this work.

REFERENCES

1. Purtilo, D. T. Defective immune surveillance in viral oncogenesis. Lab. Invest., *51*: 373–385, 1984.
2. Purtilo, D. T., Cassel, C. K., Yang, J.P.S., Harper, R., Stephenson, S. R., Landing, B. H., and Vawter, G. F. X-Linked recessive progressive combined variable immuno-deficiency (Duncan's disease). Lancet, *i*: 935–941, 1975.
3. Purtilo, D. T. Hypothesis: pathogenesis and phenotypes of an X-linked recessive lymphoproliferative syndrome. Lancet, *ii*: 882–885, 1976.
4. Purtilo, D. T., Pacquin, L. A., DeFlorio, D., Virzi, F., and Sukhuja, R. Immuno-diagnosis and immunopathogenesis of the X-linked recessive lymphoproliferative syndrome. Sem. Hematol., *16*: 309–343, 1979.
5. Grierson, H. and Purtilo, D. T. Epstein-Barr virus infections in males in the Registry of the X-Linked Lymphoproliferative Syndrome. Ann. Intern. Med., *106*: 538–545, 1987.
6. Mangi, R. J., Niederman, J. C., Kelleher, J. E., Dwyer, J. M., Evans, A. S., and Kantor, F. S. Depression of cell-mediated immunity during acute infectious mono-nucleosis. N. Engl. J. Med., *291*: 1149–1153, 1974.
7. Mroczek, E., Weisenburger, D. D., Grierson, H. L., Markin, R., and Purtilo, D. T. Fatal infectious mononucleosis and virus-associated hemophagocytic syndrome. Arch. Pathol. Lab. Med., *111*: 530–535, 1987.
8. Weisenburger, D. and Purtilo, D. T. Failures in immunological control of EB virus infection: fatal infectious mononucleosis. *In;* M. A. Epstein and B. G. Achong (eds.), The Epstein-Barr Virus: Recent Advances, pp. 127–161 William Heinemann Medical Books Ltd, London, 1986.
9. Morczek, E., Seemayer, T., Grierson, H. L., Markin, R., Linder, J., Brichacek, B., and Purtilo, D. T. Thymic lesions in fatal infectious mononucleosis. Clin. Immunol. Immunopathol., *43*: 243–255, 1987.
10. Markin, R., Mroczek, E., Weisenburger, D. D., Grierson, H., Linder, J., Davis, J., Brichacek, B., and Purtilo, D. T. Hepatitis in infectious mononucleosis. Gastroen-terology, *93*: 1210–1217, 1987.
11. Seeley, J., Svedmyr, E., Weiland, O., Klein, G., Moller, E., Eriksson, E., Andersson, K., and van der Waal, L. Epstein-Barr virus selective T cells in infectious mononu-cleosis are not restricted to HLA-A and B antigens. J. Immunol., *127*: 293–298, 1981.
12. Risdall, R. K., McKenna, R. W., Nesbit, M. E., Krivit, W., Balfour, H. H., Simons, R. L., and Brunning, R. D. Virus-associated hemophagocytic syndrome. Cancer, *44*: 993–1002, 1979.
13. Penn, I. and Starzl, T. E. Malignant tumors arising *de novo* in immunosuppressed organ transplant recipients. Transplantation, *14*: 407–417, 1972.
14. Gatti, R. A. and Good, R. A. Occurrence of malignancy and immunodeficiency diseases. Cancer, *28*: 89–98, 1971.

15. Purtilo, D. T. Epstein-Barr-virus-induced oncogenesis in immune deficient individuals. Lancet, *i*: 300–303, 1980.

16. Purtilo, D. T. and Klein, G. Introduction to Epstein-Barr virus and lymphoproliferative diseases in immunodeficient individuals. Cancer Res., *41*: 4209, 1981.

17. Harrington, D. S., Weisenburger, D. D., and Purtilo, D. T. Malignant lymphomas in the X-linked lymphoproliferative syndrome. Cancer, *59*: 1419–1429, 1987.

18. Levine, P. H., Kamaraju, L. S., Connelly, R. R., Berard, C. W., Dorfman, R. F., Magrath, I., and Easton, J. M. The American Burkitt's Lymphoma Registry: eight year's experience. Cancer, *49*: 1016–1022, 1982.

19. Ochs, H. D., Sullivan, J. L., Wedgwood, R. J., Seeley, J. K., Sakamoto, K., and Purtilo, D. T. X-linked lymphoproliferative syndrome: abnormal antibody responses to bacteriophage $\phi \times 174$. *In;* R. Wedgwood, and F. Rosen (eds.), Primary Immunodeficiency Diseases, pp. 321–323, Alan R. Liss, New York, 1983.

20. Skare, J. C., Milunsky, A., Byron, K. S., and Sullivan, J. L. Mapping the locus for X-linked lymphoproliferative syndrome. Clin. Res., *34*: 508A, 1986.

21. Purtilo, D. T., Zelkowitz, L., Harada, S., Brooks, C. D., Bechtold, T., Saemundsen, A. K., Lipscomb, H. L., Yetz, J., and Rogers, G. Delayed onset of infectious mononucleosis associated with acquired agammaglobulinemia and red cell aplasia. Ann. Intern. Med., *101*: 180–186, 1984.

22. Berenblum, B. I. and Shubik, P. A new quantitative approach to the study of stage of carcinogenesis in mouse's skin. Br. J. Cancer, *1*: 383–391, 1947.

23. Fialkow, P. J., Singer, J. W., Adamson, J. W., Vaidya, K., Dow, L. W., Ochs, J., Moor, J. W. Acute nonlymphocytic leukemia: heterogeneity of stem cell origin. Blood, *57*: 1068–1073, 1981.

24. Fearon, E. R., Burke, P. J., Schiffer, C. A., Zehnbauer, B. A., and Vogelstein, B. Differentiation of leukemia cells to polymorphonuclear leukocytes in patients with acute nonlymphocytic leukemia. N. Engl. J. Med., *315*: 15–24, 1986.

25. Cleary, M. L., Warnke, R., and Sklar, J. Monoclonality of lymphoproliferative lesions in cardiac-transplant recipients. N. Engl. J. Med., *310*: 477–523, 1984.

26. Klein, G. and Klein, E. Conditioned tumorigenicity of activated oncogenes. Cancer Res., *46*: 3211–3224, 1986.

27. Brichacek, B., Davis, J., and Purtilo, D. T. Presence of monoclonal and oligoclonal B-cell proliferation in fatal infectious mononucleosis. *In;* P. H. Levine, D. V. Ablashi, M. Nonoyama, G. R. Pearson, and R. Glaser (eds.), Epstein-Barr Virus and Human Diseases, pp. 53–54, Humana Press, Clifton, 1987.

28. Brown, N., Smith, D., Miller, G., Niederman, J., Lu, C., and Robinson, J. Infectious mononucleosis: a polyclonal B cell transformation *in vivo*. J. Infect. Dis., *150*: 517–522, 1984.

29. Watson, J. V., Sikora, K., and Evan, G. J. A simultaneous flow cytometric assay for *c-myc* oncoprotein and DNA in nuclei from paraffin-embedded material. J. Immunol. Methods, *83*: 179–192, 1985.

30. Purtilo, D. T. Prevention and treatment of Epstein-Barr virus (EBV)-associated lymphoproliferative diseases in immune deficient patients. AIDS Res., *2*: 177–182, 1986.

31. Markin, R. S., Shaw, B. W., Woods, R. P., Burnett, D. A., Brichacek, B., and Purtilo, D. T. Immunohistologic identification of Epstein-Barr virus (EBV) reactivation after OKT-3 therapy following orthotopic liver transplantation. Lab. Invest., *56*: 47A, 1987.

32. Starzl, T. E., Porter, K. A., Iwatsuki, S., Griffith, B. P., Rosenthal, J. T., Hakala, T. R., Shaw, B. W., Hardesty, R. L., Atchison, R. W., Jaffe, R., and Bahnson, H. T.

158 PURTILO ET AL.

Reversibility of lymphomas and lymphoproliferative lesions developing under cyclo-sporin-steroid therapy. Lancet, *i*: 583–587, 1984.

33. Hanto, D. W., Frizzera, G., Gajl-Peczalska, K. J., and Simmons, R. L. Epstein-Barr virus immunodeficiency, and B cell lymphoproliferation. Transplantation, *39*: 461–472, 1985.

34. Modrow, S. and Wolf, H. Characterization of two related Epstein-Barr virus-encoded membrane proteins that are differentially expressed in Burkitt lymphoma and *in-vitro*-transformed cell lines. Proc. Natl. Acad. Sci. U.S.A., *83*: 5703–5707, 1986.

35. Rooney, C. M., Edwards, C. F., Lenwar, D., Repone, H., and Rickinson, R. B. Differential activation of cytotoxic responses by Burkitt's lymphoma (BL)-cell lines: relationship to the BL-cell surface phenotypes. Cell. Immunol., *102*: 99–122, 1986.

36. Rowe, D. T., Rowe, M., Evan, G. I., Wallace, L. E., Farrell, P. J., and Rickinson, A. B. Restricted expression of EBV latent genes and T-lymphocyte-detected membrane antigen in Burkitt's lymphoma cells. EMBO J., *5*: 2599–2607, 1986.

Opportunistic Malignancies and the Acquired Immunodeficiency Syndrome

Nancy MUELLER[*1] and Angelos HATZAKIS[*2]

*Department of Epidemiology, Harvard School of Public Health, Boston, Massachusetts 02115, U.S.A.[*1]
and University of Athens School of Medicine, Department of Hygiene and Epidemiology, Athens, Greece[*2]*

Abstract: The clinical manifestations of chronic infection with the Human Immuno-deficiency Virus (HIV) fall into two broad categories: opportunistic infections and opportunistic malignancies. The initial observation of both occurring in outbreak fashion among young homosexual men led to the early identification of the present pandemic. Conversely, the identification of additional malignancies which occur in excess frequency in the presence of the immunodeficiency of HIV infection can provide insight into the role of viruses in human malignancy. The first report related to the acquired immunodeficiency syndrome (AIDS) epidemic was of a series of 5 cases of *Pneumocystis carinii* in young homosexual men in Los Angeles and was published in June 1981. This was shortly followed by the report of additional cases of *P. carinii* as well as Kaposi's sarcoma (KS) occurring among young homosexual men in California and New York City. The increased risk of KS among people with HIV infection has been confirmed since these initial reports, with 1 in 5 AIDS patients in the United States developing KS sometime in their course of disease. However, the proportion of AIDS patients with KS has decreased from 35% before 1983 to 15% in the first half of 1987. Among the recognized risk groups of AIDS patients, the proportion with KS is highest among homosexual men and female intravenous drug abusers, and lowest among children and hemophiliacs. This variation suggests that risk of KS in AIDS parallels that of sexually-transmitted infections.

A second family of opportunistic malignancy in AIDS is comprised of the non-Hodgkin's disease lymphomas (NHL). These lymphomas are typically of B-cell origin, immunoblastic or Burkitt's-like in character, and frequently present with extra-nodal involvement such as the central nervous system. These were first recognized somewhat later than KS as being associated with AIDS; together, KS and NHL account for about 95% of all neoplasms seen in AIDS patients. Additional malignancies are currently suspected to occur excessively with HIV infection. These include Hodgkin's disease, anorectal carcinoma, and testicular cancer. Validation of these associations will require extensive epidemiologic surveillance.

Since HIV infection leads to progressive loss of cellular immunity, it is probable that these malignancies result from the progressive reactivation or loss of immunologic control of latent oncogenic viruses. The cytomegalovirus has been implicated in the pathogenesis of KS, perhaps with reinfection, and the Epstein-Barr virus in the NHL. The role of papilloma viruses in anorectal carcinoma has also been proposed. The observation that opportunistic malignancies are a significant component of HIV-related disease provides evidence that altered immunologic control of latent oncogenic viruses may lead to malignancy. If true, then excess occurrence of other virus-associated malignancy such as cervical cancer and hepatocellular cancer should be anticipated as the epidemic progresses.

The epidemic of the acquired immunodeficiency syndrome (AIDS) has become a major public health problem for much of the world. The most common clinical manifestations of chronic infection with the human immunodeficiency virus (HIV), fall into two broad categories: opportunistic infections and opportunistic malignancies. The initial observation of both occurring in outbreak fashion among young American homosexual men led to the recognition of this apparently new and devastating infection. Fortuitously, the fact that a set of malignancies, all suggestive of a viral etiology, occur opportunistically in association with the progressive immunodeficiency of HIV infection provides the opportunity to gain insight into the role of viruses in human malignancy. The purpose of this paper is to briefly review the occurrence of opportunistic malignancies in AIDS and to suggest epidemiologic strategies for evaluation of their etiologies.

Kaposi's Sarcoma

The first report related to the AIDS epidemic was of 5 cases of Pneumocystis carinii occurring in young homosexual men in Los Angeles and was published in June of 1981 (*1*). This was confirmed by a subsequent report of 10 additional cases, as well as of 26 cases of Kaposi's sarcoma (KS) occurring in homosexuals elsewhere in California and in New York City (*2*).

This reported cluster of KS occurring in such a specific population with unusually aggressive clinical features was so incongruent with the established epidemiology of the disease, that it sparked the attention of a range of scientists including epidemiologists, clinicians, immunologists, and virologists. The subsequent identification of the HIV and the increasing knowledge of its pathogenesis has been a scientific achievement of immense proportion.

KS was first described in 1872 as a "multiple idiopathic pigmented sarcoma of the skin." True metastases may occur but the clinical presentation is most consistent with a multifocal origin (*3, 4*). The lesions include spindle cells and vascular structures in a network of collagen fibers (*5, 6*). Recent immunohistochemical studies suggest that the neoplastic cells are of lymphatic endothelium origin (*7–10*).

Three epidemiologic patterns of occurrence are recognized. The first involves elderly men of Mediterranean or eastern European ancestry, with a notable occurrence among Jews. Within endemic areas, foci can occur and women are also involved. Typical of this "classic" pattern is that seen in Greece as shown in Fig. 1. This type of KS appears to have a genetic component as evidenced by the association with the

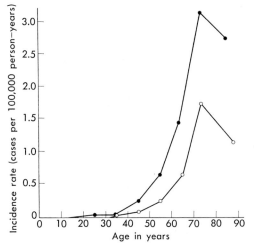

FIG. 1. Age-sex specific incidence of Kaposi's sarcoma in Greece (1976–1984). Data source: Dr. A. Kaloterakis.

● males; ○ females.

presence of DR-5 antigen of the HLA system. In a study in Italy, 67% of 12 cases had DR-5 compared to 23% of 220 controls (*11*) and in a study in Greece, 53% of 32 cases *vs.* 21% of 202 controls (*12*). In general, these patients have a relatively good prognosis with an extended survival. However, nearly one-third eventually develop a second primary malignancy, most commonly a lymphoproliferative disorder such as non-Hodgkin's lymphoma (NHL) (*13*).

A second pattern is seen in sub-Saharan Africa. There, the age distribution of KS is younger—many cases are diagnosed in young adulthood and some in child-hood—and the male predominance increases dramatically with age (*14–16*). In general, the disease follows an indolent course in these African cases. Finally, KS occurs as an iatrogenic disease following induced immunosuppression, such as for renal transplantation, in a relatively short interval of time (average=16.5 months) (*17*).

Thus, prior to the AIDS epidemic it was known that in addition to its distinctive epidemiologic features, KS was associated with an apparent genetic marker of immune function, and that acquired immunosuppression was a strong risk factor for its occurrence. These features, in addition to the observation of spontaneous regression of the multifocal lesions, have suggested that a virus may be related to its etiology (*18*).

A consistent candidate has been the cytomegalovirus (CMV). Studies evaluating this relationship have been supportive, but not conclusive. Giraldo *et al.* demonstrated the presence of herpes-like virus particles from a KS cell line and subsequently isolated human CMV (Strain K9V) (*18, 19*). Extensive seroepidemiological studies have shown a consistent association between the prevalence of CMV antibody and occurrence of KS in American and European subjects and that cases also had significantly higher titers than controls (*20, 21*). However, among African subjects, both cases and controls had elevated titers (*21*). It has been reported that CMV can replicate in endothelial cells (*22*) and Giraldo *et al.* (*23*) and Boldogh *et al.* (*24*) have reported the presence of CMV-specific nucleic acid sequences and viral-specific antigens in tumor

TABLE 1. Proportional Occurrence of Kaposi's Sarcoma at Initial Diagnosis among Major Risk Groups with AIDS in New York City, 1981–1983.

Risk group	No. of AIDS cases	KS (%)
Homosexual/bisexual men, non-IVDA	728	46.0
Homosexual/bisexual, IVDA men	97	27.8
IVDA women	72	12.5
Heterosexual men, IVDA	213	3.8

From: Des Jarlais *et al.*, N. Engl. J. Med., *310*: 1119, 1984.

biopsies. These findings have been challenged due to the presence of shared sequences of human DNA in the CMV genome and were not replicated with a smaller CMV probe (*25*).

The evaluation of the association by the comparison of the prevalence of CMV antibodies between AIDS patients with and without KS has not been informative because essentially all patients from the major risk groups have CMV antibodies (*26*). However, Marmor *et al.* have reported that the antibody titers to CMV among KS cases are significantly higher than those of the controls (*27*). Even with the use of genetic probes, the role of CMV as a passenger virus cannot be excluded among risk groups in which essentially everyone is infected.

Given this background, what have we learned about KS in relation to the AIDS epidemic? Three interesting observations are apparent. First, there is substantial variation between the major risk groups for AIDS in their risk for KS. DesJarlais *et al.* reported in 1984 that among the AIDS cases that had occurred in New York, 46% of male homosexuals who were not intravenous drug abusers (IVDA) had KS at the initial diagnosis, compared to 28% of male homosexual IVDA, 13% of female IVDA, and 4% of male heterosexual IVDA (Table 1) (*28*). Secondly, there has been a substantial secular decrease in the proportion of AIDS cases with KS—from 35% before 1983 to 15% in the first half of 1987. And thirdly, although early in the epidemic the association with DR-5 was prominent in HIV-related KS (*29–31*), it has diminished with time.

Taken together, these observations point first to a role of a sexually-transmitted infection which is common among female IVDA (many of whom are prostitutes) and promiscuous male homosexuals. The parallel decrease in number of sexual partners among male homosexuals which has been observed over the course of the epidemic and in the occurrence of KS in AIDS in this group supports this. Repeated sexual exposure to CMV could fit this model. And finally, although immunogenetic factors may heighten susceptibility to KS, these are not necessary in the presence of acquired immunosuppression. Clearly the evidence implicating a role for CMV in the etiology of KS is not conclusive, but the variation of the occurrence of KS within the AIDS epidemic allows the opportunity to pursue its role.

Non-Hodgkin's Lymphoma

The increased risk of NHL in conjunction with AIDS was recognized about a year later than that of KS. Together, KS and NHL account for 95% of all AIDS-related malignancies (*32*) and not infrequently, NHL occurs as a second malignancy in AIDS patients who initially develop KS.

One of the earliest descriptions was that of an "outbreak" of 4 cases of Burkitt's-like lymphoma diagnosed in homosexual men in San Francisco by Ziegler *et al.* (*33*). Of these, 2 presented with intraoral tumors, and a third patient had tumors "almost exclusively in the central nervous system" (CNS). All 4 had rapidly progressive disease. The authors noted the similarities of these cases to those of NHL in renal transplant patients and speculated that either CMV or the Epstein-Barr virus (EBV) was involved.

This observation was confirmed by others, and in 1984, Ziegler *et al.* reported an extended series of 90 cases of NHL in homosexual men from San Francisco, Los Angeles, Houston and New York (*34*). Nineteen (21%) of these lymphomas were preceded by KS. The histologic features of these cases differed from those seen in non-AIDS patients, with 62% being histologically defined as high-grade malignancy (mostly small non-cleaved cell or immunoblastic) and only 7% classified as low-grade. On the basis of cell-marker studies done on 35 of the cases, all but one was interpreted as of B-cell origin.

The site distribution was also striking, with 98% having extranodal involvement. Forty-three percent of patients had CNS involvement, 34% had bone marrow involvement, 17% had bowel involvement, and 16% had skin or mucosal involvement at a variety of sites. Similar to KS, the survival of these patients in comparison to non-AIDS lymphoma patients was poor, even with adjustment for histologic grade.

A series of 18 NHL cases was reported from one hospital in New York City in 1985 by Ioachim *et al.* (*35*). Seventeen of the cases were homosexual men and 1 was an IVDA. In this series, all but 1 case was histologically classified as either high or intermediate grade of malignancy. Cell typing was done on 8 specimens; all were phenotypically B-cell (*36*). Again, there was extensive extranodal involvement: 33% with bone marrow, 22% with CNS, and 67% with intra-abdominal involvement. Again, these patients had a poor survival.

In summary, the excess occurrence of NHL in conjunction with HIV infection is well established and is characterized by histologic evidence of a high grade of malignancy, B-cell origin, extensive extranodal involvement most notably of the CNS and intra-abdominal nodes, and poor prognosis. These characteristics are quite consistent with those seen in NHL occurring among therapeutically immunosuppressed patients (*37, 38*). On the basis of these observations, the clinical definition of AIDS was expanded to include persons with high grade B-cell lymphoma and HIV positivity in March of 1985 (*39*).

The role of the EBV in the pathogenesis of NHL in the presence of HIV infection has been proposed by many investigators, since EBV is closely associated with African BL and is B-cell tropic (*40*). As summarized elsewhere (*41*), a proposed model of EBV pathogenesis involves prolonged polyclonal activation of EBV-infected B cells in the presence of both defective T-cell immunity and concurrent persistent antigenic stimulation. This prolonged activation results in the chance translocation of cellular oncogenes leading to enhanced proliferation which provides a selective advantage for an abnormal monoclonal population of B-cells.

TABLE 2. Proportional Occurrence of Kaposi's Sarcoma and Non-Hodgkin's Lymphoma among Major Risk Groups with AIDS Prospectively Followed at North Shore University Hospital, 1981–1985.

Risk group	No. of AIDS cases	KS (%)	NHL (%)
Homosexuals	42	40	10
IVDA (non-homosexual)	17	6	6
Transfusion	6	17	17
Heterosexual contact	5	20	0
Caribbean origin	5	0	20

From: Kaplan *et al.*, Am. J. Med., *82*: 389–396, 1987.

Evidence in favor of this hypothesis includes the work by Sumaya *et al.* (*42*) who compared the EBV antibody response among 61 persons with AIDS or AIDS-related complex to 31 healthy controls. The HIV-infected persons had enhanced antibody response to a spectrum of EBV antigens, a pattern which is thought to characterize persistent or reactivated infection. This includes high titers to the viral capsid antigen (VCA), and increased prevalence of antibody to the early antigen (EA), predominantly the restricted component. In addition, the HIV-infected persons had a higher seroprevalence of IgA antibody against the VCA.

Rinaldo *et al.* reported a similar increase in titer against the VCA among asymptomatic HIV-positive homosexual men compared to HIV-negative homosexual men, and somewhat higher prevalence of elevated titers against EA (*43*). The authors reported that of 3 men who seroconverted to HIV, 2 had a significant concurrent increase in VCA titer. Birx *et al.* reported that cells from HIV-infected persons exhibited defective regulation of EBV infection *in vitro*, and that they had abnormally high numbers of circulating EBV-infected B-cells (*44*). Blumberg *et al.* reported that *in vitro* cytotoxic activity against EBV decreased with the extent of infection with HIV (*45*).

Thus, there is extensive data which suggest that HIV-infected persons have diminished immune capacity to control latent EBV infection. Arguing against a direct role for EBV in AIDS-related NHL is the lack of consistent observation of the presence of EBV genome (*33, 46, 47*). Finally, in contrast to AIDS-related KS, the occurrence of HIV-associated NHL does not appear to be correlated with level of sexual activity as may be inferred from risk category (Table 2) (*48*), and may also be increasing over time (*32*).

Hodgkin's Disease

In contrast to the clearly excessive incidence of both KS and NHL in association with HIV infection, there are several other malignancies which have been reported, but the validity of an association has not been established. The most common of these reports are of Hodgkin's disease (HD). The initial report concerned a 27 year old Hispanic man who was both homosexual and an IVDA who had lived in New York City and presented with advanced HD (*49*). This was followed by a report by Ioachim *et al.* of 4 cases of HD diagnosed in homosexual men in one NYC hospital between February 1982 and September 1984 (*50*). One case had previously been diagnosed with AIDS-related complex (ARC). Schoeppel *et al.* subsequently described in detail 4 cases of HD occurring in homosexual men with ARC and noted several unusual features: 3 of the 4 presented with Stage IV disease including 1 with cutaneous involvement, 1 patient had bone marrow involvement without spleen involvement, and none had mediastinal or hilar lymph node involvement (*51*). Scheib and Siegel then reported a case who presented at an advanced stage having lung parenchymal involvement, but lacking mediastinal adenopathy (*52*). Unger and Strauchen reported an additional 4 cases in homosexual men with ARC and documented the severe depletion of T-helper cells in involved tissue (*53*). Temple and Andes then reported 2 cases with confirmed HIV infection; both had advanced disease at diagnosis and were intolerant to commonly used doses of chemotherapy (*54*). Additional cases with confirmed HIV seropositivity were reported in 4 Spanish men who were IVDA (*55*) and 5 American homosexuals (*56*).

These reports suggest that risk of HD is increased among people who are apparently infected with HIV. These cases share in common the presence of unusually advanced disease with poor prognosis. Increased risk of HD has been reported in relation to immune dysfunction due to ataxia telangiectasia (*57*) and with immunosuppression for renal transplant (*58*). The mechanism for this is unclear but may relate to enhanced replication of latent EBV with immunosuppression. It has been consistently found that a larger proportion of HD patients have elevated titers against the VCA and have antibodies against the EA than expected (*59*). Recently, we have found that for extended periods of time *preceding* their diagnosis, individuals who later developed HD had enhanced antibody reactivity to the EBV (*60*). Since the immunosuppression with HIV also results in defective control of EBV, this may reflect a common pathogenesis.

Other Opportunistic Malignancies

There is only one report to our knowledge which describes the occurrence of all malignancies within a prospectively followed cohort of HIV-infected persons. This is the study by Kaplan *et al.* who followed 200 such individuals identified between 1981 and mid-1986 (*48*). Within their cohort, malignancy was diagnosed in 29 persons. KS was diagnosed in 20 patients and NHL in 7, with 3 patients having both of whom 1 also had adenocarcinoma of the colon. The authors note that all cases with KS were "sexually promiscuous". In addition, there was another case of colon cancer and 1 each of T-suppressor cell leukemia, seminoma, pancreatic cancer, and multiple myeloma. This report suggests that an array of possible opportunistic malignancies occurs in AIDS. Of interest, the patient with T-suppressor cell leukemia was co-infected with HTLV-I, as was the case of pancreatic cancer.

Logothetis *et al.* have also reported 2 cases of testicular cancer in relation to AIDS (*61*). As Newell has pointed out, testicular cancer shares many epidemiologic features with HD in young adulthood (*62*). These features suggest that for both, risk of the disease may be related to a relatively "late" and severe infection with a common virus. In a pilot study, we screened antibody titers to a range of candidate viruses in patients with testicular cancer compared to controls (*63*). We found a strong association with both prevalence and elevated titers to CMV. This was also present in a similar study by Newell, but a stronger association was present for EBV (*64*).

Finally, there is one additional malignancy which has received attention: anorectal cancer. There had been several initial reports of relatively high rates of anorectal cancer occurring among men who had never married, suggesting that risk may be associated with homosexuality (*65, 66*). A recent case-control study has confirmed this association, with risk strongly related to reported history of anal intercourse (*67*). In addition, among both men and women, history of genital warts was an extremely strong risk factor as were other indicators of sexually-transmitted disease. This report had no data on HIV status nor direct evidence of papilloma virus infection (HPV). However, a study involving cytologic screening for dysplasia and for evidence of HPV infection was carried out on 61 homosexual men as part of a prospective study on the natural history of HIV infection (*68*). In this study, anorectal dysplasia was associated with a history of anal warts, frequent receptive anal intercourse, and HIV seropositivity.

In summary, of all of the malignancies which are either conclusively associated with HIV infection or are suspected as such, most also are thought to have viral etiologies. Some—but not all—have previously been observed in conjunction with either acquired or induced immunosuppression. In AIDS, these malignancies tend to behave more aggressively than in non-AIDS patients, and often have unusual site distributions. All of the candidate viruses which have gained attention as possible agents are latent infections which are normally kept under control by cellular immunity. With the progressive depletion of T-helper cells which is the hallmark of HIV infection, there is a simultaneous loosening of control of an individual's inventory of acquired latent infections, with increased likelihood of reactivation (*69*). For a virus such as the EBV, this enhanced replication and stimulation of immunoglobulin gene rearrangement may increase the chances for oncogene rearrangements as is postulated to occur in African BL (*70*). With the family of HPV, there may be increased chance for viral integration and apparent increased risk of malignancy as is suspected for anorectal cancer and perhaps in relation with herpes simplex virus, for genital cancer (*71, 72*).

The epidemiologic problems in evaluating these opportunistic malignancies fall into several categories. The first will be to establish the likelihood that the malignancies which appear to cluster with AIDS are in fact associated. For both KS and NHL, the data are persuasive. For others such as HD and testicular cancer, the data are not. The problem is confounded by the fact that AIDS is occurring in the age group where both are normally seen. For anorectal and cervical cancer (if it increases), the problem will be confounded by the fact that both are associated with sexual exposure.

The second problem will be to establish the specificity of these associations. Strategies which may be relevant include evaluation of a variety of measures of antibody response, such as titer level, antibody class, but also to an array of antigens which may reflect viral replication. This would be particularly useful when serial serum specimens are available, as are now being collected in the large prospective cohort studies. More persuasive evidence of specificity may come with the identification of HIV-infected populations in which substantial numbers lack the virus(es) of interest; for example, male homosexuals without CMV infection, or less likely, EBV.

The observation that most of the opportunistic malignancies that have been seen in AIDS are hematopoietic or are associated with a viral infection argues against the broad role of immune surveillance as a protection against cancer (73). However, these malignancies may provide insight into the mechanisms by which latent viral infections influence oncogenesis. It is likely that there is a cascade of these malignancies which occur in the natural history of HIV infection within a population, where the risk of each is related both to the biologic nature of the latent virus—such as the frequency of reactivation—as well as to the influence of other factors—such as nutritional status, co-existing infections, and initial host-viral balance. This cascade may have a protracted time-course with early outcomes being KS and NHL, and more long term outcomes such as hepatocellular carcinoma in association with chronic hepatitis B virus infection. We can anticipate an upsurge in the occurrence of cervical cancer, as a larger number of women become infected with HIV. Another possible outcome may be increased skin cancer, as these are seen in conjunction with renal transplant (74), and have been postulated to involve HPV infection (75).

In summary, the pandemic of HIV infection affords an unheralded opportunity to gain understanding of the role of latent viral infections in the etiology of human malignancy. It should also illuminate our understanding of how these latent infections are normally controlled by the immune system. As epidemiologists and virologists alike, it is both our privilege and obligation to explore these questions.

ACKNOWLEDGMENTS

This work is supported by a grant from the Helena Rubenstein Foundation, and grant ROl AI 2643 from the U.S. National Institute of Health.

REFERENCES

1. Centers for Disease Control. *Pneumocystis* pneumonia—Los Angeles. MMWR, *30*: 250–252, 1981.
2. Centers for Disease Control. Follow-up on Kaposi's sarcoma and *pneumocystis* pneumonia. MMWR, *30*: 409–410, 1981.
3. Safai, B. and Good, R. A. Kaposi's sarcoma: A review and recent developments. Clin. Bull., *10*: 62–69, 1980.
4. Costa, J. and Rabson, A. S. Generalized Kaposi's sarcoma is not a neoplasm. Lancet, *i*: 58, 1983.
5. Lothe, F. Kaposi's sarcoma in Ugandan Africans. Acta Pathol. Microbiol. Scand., *161*: Suppl., 7–8, 1963.
6. Krigel, R., Laubenstein, L. J., and Muggia, F. Kaposi's sarcoma: A new staging classification. Cancer Treat. Rep., *67*: 531–534, 1983.
7. Nadji, M., Morales, A. R., Ziegler-Weissman, J., and Penneys, N. S. Kaposi's sarcoma: Immunohistologic evidence or an endothelial origin. Arch Pathol. Lab. Med., *105*: 274–275, 1981.
8. Modlin, R. L., Hofman, F. M., Kempt, R. A., Taylor, C. R., Conant, M. A., and Rea, T. H. Kaposi's sarcoma in homosexual men: an immunohistochemical study. J. Am. Acad. Dermatol., *8*: 620–627, 1983.
9. Flotte, T. J., Hatcher, V. A., and Friedman-Kein, A. E. Factor VIII-related antigen in Kaposi's sarcoma in young homosexual men. Arch Dermatol., *120*: 180–182, 1984.
10. Beckstead, J. H., Wood, G. S., and Fletcher, V. Evidence for the origin of Kaposi's

sarcoma from lymphatic endothelium. Am. J. Pathol., *119*: 294–300, 1985.

11. Contu, L., Cerimele, D., Pintus, A., Cottoni, F., and LaNasa, G. HLA and Kaposi's sarcoma in Sardinia. Tissue Antigens, *23*: 240–245, 1984.

12. Papasteriades, C., Kaloterakis, A., Filiotou, A., Economidou, J., Nicolis, G., Trichopoulos, D., and Stratigos, J. Histocompatibility antigens HLA-A, -B, -DR in Greek patients with Kaposi's sarcoma. Tissue Antigens, *24*: 313–315, 1984.

13. Safai, B., Mike, V., Giraldo, G., Beth, E., and Good, R. A. Association of Kaposi's sarcoma with second primary malignancies. Possible etiopathogenetic implications. Cancer, *45*: 1472–1479, 1980.

14. Hutt, M.S.R. and Burkitt, D. P. Geographical distribution of cancer in East Africa. Br. Med. J., *2*: 719–722, 1965.

15. Taylor, J. F., Smith, P. G., Bull, D., and Pike, M. C. Kaposi's sarcoma in Uganda. Geographic and ethnic distribution. Br. J. Cancer, *26*: 483–496, 1972.

16. Olweny, C.L.M. Epidemiology and clinical features of Kaposi's sarcoma in tropical Africa. *In;* A. E. Friedman-Kien and L. J. Laubenstein (eds.), AIDS: The Epidemic of Kaposi's Sarcoma and Opportunistic Infections, pp. 35–40, Masson Publishing, New York, 1963.

17. Penn, I. Kaposi's sarcoma in immunosuppressed patients. J. Clin. Lab. Immunol., *12*: 1–10, 1983.

18. Giraldo, G., Beth, E., Coeur, P., Vogel, Ch. L., and Dhru, D. S. Kaposi's sarcoma: a new model in the search for viruses associated with human malignancies. JNCI, *49*: 1495–1507, 1972.

19. Giraldo, G., Beth, E., and Hagueman, F. Herpes-type virus particles in tissue culture of Kaposi's sarcoma from different geographic regions. JNCI, *49*: 1509–1526, 1972.

20. Giraldo, G., Beth, E., Henle, W., Henle, G., Mike, V., Safai, B., Huraux, J. M., McHardy, J., and DeThe, G. Antibody patterns to herpes viruses in Kaposi's sarcoma. II. Serologic association of American Kaposi's sarcoma with cytomegalovirus. Int. J. Cancer, *22*: 126–131, 1978.

21. Giraldo, G., Beth, E., Kourilsky, I., Henle, W., Henle, G., Mike, V., Huraux, J. M., Andersen, H. K., Gharbi, M. R., Kyalwazi, S. K., and Puissant, A. Antibody patterns of herpes viruses in Kaposi's sarcoma: serologic association of European Kaposi's sarcoma with cytomegalovirus. Int. J. Cancer, *15*: 839–848, 1975.

22. Ho, D. D., Rota, T. R., Andrews, C. A., and Hirsch, M. S. Replication of human cytomegalovirus in endothelial cells. J. Inf. Dis., *150*: 956–957, 1984.

23. Giraldo, G., Beth, E., and Huang, E. S. Kaposi's sarcoma and its relationship to cytomegalovirus (CMV) III. CMV-DNA and CMV early antigens in Kaposi's sarcoma. Int. J. Cancer, *26*: 23–29, 1980.

24. Boldogh, I., Beth, E., Huang, E. S., Kyalwazi, S. K., and Giraldo, G. Kaposi's sarcoma. II. Detection of CMV-DNA, CMV-RNA and CMNA in tumor biopsies. Int. J. Cancer, *28*: 469–474, 1981.

25. Runger, R., Colimon, R., and Fleckenstein, B. Search for DNA sequences of human cytomegalovirus in Kaposi's sarcoma tissues with cloned probes. Preliminary report. Antibiot. Chemother., *32*: 43–47, 1984.

26. Zollo-Pazner, S. Serology. *In;* P. Ebbesen, R. Biggar, and M. Melbye (eds.), AIDS: A Basic Guide for Clinicians, pp. 151–172, Munkgaard, Copenhagen, 1984.

27. Marmor, M., Friedman-Kien, A. E., Zolla-Pazner, S., Stahl, R. E., Rubinstein, P., Laubenstein, L., William, D. C., Kjlein, R. J., and Spigland, I. Kaposi's sarcoma in homosexual men. Ann. Intern. Med., *100*: 809–815, 1984.

28. DesJarlais, D. C., Marmor, M., Thomas, P., Chamberland, M., Zolla-Pozner, S., and Spencer, D. J. Kaposi's sarcoma among four different AIDS risk groups. N. Engl.

J. Med., *310*: 1119, 1984.

29. Friedman-Kien, A. E., Laubenstein, L. J., Rubinstein, P., Buimovici-Klein, E., Marmor, M., Stahl, R., Spigland, I., Kim, K. S., and Zolla-Pazner, S. Disseminated Kaposi's sarcoma in homosexual men. Ann. Intern. Med., *96*: 693–700, 1982.

30. Pollack, M. S., Safai, B., Myskowski, P. L., Gold, J.W.M., Pandey, J., and Dupont, B. Frequencies of HLA and Gm immunogenetic markers in Kaposi's sarcoma. Tissue Antigens, *21*: 1–8, 1983.

31. Prince, H. E., Schroff, R. W., Ayoub, G., Han, S., Gottlieb, M. S., and Fahey, J. L. HLA studies in acquired immunodeficiency syndrome patients with Kaposi's sarcoma. J. Clin. Immunol., *4*: 242–245, 1984.

32. Levine, A. M. Non-Hodgkin's lymphomas and other malignancies in the acquired immunodeficiency syndrome. Sem. Oncol., *14* (Suppl. 3): 34–39, 1987.

33. Ziegler, J. L., Drew, W. L., Miner, R. C., Mintz, L., Rosenbaum, E., Gershow, J., Lennette, E. T., Greenspan, J., Shillitoe, E., Beckstead, J., Casavant, C., and Yamamoto, K. Outbreak of Burkitt's-like lymphoma in homosexual men. Lancet, *2*: 631–633, 1982.

34. Ziegler, J. L., Beckstead, J. A., Volberding, P. A., Abrams, D. I., Levine, A. M., Lukes, R. J., Gill, P. S., Burkes, R. L., Meyer, P. R., Metroka, G. E., Mouradian, J., Moore, A., Riggs, S. A., Butler, J. J., Cabanillas, F. C., Hersh, E., Newell, G. R., Laubenstein, L. J., Knowles, D., Odajnyk, C., Raphael, B., Koziner, B., Urmacher, C., and Clarkson, B. D. Non-Hodgkin's lymphoma in 90 homosexual men. N. Engl. J. Med., *311*: 565–570, 1984.

35. Ioachim, H. L., Cooper, M. C., and Hellman, G. C. Lymphomas in men at high risk for acquired immune deficiency syndrome (AIDS): A study of 21 cases. Cancer, *56*: 2831–2842, 1985.

36. Ioachim, H. L. and Cooper, M. C. Lymphomas of AIDS. Lancet, *1*: 96, 1986.

37. Penn, I. Malignant lymphomas in organ transplant recipient. Transplant. Proc., *13*: 736–738, 1981.

38. Cleary, M. L., Warnke, R., and Sklar, J. Monoclonality of lymphoproliferative lesions in cardiac transplant recipients: Clonal analysis based on immunoglobulin-gene rearrangements. N. Engl. J. Med., *310*: 477–482, 1984.

39. Centers of Disease Control. Diffuse, undifferentiated non-Hodgkin's lymphoma among homosexual males—United States. MMWR, *31*: 277, 1982.

40. Miller, G. Burkitt's Lymphoma. *In;* A. S. Evans (ed.), Viral Infections of Humans: Epidemiology and Control, pp. 599–620, Plenum Medical Book, New York, 1982.

41. Anon. Malignant lymphomas in homosexuals. Lancet, *1*: 193–194, 1986.

42. Sumaya, C. V., Boswell, R. N., Ench, Y., Kisner, D. L., Hersh, E. M., Reuben, J. M., and Mansell, P.W.A. Enhanced serologic and virological findings of Epstein-Barr virus in patients with AIDS and AIDS-related complex. J. Infect. Dis., *154*: 864–870, 1986.

43. Rinaldo, C. R., Jr., Kingsley, L. A., Lyter, D. W., Rabin, B. S., Atchison, R. W., Bodner, A. J., Weiss, S. H., and Saxinger, W. C. Association of HTLV-III with Epstein-Barr virus infection and abnormalities of T lymphocytes in homosexual men. J. Infect. Dis., *154*: 556–561, 1986.

44. Birx, D. L., Redfield, R. R., and Tosato, G. Defective regulation of Epstein-Barr virus infection in patients with acquired immunodeficiency syndrome (AIDS) or AIDS-related disorders. N. Engl. J. Med., *314*: 874–879, 1986.

45. Blumberg, R. S., Paradis, T., Byington, R., Henle, W., Hirsch, M. S., and Schooley, R. T. Effects of human immunodeficiency virus on the cellular immune response to Epstein-Barr virus in homosexual men: Characterization of the cytotoxic response and lymphokine production. J. Infect. Dis., *155*: 877–890, 1987.

46. Levine, A. M., Parkash, S. G., Meyer, P. R., Burkes, R. L., Ross, R., Dworsky, R. D., Krailo, M., Parker, J. W., Lukes, R. J., and Rasheed, S. Retrovirus and malignant lymphoma in homosexual men. JAMA, *254*: 1921–1925, 1985.

47. Abrams, D. I., Kaplan, L. D., McGrath, M. S., and Volberding, P. A. AIDS-related benign lymphadenopathy and malignant lymphoma: Clinical aspects and virologic interactions. AIDS Res., *2* (Suppl. 1): S131–140, 1986.

48. Kaplan, M. H., Susin, M., Pahwa, S. G., Fetten, J., Allen, S. L., Lichtman, S., Sarngadharan, M. G., and Gallo, R. C. Neoplastic complications of HTLV-III infection: Lymphomas and solid tumors. Am. J. Med., *82*: 389–396, 1987.

49. Robert, N. J. and Schneiderman, H. Hodgkin's disease and the acquired immunodeficiency syndrome. Ann. Intern. Med., *101*: 142–143, 1984.

50. Ioachim, H. L., Cooper, M. C., and Hellman, G. C. Hodgkin's disease and the acquired immunodeficiency syndrome. Ann. Intern. Med., *101*: 876–877, 1984.

51. Schoeppel, S. L., Hoppe, R. T., Dorfman, R. F., Horning, S. J., Collier, A. C., Chew, T. G., and Weiss, L. M. Hodgkin's disease in homosexual men with generalized lymphadenopathy. Ann. Intern. Med., *102*: 68–70, 1985.

52. Scheib, R. G. and Siegel, R. S. A typical Hodgkin's disease and the acquired immunodeficiency syndrome. Ann. Intern. Med., *102*: 554, 1985.

53. Unger, P. D. and Strauchen, J. A. Hodgkin's disease in AIDS complex patients: Report of four cases and tissue immunologic marker studies. Cancer, *58*: 821–825, 1986.

54. Temple, J. J. and Andes, W. A. AIDS and Hodgkin's disease. Lancet, *2*: 455–456, 1986.

55. Lopez-Herce, Cid. J. A., Loez-Herce, Cid. J., Sanudo, E. F., Menarguez, J., and Ochaita, J. C. AIDS and Hodgkin's disease. Lancet, *2*: 1104–1105, 1986.

56. Prior, E., Goldberg, A. F., Conjalka, M. S., Chapman, W. E., Tay, S., and Ames, E. A. Hodgkin's disease in homosexual men: An AIDS-related phenomenon? Am. J. Med., *81*: 1085–1088, 1986.

57. Frizzera, G., Rosai, J., Dehner, L. P., Spector, B. D., and Kersey, J. H. Lymphoreticular disorders in primary immunodeficiencies. Cancer, *46*: 692–699, 1980.

58. Doyle, T. J., Venkatachalam, K. K., Maeda, K., Saeed, S. M., and Tilchen, E. J. Hodgkin's disease in renal transplant recipients. Cancer, *51*: 245–247, 1983.

59. Evans, A. S. and Gutensohn (Mueller), N. M. A population-based case-control study of EBV and other viral antibodies among persons with Hodgkin's disease and their siblings. Int. J. Cancer, *34*: 149–157, 1984.

60. Mueller, N. Epidemiologic studies assessing the role of the Epstein-Barr virus in Hodgkin's disease. Yale J. Biol. Med., *60*: 321–327, 1987.

61. Logothetis, C. J., Newell, G. R., and Samuels, M. L. Testicular cancer in homosexual men and cellular immune deficiency: report of 2 cases. J. Urol., *133*: 484–486, 1985.

62. Newell, G. R., Mills, P. K., and Johnson, D. E. Epidemiologic comparison of cancer of the testis and Hodgkin's disease among young males. Cancer, *54*: 1117–1123, 1984.

63. Mueller, N., Hinkula, J., and Wahren, B. Elevated antibody titers against cytomegalovirus among patients with testicular cancer. Int. J. Cancer, *41*: 399–403, 1988.

64. Algood, C. B., Newell, G. R., and Johnson, D. E. Viral etiology of testicular tumors. J. Urol., in press.

65. Daling, J. R., Weiss, N. S., Klopfenstein, L. L., Cochran, L. E., Chow, W. H., and Daifuku, R. Correlates of homosexual behavior and the incidence of anal cancer. JAMA, *247*: 1988–1990, 1982.

66. Peters, R. K. and Mack, T. M. Patterns of anal carcinoma by gender and marital status in Los Angeles county. Br. J. Cancer, *48*: 629–636, 1983.

67. Daling, J. R., Weiss, N. S., Hislop, T. H., Maden, C., Coates, R. L., Sherman, K. J., Ashley, R. L., Beagrie, M., Ryan, J. A., and Corey, L. Sexual practice, sexually transmitted diseases, and the incidence of anal cancer. N. Engl. J. Med., *317*: 973–977, 1987.

68. Frazer, I. H., Medley, G., Crapper, R. M., Brown, T. C., and MacKay, I. R. Association between anorectal dysplasia, human papillomavirus, and human immunodeficiency virus infection in homosexual men. Lancet, *2*: 657–660, 1986.

69. Evans, A. S. Hypothesis: the pathogenesis of AIDS. Activation of the T- and B-cell cascades. Yale J. Biol. Med., *57*: 317–327, 1984.

70. Leder, P., Battey, J., Lenoir, G., Moulding, G., Murphy, W., Potter, H., Stewart, T., and Taub, R. Translocations among antibody genes in human cancer. Science, *222*: 765–771, 1983.

71. zur Hausen, H., deVilliers, E. M., and Gissmann, L. Papillovirus infections and human genital cancer. Gynecol. Oncol., *12*: 124–128, 1981.

72. Bradbeer, C. Is infection with HIV a risk factor for cervical intraepithelial neoplasia? Lancet, *ii*: 1277–1278, 1987.

73. Ehrlich P. *In;* S. Himmelweit (ed.), The Collected Papers of Paul Ehrlich, Vol 2, p. 561, Pergamon Press, Oxford, 1957.

74. Hoover, R. and Fraumeni, J. F., Jr. Risk of cancer in renal-transplant recipients. Lancet, *ii*: 55–57, 1973.

75. Bunney, M. H., Barr, B. B., McLaren, K., Smith, I. W., Benton, E. C., Anderton, J. L., and Hunter, J.A.A. Human papillomavirus type 5 anal skin cancer in renal allograft recipients. Lancet, *ii*: 181–182, 1987.

Epidemiologic Similarities Leading to Etiologic Hypotheses

Guy R. Newell, Margaret R. Spitz, and Douglas E. Johnson

Departments of Cancer Prevention and Control and Urology, The University of Texas M. D. Anderson Hospital and Tumor Institute, Houston, Texas 77030, U.S.A.

Abstract: Analogy is a useful means of generating etiologic hypotheses which can be tested by epidemiologic, clinical, or laboratory studies. We describe how the use of analogy has furthered the understanding of three disease entities—Hodgkin's disease (HD), testicular cancer (TC), and acquired immune deficiency syndrome (AIDS). HD is probably caused by a virus of low pathogenicity with clinical expression dependent on social factors. TC may have a viral etiology, although clinical disease may be triggered by other factors. AIDS is caused by a virus which may act as an initiator. AIDS-related Kaposi's sarcoma (KS) may be the result of exposure to a carcinogenic chemical acting as a promoter. In all three diseases, the clinical manifestation could be regarded as varying expressions of host response to a viral agent, modified by an array of socioeconomic and/or biologic cofactors.

Uses of Analogy

Epidemiologic similarities can be drawn between patterns of disease occurrence in humans (*1, 2*); between animal diseases of known etiology and human diseases of unknown etiology (*3*); or between syndromes in animals known to be induced virally or chemically, and thus likely to occur in humans as well (*4*). The presence of shared characteristics suggests that the diseases also share the same or similar etiologies. This should be interpreted in its broadest sense. The shared etiology may exert a direct causal association. However, there may be different etiologies, exerting their effect through an indirect association, but manifested through common pathways of expression, such as socioeconomic status. In either case, the diseases will share similar characteristic distributions.

In almost all uses of analogy, selected items are chosen for the purpose of drawing a comparison and do not necessarily account for all of the observations that have been made (*2*). Some of the selected items may not have been confirmed by all the reported studies or not all items may have been studied for both diseases being compared. Finally, each disease may have a set of unique features, such as the case with HD and TC. None of these limitations detract from the usefulness of analogy in generating etiologic hypotheses, provided that their limitations are recognized and results are interpreted cautiously.

Hodgkin's Disease

The similar epidemiologic features of HD and multiple sclerosis (MS) are consistent with the hypothesis of a prevalent infection of low pathogenicity. Gutensohn and Cole expanded on the similarities of this model with that of paralytic poliomyelitis (PP) (5). In addition, this model shares characteristics with tuberculosis, sarcoidosis, and infectious mononucleosis (6). The incidence of Hodgkin's disease is characterized by substantial variations internationally that differ by age, socioeconomic status, ethnicity and histologic subtype. These patterns strongly support the role of environmental factors in the etiology of the disease (7).

1. International variation and ethnic differences

In 1971, Correa and O'Conor contrasted the histologic and age patterns of Hodgkin's disease occurrence in underdeveloped countries (Pattern I) with that occurring in developed, industrialized countries (Pattern III) (6). Pattern I was characterized by high rates in childhood and predominance of histologic subtypes having poor prognosis. HD in Latin America is characterized by such a pattern (8). Pattern III was characterized by high rates in young adults and predominance of histologic subtypes associated with better prognosis.

Patterns of HD observed internationally are also evident within ethnic groups nationally. The state of Connecticut has the characteristic distribution of Pattern III (9). Vianna et al. reported that the pattern among blacks in Washington, D.C., resembled Pattern III whereas in New Jersey and parts of New York state an intermediate pattern was evident (10). Analysis of SEER data for the time period 1973 through 1982 revealed that during childhood and adolescence, whites exhibited the highest percentage of nodular sclerosis subtype (65%) and Hispanics the lowest (45%). Conversely, Hispanics had higher percentages of histologic subtypes associated with a poorer prognosis—mixed cellularity and lymphocyte depletion (11). Similarly, among adults the pattern for Hispanics in Puerto Rico was representative of that seen in populations in developing countries, while the pattern among Mexican-Americans in the continental U.S. more closely approximated that seen among US whites (12). These differences by age, sex, ethnicity, and histology are in perfect accord with the hypothesis of Correa and O'Conor (6).

2. Age at onset and social environment

The striking bimodality of Hodgkin's disease led to MacMahon's two-disease hypothesis (13). He suggested that the young adult disease component "is probably infectious in nature, though of very low infectivity." HD incidence in childhood is characterized by a male preponderance, particularly among blacks. Washburn et al. noted that during the first years of life, male children were more susceptible to infection (14). In 1981, Gutensohn and Cole reported a set of factors in the childhood social environment which tended to decrease or delay early exposures to infection (15). These included sibship size, housing units, and maternal education. They suggested that these patterns might be explained by a viral origin of the disease, with age at infection as a major modifier of risk. We have recently demonstrated that white adolescents 15–19 years old have the highest incidence rates compared with blacks and Hispanic adolescents (11). Highest adolescent-to-childhood ratios of incidence rates were found for females compared to males and for whites compared to blacks and Hispanics. These data support Gutensohn and Cole's hypothesis.

3. Variations with time

There is a reciprocal relationship between HD incidence in childhood and young adulthood. As living conditions improve there is a decline in the childhood component of the disease and a corresponding increase in young adulthood incidence. This pattern, too, is compatible with the proposed infectious etiology model.

Reports of a seasonal pattern of clinical onset of Hodgkin's disease have been inconsistent. We found significant fluctuations of month of diagnosis for young adults (15–39 years) but not older adults (16). February was the month of peak diagnosis both among young men and women. The use of seasonal variation of disease onset as a surrogate for patterns of etiology is questionable. Other types of time-space clusterings were found only among young adults (17). These findings are consistent with the prevailing hypothesis of a rare manifestation of a prevalent infection with a virus of low pathogenicity.

Testicular Cancer

The epidemiology of testicular cancer has most often been contrasted with other endocrine-dependent cancers such as prostate and breast cancer (18). However, testicular cancer shares similar epidemiologic features with Hodgkin's disease, which suggests that it may also have a viral-related etiology (2).

1. International variation and ethnic differences

There are distinct ethnic risk differentials in SEER incidence data for TC. White men have significantly higher rates than their black, Puerto Rico, and New Mexican Hispanic counterparts (19). Higher rates of TC among indigenous U.S. Hispanics relative to their migrant counterparts indicate that environmental factors are important in this disease etiology (20). However, testicular cancer is rare among all black populations of the world, suggesting a genetic resistance to this tumor among these persons (21).

2. Age at onset and social environment

Testicular cancer occurs more frequently in men of higher rather than lower social class, even within the same ethnic group (22). Most studies report a positive relationship between testicular cancer incidence and several indicators of social class. In the lowest social class the curve is bimodal, but assumes a unimodal peak in young adults in the highest social class (18). Protection is also afforded by large sibship size (23). This is consistent with the hypothesis of a highly prevalent infection for which early immunization is protective in later life, much like paralytic poliomyelitis (2).

In this country and in England and Wales, the increase in testicular cancer in young men has been followed by a decrease in older men (*19, 22*). This shift among age groups could occur as susceptible individuals in one age group increase while those in another age group decreased. This pattern would be consistent with widespread infection with an agent of low pathogenicity, similar to paralytic poliomyelitis (*2*). As noted for Hodgkin's disease, susceptibility to primary infection is directly related to improvements in social and economic conditions.

The sharing of several indicators of social class between testicular cancer and Hodgkin's disease could reflect an indirect association with social status. Social class is a general term that includes a complex set of interrelating factors, as noted previously.

3. Time trends

The most striking feature of the epidemiology of testicular cancer is its rapidly increasing occurrence. It has been increasing in young white men in this country and in England and Wales for the last 40 years or more (*22*). More recently, it may have begun to increase in Hispanic Americans as well (*20*). In England and Wales, this increase occurred first among men of higher social class. Davies attributes this to features of modern life which have always affected men in higher social classes and which are becoming more common throughout society (*22*). She argues against occupation, exposure *in utero* or in childhood, or cryptorchidism as contributing substantially to this increase.

4. Possible association with Epstein-Barr virus (EBV)

EBV antibodies have been reported in Hodgkin's disease both after and before its onset (*24*). Persons with serologically confirmed infectious mononucleosis have an approximately threefold increased risk for developing Hodgkin's disease. In a small preliminary serologic survey, we found significantly elevated EBV titers among untreated patients with TC compared with a group of physicians and another group of non-physicians (*25*). Titers to cytomegalovirus (CMV), hepatitis A and hepatitis B viruses were not elevated in the patients compared with the controls. We stress that this represents a preliminary observation requiring further investigation.

5. Testicular cancer in AIDS patients

We reported the first two cases of testicular cancer occurring in patients with AIDS (*26*). One patient had taken marijuana, volatile nitrites, and methyl-dextroamphetamines regularly. The other patient had been a service supervisor for a large local pest control company for the last one-and-a-half years and had sprayed chemicals for insect control for two years. Chemical exposure is not necessarily incompatible with a viral etiology, as described further below.

Acquired Immune Deficiency Syndrome (AIDS)

Investigators have used epidemiologic similarities to generate etiologic hypotheses pertaining to the cause(s) of AIDS as well. These have expedited elucidation of the etiologic virus associated with AIDS.

1.   Analogy with known diseases

In 1983, Francis *et al.* reviewed the epidemiologic characteristics of hepatitis B virus (HBV) transmission in humans and clinical manifestations of feline leukemia virus (FeLV) in cats to help elucidate the etiology of acquired immune deficiency syndrome (*3*). They noted that the epidemiologic similarities between HBV and the descriptions of the putative AIDS virus based on available epidemiology were striking. Equally as striking were the similarities between the clinical disease produced in cats by the FeLV and clinical manifestation of AIDS. Their ability to predict epidemiologic and clinical characteristics of an unknown virus based on analogy provides an excellent example of how this technique can contribute to disease understanding. They also suggested that the responsible agent might be both immunosuppressive and oncogenic.

2.   Volatile nitrites as a cofactor

In 1985, we proposed nitrite inhalation as a possible cofactor in the cause of KS associated with AIDS in young male homosexuals (*4*). Evidence which suggested this was a reasonable hypothesis included: (a) nitroso compounds are among the most potent known chemical carcinogens in animals; (b) nitrites can be converted to nitroso compounds by amines and amides naturally occurring in human saliva and gastric juice; (c) street variety volatile nitrites were shown to have deleterious effects on human lymphocytes both *in vivo* and *in vitro*; (d) the timing of the production and sale of street variety nitrite inhalants coincided with their increased use among male homosexuals particularly; (e) in the early studies of risk factors for the new syndrome now called AIDS the majority of patients had KS as a manifestation; (f) among the patients with KS, with or without associated pneumonia, the use of volatile nitrites was very prevalent and there was a clear dose-response demonstrable; (g) the age group of young men presenting with KS was consistent with a cohort initially exposed seven to 10 years previously. Mirvish and Ramm recently demonstrated that relatively large amounts of at least one nitrosamine can be produced *in vivo* from simple nitrite esters (*27*). This adds biologic plausibility to the suggested association of inhaled nitrites with KS.

3.   Initiation-promotion hypothesis

Haverkos *et al.* analysed results from 87 homosexual men with KS and/or *Pneumocystis carinii* pneumonia (PCP) interviewed by Centers for Disease Control personnel during early studies (*28*). They compared the results for patients having KS (with or without PCP) with patients having PCP only. In multivariate analysis, total days of nitrite use more significantly differentiated KS (with or without PCP) from PCP only patients than did any other variable. Among patients for whom matched controls were interviewed, nitrite use was the only significant variable among KS only patients and KS plus PCP patients but not for PCP only patients. Not all subsequent studies have found an association between nitrite use and KS. This could be due either to methodologic problems or the decreasing occurrence of KS among patients with AIDS (*28*).

Haverkos *et al.* postulated a unifying hypothesis to reconcile the existence of a proven etiologic virus with strong evidence for use of immunosuppressive and carcinogenic chemicals. They suggested that the natural history of AIDS begins with immune dysfunction, most likely as a result of infection of T-helper lymphocytes with the HIV as an initiator. One or several cofactors, present in some but not necessarily all patients, determine clinical manifestations of the syndrome. A promoter for development of KS may be the use of nitrite inhalants, for the many reasons we described (4) along with new information provided by Haverkos et al. (28).

There is sufficient evidence that chemicals act as tumor promoters for the induction of human cancers having viral etiologies to lend biologic plausibility to the initiation-promotion hypothesis of Haverkos et al.. Tumor promoters have been extensively studied by the Japanese (29). Ito reported the induction of Epstein-Barr virus antigen from Raji cells by TPA, and this observation was confirmed with newer tumor promoters (30). It was suggested that the exposure to various tumor promoters in traditional herb remedies may be partly related to the incidence of nasopharyngeal cancers in Southeast Asia and of Burkitt's lymphoma in Africa (29).

Conclusions

1. The hypothesis has been sustained that Hodgkin's disease is a manifestation of infection with a widespread virus of low infectivity and pathogenicity. The clinical disease reflects host responses modified by social factors.

2. The hypothesis that testicular cancer may also have a viral etiology based on the same model as Hodgkin's disease is plausible, although additional studies directed toward testing this hypothesis are required. There is some speculation that chemical exposure may also have an etiologic role in testicular cancer. The contributions of both viruses and chemicals are not necessarily mutually exclusive.

3. There is good evidence to sustain the hypothesis that volatile nitrite use is causally associated with the expression of Kaposi's sarcoma in AIDS. Nitrites can be converted in vivo to nitrosamines, and there is precedent for chemicals, acting as promoters, to activate oncogenic viruses, acting as initiators. This sustains the initiation-promotion explanation offered by Haverkos and colleagues.

REFERENCES

1. Newell, G. R. Etiology of multiple sclerosis and Hodgkin's disease. Am. J. Epidemiol., 2: 119–122, 1970.
2. Newell, G. R., Mills, P. K., and Johnson, D. E. Epidemiologic comparison of cancer of the testis and Hodgkin's disease among young males. Cancer, 54: 1117–1123, 1984.
3. Francis, D. P., Curran, J. W., and Essex, M. Epidemic acquired immune deficiency syndrome: Epidemiologic evidence for a transmissible agent. J. Natl. Cancer Inst., 71: 1–4, 1983.
4. Newell, G. R., Mansell, P.W.A., Spitz, M. R., Reuben, J. M., and Hersh, E. M. Volatile nitrites. Use and adverse effects related to the current epidemic of the acquired immune deficiency syndrome. Am. J. Med., 78: 811–816, 1985.
5. Gutensohn, N. and Cole, P. Epidemiology of Hodgkin's disease in the young. Int. J. Cancer, 19: 595–604, 1977.
6. Correa, P. and O'Conor, G. T. Epidemiologic patterns of Hodgkin's disease. Int. J. Cancer, 8: 192–201, 1971.

7. Newell, G. R. and Rawlings, W. Evidence for environmental factors in the etiology of Hodgkin's disease. J. Chron. Dis., *25*: 261–267, 1972.

8. Correa, P. Hodgkin's disease in Latin America. Natl. Cancer Inst. Monogr., *36*: 9–14, 1973.

9. O'Conor, G. T., Correa, P., Christine, B., Axtell, L., and Myers, M. Hodgkin's disease in Connecticut: Histology and age distribution. Natl. Cancer Inst. Monogr., *36*: 3–8, 1973.

10. Vianna, N. J., Thind, I. S., Louria, D. B., Polan, A., Kirmss, V., and Davies, J.N.P. Epidemiologic and histologic patterns of Hodgkin's disease in blacks. Cancer, *40*: 3133–3139, 1977.

11. Spitz, M. R., Sider, J. G., Johnson, C. C., Butler, J. J., Pollack, E. S., and Newell, G. R. Ethnic patterns of Hodgkin's disease incidence among children and adolescents in the United States, 1973–82. J. Natl. Cancer Inst., *76*: 235–239, 1986.

12. Spitz, M. R., Pollack, E. S., Butler, J. J., Sider, J. G., Lynch, H. K., and Newell, G. R. Incidence of Hodgkin's disease among Hispanics in the United States, 1973–82. Cancer J., *1*: 30–33, 1986.

13. MacMahon, B. Epidemiology of Hodgkin's disease. Cancer Res., *26*: 1189–1200, 1966.

14. Washburn, T. C., Medearis, D. N., Jr., and Childs, B. Sex differences in susceptibility to infections. Pediatrics, *35*: 57–64, 1965.

15. Gutensohn, N. and Cole, P. Childhood social environment and Hodgkin's disease. N. Engl. J. Med., *304*: 135–140, 1981.

16. Newell, G. R., Lynch, H. K., Gibeau, J. M., and Spitz, M. R. Seasonal diagnosis of Hodgkin's disease among young adults. J. Natl. Cancer Inst., *74*: 53–56, 1985.

17. Greenberg, R. S., Grufferman, S., and Cole, P. An evaluation of space-time clustering in Hodgkin's disease. J. Chronic Dis., *36*: 257–262, 1983.

18. Ross, R. K., McCurtis, J. W., Henderson, B. E., Menck, H. R., Mack, T. M., and Martin, S. P. Descriptive epidemiology of testicular and prostate cancer in Los Angeles. Br. J. Cancer, *39*: 284–292, 1979.

19. Spitz, M. R., Sider, J. G., Pollack, E. S., Lynch, H. K., and Newell, G. R. Incidence and descriptive features of testicular cancer among United States whites, blacks, and Hispanics, 1973–82. Cancer, *58*: 1785–1790, 1986.

20. Thomas, D. B. Epidemiologic studies of cancer in minority groups in the Western United States. Natl. Cancer Inst. Monogr., *53*: 103–113, 1979.

21. Tulinius, H., Day, N., and Muir, C. S. Rarity of testis cancer in Negroes. Lancet, *1*: 35–36, 1973.

22. Davies, J. M. Testicular cancer in England and Wales: Some epidemiological aspects. Lancet, *1*: 928–932, 1981.

23. Henderson, B. E., Benton, B., Jing, J., Yu, M. C., and Pike, M. C. Risk factors for cancer of the testis in young men. Int. J. Cancer, *23*: 598–602, 1979.

24. Evans, A. S. and Comstock, G. W. Presence of elevated antibody titers to Epstein-Barr virus before Hodgkin's disease. Lancet, *1*: 1183–1186, 1981.

25. Algood, C. B., Newell, G. R., and Johnson, D. E. Viral etiology of testicular tumors. J. Urol., *139*: 308–310, 1988.

26. Logothetis, C. J., Newell, G. R., and Samuels, M. L. Testicular cancer in homosexual men with cellular immune deficiency: Report of two cases. J. Urology, *113*: 484–486, 1985.

27. Mirvish, S. S. and Ramm, M. D. Demonstration of *in vivo* formation of the nitrosamine N-nitroso-N-methylaniline from amyl nitrite. Cancer Lett., *36*: 126–129, 1987.

28. Haverkos, H. W., Pinsky, P. F., Drotman, D. P., and Bregman, D. J. Disease manifestation among homosexual men with acquired immunodeficiency syndrome: A pos-

sible role of nitrites in Kaposi's sarcoma. Sex. Trans. Dis., *12*: 203–208, 1985.

29. Sugimura, T. Studies on environmental chemical carcinogenesis in Japan. Science, *233*: 312–318, 1986.

30. Ito, Y., Tokuda, H., Ohigashi, H., and Koshimizu, K. *In;* H. Fujiki, E. Hecker, R. E. Moore, T. Sugimura, and I. B. Weinstein, (eds.), Cellular Interactions by Environmental Tumor Promoters, pp. 125–127, Japan Sci. Soc. Press, Tokyo, 1984.

UNUSUAL OCCURRENCES AS CLUES TO CANCER ETIOLOGY, R. W. MILLER ET AL. (EDS.),
JAPAN SCI. SOC. PRESS, TOKYO/TAYLOR & FRANCIS, LTD., PP. 181–186, 1988

HTLV-I-associated Myelopathy: An Overview

Akihiro IGATA

Kagoshima University, Kagoshima 890, Japan

Abstract: From our past clinical observations, we have identified a cluster of cases with distinct neurological manifestations and, together with our viral studies, it has been proven that in fact these cases belong to a new clinical entity. The association of this slowly progressive spastic paraparesis with human T-cell lymphotropic virus type I (HTLV-I) enabled us to designate this clinical entity as HTLV-I-associated myelopathy or HAM. Later studies showed that 1) the geographical distribution of HAM follows that of adult T-cell leukemia (ATL) and 2) viruses detected in both disorders were identical by DNA blotting assay, but HAM and ATL are definitely expressed clinically as distinct from the other. In this regard, human leukocyte antigen (HLA) studies and the pattern of immune responsiveness seem to show a clear segregation of one from the other. As many initially studied cases have responded favorably to cor-ticosteroids and had frequent perivascular cuffing in the spinal cord of a necropsied case, it is likely that, in part, immune events play a role in the pathogenesis. Our efforts are now directed to determining whether a) HAM is purely an autoimmune process, or b) a slow virus infection with a long incubation period may be the culprit.

History of the Discovery of a New Clinical Entity: HAM

By virtue of clinical observation, it struck the author's attention 15 years ago that our cases with spinal spastic paraparesis not only had a high incidence, but also they tended to cluster with characteristic clinical features (*1*). While it was prema-ture at that time to draw conclusions, our survey proved such an occurrence back in 1975 (*2*). The goal in the search for an etiology for this clinical syndrome was realized just 3 years ago, when we noted lymphocytes with lobulated nuclei which had similar appearances to leukemic cells in adult T-cell leukemia (ATL) (ATL-like cells) in blood and cerebrospinal fluid (CSF). Hence, we concentrated our efforts in trying to prove whether or not these cases had ATL. The results indicated that they differed from ATL both clinically and hematologically, enabling us to conclude that they were, after all, carriers of human T-cell lymphotropic virus type I (HTLV-I).

We also observed that the antibody titers to HTLV-I were positive both in the serum and CSF. Further, these cases showed the presence of immunoglobulin G (IgG) which reacted with the p24 and p32 bands of HTLV-I evident by Western blot analysis. Our computations using Tourtellotte's method (3) indicated that the blood-brain-barrier was intact and that there were elevated intrathecal IgG synthesis rates (4). Through the analysis of 287 stored CSF samples of various neurological disorders in our laboratory, 12 were confirmed positive for HTLV-I antibody, and 6 with high titers were eventually found to have the characteristic clinical features of HAM. Notably, many of these cases having the same clinical features showed favorable responses to corticosteroids. Summing up all our original data, we reached the conclusion that these cases presenting with characteristic clinical features are associated with HTLV-I. Henceforth, we designated them as a new clinical entity, nosologically termed HTLV-I associated myelopathy (HAM).

Then we found a report (5) stating that in the clinical syndrome, tropical spastic paraparesis (TSP), later thought to have similar clinical features as HAM, has been, in part, associated with elevated antibodies to HTLV-I. This prompted us to express our firm belief that HAM is clinically identical with TSP (6). However, TSP cannot be fully applied to our cases because, for one, Japan is not tropical and some cases of TSP are actually seronegative for the antibody. We believe that HAM is essentially the same as HTLV-I-associated TSP (7) and can be used as a nosological term which includes both tropical and non-tropical myelopathies associated with HTLV-I.

Clinical Features

Cases with HAM give a history of a slow progressive course. The initial complaints are urinary and gait disturbances. Rarely are radicular pains observed. It is more frequent in females with an approximate ratio of 1M: 2F (1, 4, 6, 8). On examination (Table 1), a spastic gait is usually seen which is manifested neurologically by prominent pyramidal tract signs. Some may complain of mild sensory disturbance in the distal extremities but examination will reveal mostly a distal vibratory sense disturbance, and only few will show pain-temperature sense impairment, and less

TABLE 1.   Summary of Neurological Findings in HAM Patients

Neurological findings	Percentage (%)
Pyramidal tract signs	
Spasticity	85.1
Hyperreflexia UE	69.3
LE	97.8
Urinary disturbance	93.8
Muscle weakness UE	34.2
LE	88.2
Sensory disturbances	56.2
Finger tremors	27.2
Transient cranial nerve deficits	11.6
Hyporeflexia of LE	9.7

UE, upper extremities, bilaterally; LE, lower extremities, bilaterally.

often indistinct sensory levels. Some patients will complain of muscle weakness which is predominantly in the lower extremities and distal in distribution. Less than 10% of cases will have decreased to absent ankle jerks. Jaw jerks are not usually increased. Bladder testing will reveal abnormalities in the majority of cases (9). A few will show transient focal cranial nerve deficits, most of which are referred to as eye movement disturbance (1, 10). As yet, there are no cases to suggest impairment of cerebral functions and/or higher cortical functions. A proportion will have pulmonary signs mostly on account of diffuse lung infiltrates as seen radiologically.

Clinical Classification

Previous studies indicated that patients with HAM can be clinically segregated into two groups with reference to the history of blood transfusion (11). About 39% of HAM patients had previous history of blood transfusion, and analysis of these cases revealed that it took approximately 3 years from transfusion to onset of symptoms (Fig. 1) (10). Among those without any history of previous transfusion, cases with HAM had a younger age of onset. All of the tested mothers of patients with

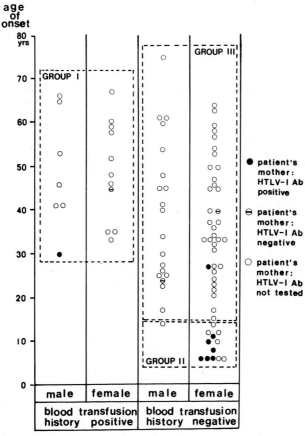

FIG. 1.   Ages of onset of 85 HAM cases. Group I, blood transfusion history; group II, no blood transfusion (age of onset below 15); group III, no blood transfusion (age of onset 15 or older).

onset under 15 years revealed positive antibody titers to HTLV-I, supporting the existence of a subgroup we called mother-to-child transmission cases (*12*). The remaining cases from the group with no history of transfusion are probably a mixture of vertical and other horizontal modes (*e.g.*, *via* sexual contact). Symptom progression appears slower in HAM patients with no history of blood transfusion, indicating that blood transfusion may be an important factor in the incubation period of the virus.

Laboratory Tests

Important blood tests reveal that there is elevation of OKT4/OKT8, OKT10, and OKIal positive cells and decreased Leu7 and activity of NK cells (*1*). The elevated OKT10 positive cells may indicate increased numbers of activated T-cell lymphocytes. Increased OKT4/OKT8 may be derived from increased OKT4 positive cells and/or decreased OKT8 positive cells. These data would mean increased inducer/helper T-cell and/or decreased suppressor cytotoxic T-cell in cases with HAM. The CSF revealed mild pleocytosis in many, with increased protein and β_2-microglobulin. Myelin basic protein was not present in all of 15 cases tested. In some cases, oligoclonal bands in CSF were identified.

Electrophysiologic Tests

Except for a few derangements in proximal nerve conduction studies (F-responses) of some HAM patients, no abnormalities were shown by other motor and sensory conduction tests of peripheral nerves (*13*). Routine electromyography of sampled muscles revealed polyphasic potentials, and some had giant spikes especially in the distally located muscles. Multimodal evoked potential (EP) studies revealed abnormalities predominantly in the somatosensory function, and only a few had changes in visual EPs and brainstem auditory EPs. Since somatosensory EPs showed most of the involvement to be in the tested tibial nerves as against that of the tested median nerves, and that abnormalities were in central conduction, it appears that the main pathologic correlates in HAM are located in the spinal cord, most likely below the cervical cord (*13*). The pattern of changes in the F-responses of electromyography suggest involvement of the anterior horn cells or the anterior roots, most probably the intraspinal segments of the motor root. However, involvement of areas above the spinal cord may exist in a few cases with HAM, as evidenced by changes in brainstem auditory EPs and visual EPs and electrooculography (*10*).

Pathology

Neuropathologic studies of one case showed atrophy of the spinal cord, especially at the thoracic level (*14*). In the white and grey matter, there was marked proliferation of capillaries and perivascular cuffing with lymphocytes. Loss of myelin and axons were notable in the anterolateral columns, although the dorsal columns were not completely spared. Rarely were the anterior horn cells involved (mainly central chromatolysis). Perivascular cuffing with lymphocytes was seen in the medulla, pons, cerebellum, and cerebral white matter. These neuropathologic findings confirm results of our electrophysiologic studies.

HLA Studies

HTLV-I is a retrovirus known to cause ATL. Recent findings indicate that the genomic composition of the viruses isolated from patients with HAM appears to be identical to that of viruses isolated from patients with ATL using restriction enzyme analysis (15). The apparent similarity in this respect, with obvious disparity clinically, makes one look on the circumstances around the host. By HLA studies, the noted "HAM-associated haplotypes" were not found in cases with ATL (16). Either AllBw54Cw1DR4DQw3, A24Bw54Cw1DR4DQ-, A24B7Cw7DR1DQw1, or A24Bw-52Cw-DR2DQw1 and related haplotypes were found in 70% of cases with HAM. The in vitro cultures of peripheral blood lymphocytes with HTLV-I virion antigens revealed that the proliferative response with HAM peripheral blood lymphocytes was remarkably higher than that with ATL in patients with ATL. The high immune response to HTLV-I can thus be an important factor in the development of HAM, although we have no direct evidence to prove this assumption at the moment.

Conclusion

As we move forward toward understanding of HAM, especially of the extent to which the infectious agent, HTLV-I, participates, the apparent association with TSP has become clarified. HTLV-I-associated TSP (7) has now been described in several areas in the tropics and the latest studies indicate that HAM and HTLV-I-associated TSP may be one and the same disorder (17). Whether these HTLV-I-associated myelopathies can only be understood on the basis of an autoimmune process or of a slow viral infection with a long incubation period remains to be determined, and should be the direction of investigations.

ACKNOWLEDGMENTS

The author is grateful for the kind assistance of Professor Mitsuhiro Osame, Dr. Raymond L. Rosales, and the Staff of the Third Department of Internal Medicine, Kagoshima University, whose efforts made the research and this overview possible.

REFERENCES

1. Osame, M., Igata, A., Matsumoto, M., Usuku, K., Kitajima, I., and Takahashi, K. On the discovery of a new clinical entity: human T-cell lymphotropic virus type I-associated myelopathy (HAM). Adv. Neurol. Sci., 31 (5): 727–745, 1987.
2. Osame, M., Arima, H., Norimatsu, K., Kawahira, M., Okatsu, Y., Nagamatsu, K., and Igata, A. Epidemiostatistical studies of muscular atrophy in Southern Kyushu (Kagoshima and Okinawa prefectures). Jpn. J. Med., 14: 230–231, 1975.
3. Tourtellotte, W. W., Staugaitis, S. M., Walsh, M. J., Shapshak, P., Baumhefner, R. W., Potvin, A. R., and Syndulko, K. The basis of intra-blood-brain-barrier IgG synthesis. Ann. Neurol., 17: 21–27, 1985.

4. Osame, M., Matsumoto, M., Usuku, K., Izumo, S., Ijichi, N., Amitani, H., Tara, M., and Igata, A. Chronic progressive myelopathy associated with elevated antibodies to HTLV-I and adult T-cell leukemia-like cells. Ann. Neurol., *21*: 117–122, 1987.

5. Gessain, A., Francis, H., Sonan, T., Giordano, C., Akani, F., Piquemal, M., Claudie, C., Malone, G., Essex, M., and de-Thé, G. HTLV-I and tropical spastic paraparesis in Africa. Lancet, *ii*: 698, 1986.

6. Osame, M., Usuku, K., Izumo, S., Ijichi, N., Amitani, H., Igata, A., Matsumoto, M., and Tara, M. HTLV-I associated myelopathy, a new clinical entity. Lancet, *i*: 1031–1032, 1986.

7. Vernant, J. C., Maurs, L., Gessain, A., Barin, F., Gout, O., Delaporte, J. M., Sanhadji, K., Buisson, G., and de-Thé, G. Endemic tropical spastic paraparesis associated with human T-lymphotropic virus type I: a clinical and seroepidemiological study of 25 cases. Ann. Neurol., *21*: 124–130, 1987.

8. Osame, M., Igata, A., Matsumoto, M., Usuku, K., Izumo, S., and Kosaka, K. HTLV-I-associated myelopathy: a report of 85 cases. Ann. Neurol., *22*: 116, 1987.

9. Hiyoshi, T., Osame, M., Moritoyo, T., Takahashi, K., Nakamura, K., Kubota, R., Yamano, T., Rosales, R., Igata, A., Kawahira, K., Tanaka, N., and Ohi, Y. Cystometric analysis of the urinary function of HTLV-I-associated myelopathy: a preliminary report. Acta Med. Univ. Kagoshima, *29*: 19–27, 1987.

10. Arimura, Y., Arimura, K., Osame, M., and Igata, A. Neuro-ophthalmological abnormalities in HTLV-I associated myelopathy. Neuro-opthalmology, *7* (4): 243–248, 1987.

11. Osame, M., Izumo, S., Igata, A., Matsumoto, M., Matsumoto, T., Sonoda, S., Tara, M., and Sibata, Y. Blood transfusion and HTLV-I associated myelopathy. Lancet, *ii*: 104–105, 1986.

12. Osame, M., Igata, A., Usuku, K., Rosales, R., and Matsumoto, M. Mother-to-child transmission in HTLV-I associated myelopathy. Lancet, *ii*: 106, 1986.

13. Arimura, K., Rosales, R., Osame, M., and Igata, A. Clinical electrophysiologic studies of HTLV-I associated myelopathy. Arch. Neurol., *44*: 609–612, 1987.

14. Akizuki, S., Nakazato, Y., Higuchi, Y., and Tanabe, K. Necropsy findings in HTLV-I associated myelopathy. Lancet, *i*: 156–157, 1987.

15. Yoshida, M., Osame, M., Usuku, K., Matsumoto, M., and Igata, A. Viruses detected in HTLV-I associated myelopathy and adult T-cell leukemia are identical on DNA blotting. Lancet, *i*: 1085–1086, 1987.

16. Usuku, K., Sonoda, S., Osame, M., Yashiki, S., Takahashi, K., Matsumoto, M., Sawada, T., Tsuji, K., Tara, M., and Igata, A. HLA haplotype-linked high immune responsiveness against HTLV-I in HTLV-I-associated myelopathy—comparison with adult T-cell leukemia/lymphoma. Ann. Neurol., *23*: 143–150, 1988.

17. Roman, G. S. Retrovirus-associated myelopathies. Arch. Neurol., *44*: 659–663, 1987.

UNUSUAL OCCURRENCES AS CLUES TO CANCER ETIOLOGY, R. W. MILLER ET AL. (EDS.),
JAPAN SCI. SOC. PRESS, TOKYO/TAYLOR & FRANCIS, LTD., PP. 187–195, 1988

Cutaneous Ki-1 Lymphoma: Pathology, Immunology and Clinical Characteristics

Marshall E. Kadin

Department of Pathology and Charles A. Dana Research Institute, Beth Israel Hospital and Harvard Medical School, Boston, Massachusetts 02115, U.S.A.

Abstract: This paper describes a newly recognized clinicopathologic syndrome of regressing cutaneous nodules, peripheral lymphadenopathy and fever occurring mainly in children and adolescents. Skin lesions show pseudoepitheliomatous hyperplasia, absence of epidermotropism and pleomorphic large lymphoma cells infiltrating the dermis and subcutaneous fat. Lymph nodes have a distinctive appearance with lymphoma cells in sinuses and paracortex. Despite their usual histiocyte-like appearance, the lymphoma cells in most cases have an aberrant T-cell phenotype, expressing several activation antigens including Hodgkin's disease associated antigen Ki-1 (CD30). Clonal rearrangements of the beta chain genes for the T-cell antigen receptor (TCR) were found and revealed a T-cell origin in one case lacking T-cell surface antigens. Identical rearrangements of the TCR genes indicated a monoclonal origin for separate lesions on the arm and leg of another patient. Treatment results in the first group of patients indicate that radiation treatment of an affected area is associated with frequent relapse at other sites, but multiagent chemotherapy (COMP or D-COMP) produces durable remissions in nearly all patients. Bone marrow transplantation was effective salvage therapy for treatment failures. Further studies are underway to investigate the mechanism(s) of tumor regression, the epidemiology, and etiology of Ki-1+ lymphomas which appear to be relatively more frequent in Oriental and Black patients, and in which the first lesion may resemble an insect bite.

In 1985, Stein and co-workers introduced the concept that many cases previously diagnosed as malignant histiocytosis were actually tumors of activated lymphoid cells (*1*). Their conclusion was based on the observation that activated lymphoid cells express a unique antigen Ki-1 (CD30) which permits their identification in tissue sections (*2*). These Ki-1+ lymphomas were all of pleomorphic large cell type. They infiltrated lymph nodes in a distinctive pattern of sinus and paracortical involvement characteristic of malignant histiocytosis (*3*).

A few years ago we saw three patients whose skin lesions had the same unusual immunological phenotype. This abnormality led us in 1986 to recognize a syndrome of frequently regressing skin lesions and peripheral lymphadenopathy among children and adolescents with Ki-1+ large cell lymphoma (4). These cases often presented a diagnostic dilemma because of their unusual clinical manifestations and histology which were unfamiliar to clinicians and pathologists. Earlier recognition of this clinical entity and treatment with multiagent chemotherapy has led to improved survival and freedom from relapse (5). However many questions remain to be answered regarding the etiology, mechanism of regression of skin lesions, and epidemiology in which a disproportionately large number of Oriental and Black patients are represented among about 25 North American patients. Clearly more information is needed in studies from other regions of the world including Japan.

Clinical Features

As summarized in Table 1, patients with cutaneous Ki-1 lymphoma frequently present with the abrupt onset of one or several skin and/or subcutaneous nodules. A typical patient is shown in Fig. 1. Several patients have described the onset of their lesions in association with outdoor activities such as camping trips, and have attributed the cause of the lesions to possible insect bites. This may be a misleading impression resulting from the young age of most patients who are commonly involved in outdoor activities. Some older patients have reported a history of several or numerous small lesions which have regressed spontaneously. In many cases regression of the early lesion(s) has led to uncertainty about a diagnosis of malignancy, and thereby appropriate unwillingness of clinicians to treat the lesions with cytotoxic therapy. In most cases, the lesions will recur in the original and/or other sites, and

TABLE 1. Cutaneous Ki-1 Lymphoma—Clinical Features

1. Abrupt onset with skin (subcutaneous) nodules, peripheral lymphadenopathy, fever
2. Regressing character of skin lesions
3. Possibly related to insect bite
4. Peak incidence in childhood and adolescence (second decade)

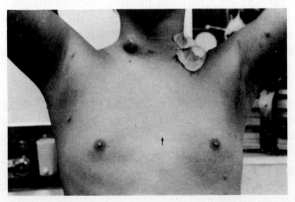

FIG. 1. 11 year old boy with cutaneous nodules, largest on right side on neck. Bandaged biopsy site on left side of neck showed Ki-1+ large cell lymphoma. A lesion which regressed spontaneously is revealed by a depigmented area on the chest (arrow).

eventually will be associated with peripheral lymphadenopathy. At this time the diagnosis of malignant lymphoma can be established.

Histology

Biopsy of the skin and/or lymph nodes will often result in a final diagnosis of lymphoma. However preceding this final diagnosis are usually numerous consultations with other pathologists, including hematopathologists, because of current unfamiliarity with the histology of Ki-1 lymphoma. Most common initial diagnoses, other than malignant non-Hodgkin's lymphoma, are malignant histiocytosis; regressing atypical histiocytosis, a reasonable diagnosis made in the context of the clinically regressing skin lesions; inflammation, when malignant cells are infrequent or not very atypical in appearance; metastatic carcinoma when lymph node sinus infiltration is prominent; or Hodgkin's disease when Reed-Sternberg-like cells are present.

Table 2 describes the most typical histologic features of cutaneous Ki-1 lymphoma which permit the correct diagnosis to be made. The appearance of pseudoepitheliomatous epidermal hyperplasia and atypical histiocytes, as shown in Figs. 2 and 3, were described as the characteristic features of regressing atypical histiocytosis (6). We believe that most if not all cases of regressing atypical histiocytosis represent Ki-1 lymphomas.

The skin lesions may initially be confined to the deep dermis and subcutaneous fat (non-epidermotropic). However with enlargement and expansion, the overlying epidermis often becomes ulcerated. A cuff of small reactive lymphocytes is sometimes found at the periphery, raising the possibility of a cellular immune response to the tumor. This may be a contributing factor to the spontaneous regression of some lesions.

The tumor cells vary somewhat in appearance from case to case, but are usually the same in different lesions from an individual patient. The term pleomorphic refers to the non-uniform size and shape of nuclei in the tumor cells. Tumor cells can have kidney-shaped nuclei with abundant cytoplasm resulting in a histiocyte-like appearance. In other cases, the nuclei are oval with prominent nucleoli resembling immunoblasts. Nuclear convolutions with intra-nuclear cytoplasmic inclusions are an infrequent but characteristic feature. Multinucleated cells can have a peripheral wreath-like arrangement, resembling histiocytes in granulomatous inflammation, or two to several nuclei with inclusion-like nuclei resembling Reed-Sternberg cells of Hodgkin's disease.

In lymph nodes, there is usual sparing of germinal centers of primary follicles. The node is often focally involved by groups of tumor cells resulting in an appearance similar to metastatic carcinoma. Lymph node sinus infiltration by tumor cells is the

TABLE 2.   Cutaneous Ki-1 Lymphoma—Histology

1. Skin lesions with pseudoepitheliomatous hyperplasia and atypical "histiocytes"
2. Pleomorphic tumor cells including immunoblasts, multinucleated cells and Reed-Sternberg-like cells
3. Subcutaneous location, non-epidermotropic
4. Cuff of reactive lymphocytes
5. Lymph node sinus and paracortical infiltration

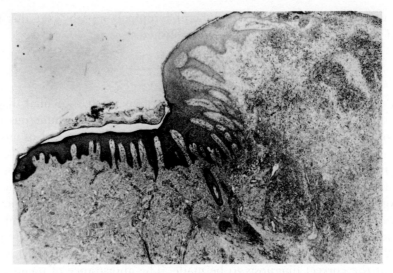

FIG. 2. Cutaneous lesion of Ki-1+ lymphoma showing pseudoepitheliomatous epidermal hyperplasia and ulcerated surface overlying sheets of tumor cells.

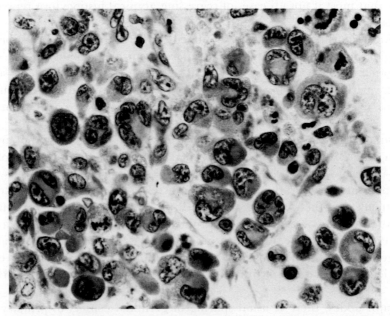

FIG. 3. Markedly pleomorphic tumor cells in skin lesion of Ki-1+ large cell lymphoma. Tumor cells have abundant cytoplasm and kidney-shaped, sometimes multiple, nuclei giving the appearance of atypical "histiocytes".

main feature leading to the impression of malignant histiocytosis. This impression may be supported by tumor cell erythrophagocytosis evident in tissue sections or in imprint preparations.

Immunology

Table 3 lists the usual immunological features of tumor cells in Ki-1 lymphoma. The most consistent feature is tumor cell expression of several activation antigens including Ki-1 (CD30), a Hodgkin's disease associated antigen, Tac (CD25) corresponding to the receptor for Interleukin-2 or T-cell growth factor, Ia (DR) class II-histocompatibility antigens, and T9, the receptor for transferrin, a lymphocyte growth factor.

The tumor cells in Ki-1 non-Hodgkin's lymphoma can be distinguished from Hodgkin/Reed-Sternberg cells by the absence of Leu-M1 (CD15), an antigen expressed by Reed-Sternberg cells in the most common types of Hodgkin's disease. In addition the tumor cells of Ki-1 lymphoma express leukocyte common antigen (CD45), which is usually absent or expressed only weakly by Reed-Sternberg cells.

Despite the histiocyte-like appearance of tumor cells in many cases, the cells of Ki-1 lymphoma were found to lack entirely or show only focal staining for nonspecific esterase, a marker of histiocytes. In addition they lacked several surface antigens of the histiocyte lineage. Their true T-cell derivation was shown in most cases by the expression of T-cell specific antigens, most commonly T4 (CD4) or T11 (CD5). In all cases, the tumor cells showed aberrant expression of T-cell antigens consistent with a malignant phenotype (7).

Unexpectedly the tumor cells in some cases marked for epithelial membrane antigen (EMA), which could contribute toward confusion of Ki-1 lymphoma with metastatic carcinoma. In two cases myeloid surface antigens were also detected. This is interesting because myeloid antigens have been found on Reed-Sternberg cells (8). Finally numerous vimentin intermediate filaments, which are prominent in some peripheral T-cell lymphomas (9), were also present in some Ki-1 lymphoma cells.

Genetics

In the first and therefore most puzzling case of Ki-1 lymphoma studied, we found no surface markers of T or B cells. It was at first surprising that we found clonal rearrangement of the T-cell antigen receptor beta chain genes in this case (4). The same has been true of five Ki-1 lymphomas studied subsequently. In one of these cases, an identical T-beta gene rearrangement pattern was found in each of two separate lesions, one from the leg and the other from the arm, of a patient with Ki-1 lymphoma, indicating that both lesions were derived from the same T-cell clone (Fig. 4). However, no circulating T-cell clone could be detected in the peripheral blood of this pa-

TABLE 3.   Cutaneous Ki-1 Lymphoma—Immunology

1. Tumor cells express lymphoid activation antigens Ki-1 (CD30), Tac (CD25), Ia (DR), T9 (transferrin receptor)
2. Absence of Leu M1 (CD15) and expression of LCA (CD45) distinguishes tumor cells from Hodgkin/Reed-Sternberg cells.
3. Absence of non-specific esterase, histiocyte-macrophage surface markers
4. Expression of T-cell antigens in 75 percent of cases
5. Vimentin, epithelial membrane antigen, myeloid surface antigens

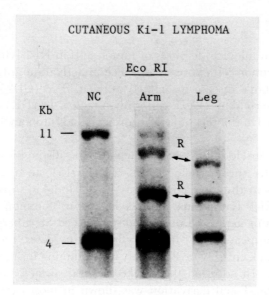

FIG. 4.   Identical T-cell antigen receptor beta chain gene rearrangements (R) indicate mono-clonal origin for arm and leg skin nodules of patient with Ki-1+ lymphoma.

TABLE 4.   Cutaneous Ki-1 Lymphoma—Genetics

1.	Clonal rearrangement of T-cell antigen receptor beta chain genes
2.	Same rearrangement present in anatomically separate lesions
3.	Chromosomal abnormalities under investigation

tient. There are two likely explanations for the inability to detect a circulating clone of T-cells in this case. First the separate skin lesions were most likely seeded at an earlier time when a circulating clone might have been found. Second, the sensitivity of the method to detect clonal T-cells requires at least 1 to 5 percent of cells from the same clone to be present, and the actual frequency of clonal T-cells in the blood could be much lower than that.

The next important step is to perform cytogenetics on fresh Ki-1 lymphoma cells to learn whether specific chromosome abnormalities may be associated with the pathogenesis of this disease. Since beta chain gene rearrangements are frequently found, deletions, rearrangements and/or translocations affecting chromosome 7, the site of the beta chain genes are likely to be encountered (10).

Treatment

Analysis of the results of treatment for the first 6 cutaneous Ki-1 lymphoma patients suggest that radiation alone to involved sites is not adequate for control of this disease. Several patients relapsed at sites outside the radiation field. Delay of treatment, due to difficulty of diagnosis, may also contribute to these poor treatment results. In contrast to the poor results recorded for radiation alone, patients who received prompt multiagent chemotherapy with cyclophosphamide, vincristine, methotrexate and prednisone (COMP) have experienced complete and durable remissions.

TABLE 5. Cutaneous Ki-1 Lymphoma—Treatment

1. Often delayed due to difficulty of diagnosis
2. Local radiation inadequate
3. Multiagent chemotherapy (COMP or D-COMP) effective
4. Bone marrow transplantation effective as salvage therapy

The efficacy of the COMP regimen for treatment of Ki-1+ large cell lymphoma seems to be supported by preliminary analysis of results for children enrolled in protocols for non-lymphoblastic lymphoma in the Children's Cancer Study Group in the United States. Preliminary results show each of 14 patients with Ki-1+ large cell lymphoma to be free of disease with a median survival of 19 months (5). A good response to chemotherapy for children with primary Ki-1+ large cell lymphoma has also been found by German investigators (11). Interestingly two of our first 6 patients who relapsed after extensive therapy, have experienced durable remissions following allogeneic bone marrow transplantation therapy. It is suggested that autologous bone marrow transplantation may be feasible in future refractory cases, since bone marrow involvement appears to be rare in primary Ki-1 lymphoma.

Future Directions

Mechanism of tumor regression: It would seem to be most important to investigate the mechanism(s) of spontaneous tumor regression in Ki-1 lymphomas. The most likely alternatives are: (1) host immune response to the tumor and (2) growth factor regulation of tumor cells. Host infiltrates of T-helper cells were found to correlate with treatment response in B-cell lymphoma patients treated with anti-idiotype antibodies (12). Therefore, it is interesting to note the appearance of small lymphocytes at the periphery of tumor nodules in some cases of Ki-1 lymphoma. Phenotyping of these reactive cells is in progress.

Recently we have demonstrated that growth factors may be important in regulating the *in vitro* proliferation of Ki-1+ lymphomas. Ki-1 positive tumor cells which express receptors for T-cell growth factor or IL-2 remain partially dependent on IL-2. Their growth can be inhibited by suppression of IL-2 receptors which can be mediated by transforming growth factor-beta (13). In contrast Ki-1+ tumor cells which lack IL-2 receptors grew autonomously of IL-2 and were unaffected by exogenous transforming growth factor-beta (14).

Etiology: It is attractive to speculate that a retrovirus in the HTLV family could play a role in the pathogenesis of this tumor of activated T-cells. The early

TABLE 6. Cutaneous Ki-1 Lymphoma—Future Directions

1. Investigate mechanism of tumor regression
     role of growth factors and receptors
2. Investigate etiologic agents
     similarity to insect (mosquito) bite (vector?)
     epidemiological studies
     genetic (racial) background
     viral antibodies

age of onset for most patients is however dissimilar from the course of adult T-cell leukemia in which HTLV-I is thought to play a causative role (*15, 16*).

The theory of an infectious agent is compatible with the acute inflammatory nature of some early Ki-1 lymphoma lesions. An insect could provide the vector for transmission of this agent. It is interesting that hypersensitivity to mosquito bites has been postulated to be the cause of seven fatal cases of malignant histiocytosis (*17*). The affected patients were Japanese who were 3 to 19 years of age at the onset of their disease. Four patients had subcutaneous nodules and swelling of lymph nodes initially, or in the final stages of their disease. The Japanese cases seem to differ from American cases in their rapid downhill course to death after the first symptoms of malignancy appeared. Nevertheless a comparison between American and Japanese cases of "malignant histiocytosis" should be made to learn more about the etiology and epidemiology of both diseases.

Future studies of cutaneous Ki-1+ lymphomas could provide important clues to understand the mechanism of spontaneous regression sometimes observed in human lymphomas (*18–21*). This could lead to a rationale for treatment with non-cytotoxic biological response modifiers. Hodgkin's disease might be among the lymphomas affected because of its morphologic and immunologic similarities to Ki-1+ lymphoma.

ACKNOWLEDGMENT

This work was supported by Grant C254A from the American Cancer Society.

REFERENCES

1. Stein, H., Mason, D. Y., Gerdes, J., O'Connor, N., Wainscoat, J., Pallesen, G., Gatter, K., Falini, B., Delsol, G., Lemke, H., Schwarting, R., and Lennert, K. The expression of the Hodgkin's disease associated antigen Ki-1 in reactive and neoplastic tissue. Evidence that Reed-Sternberg cells and histiocytic malignancies are derived from activated lymphoid cells. Blood, *66*: 848–858, 1985.
2. Schwab, V., Stein, H., Gerdes, J., Lemke, H., Kirchner, H., Schaadt, M., and Diehl, V. Production of a monoclonal antibody specific for Hodgkin and Sternberg-Reed cells of Hodgkin's disease and a subset on normal lymphoid cells. Nature, *299*: 65–67, 1982.
3. Byrne, G. E. and Rappaport, H. Malignant histiocytosis. Gann Monogr. Cancer Res., *15*: 145–162, 1973.
4. Kadin, M. E., Sako, D., Berliner, N., Franklin, W., Woda, B., Borowitz, M., Ireland, K., Schweid, A., Herzog, P., Lange, B., and Dorfman, R. F. Childhood Ki-1 lymphoma presenting with skin lesions and peripheral lymphadenopathy. Blood, *68*: 1042–1049, 1986.
5. Kadin, M. E., Sposto, R., Agnarsson, B. A., Kjeldsberg, C. A., Meadows, A., Siegel, S., Chilcote, R., and Hammond, D. Ki-1 antigen expression in childhood non-Hodgkin's lymphoma. Blood, 1988, in press.
6. Flynn, K. J., Dehner, L. P., Gajl-Peczalska, K. J., Dahl, M. V., Ramsay, N., and Wang, N. Regressing atypical histiocytosis: A cutaneous proliferation of atypical neoplastic histiocytes with unexpectedly indolent biologic behavior. Cancer, *49*: 959–970, 1982.
7. Picker, L. J., Weiss, L. M., Medeiros, L. J., Wood, G. S., and Warnke, R. A. Immunophenotypic criteria for the diagnosis of non-Hodgkin's lymphoma. Am. J. Pathol.,

128: 181–201, 1987.

8. Stein, H., Uchanska-Ziegler, B., Gerdes, J., Ziegler, A., and Wernet, P. Hodgkin and Sternberg-Reed cells contain antigens specific to late cells of granulopoiesis. Int. J. Cancer, *29*: 283–290, 1982.

9. Bolen, J. B. and Kadin, M. E. Peripheral T-cell lymphoma with Reed-Sternberg-like cells. Ultrastruct. Pathol., *9*: 225–231, 1985.

10. Caccia, N., Kronenberg, M., Saxe, D., Haars, R., Bruns, G.A.P., Goverman, J., Malissen, M., Hunt, W., Yoshikai, Y., Simon, M., Hood, L., and Mak, T. W. The T cell receptor beta chain genes are located on chromosome 6 in mice and chromosome 7 in humans. Cell, *37*: 1091–1099, 1984.

11. Engelhard and others. Proceedings of International Symposium on Hodgkin's Disease, Cologne, West Germany, Oct. 2–3, 1987.

12. Garcia, C. F., Lowder, J., Meeker, T. C., Bindl, J., Levy, R., and Warnke, R. A. Differences in "host infiltrates" among lymphoma patients treated with anti-idiotype antibodies: Correlation with treatment response. J. Immunol., *135*: 4252–4260, 1985.

13. Kehrl, J. F., Wakefield, L. M., Roberts, A. M., Jakowlew, M., Alvarez-Mon, M., Derynck, R., Sporn, M. R., and Fauci, A. S. Production of transforming growth factor beta by human T lymphocytes and its potential role in the regulation of T cell growth. J. Exp. Med., *163*: 1037–1050, 1986.

14. Newcom, S. R. and Kadin, M. E. Production of transforming growth factor beta activity by Ki-1 positive lymphoma cells and analysis of its role in the regulation of Ki-1 positive lymphoma growth, Blood, *70* (Suppl.): 265a.

15. Hinuma, Y., Kodama, H., Chosa, T., and others. Antibodies to adult T-cell leukemia virus-associated antigen (ATLA) in sera from patients and controls in Japan: A nationwide epidemiologic survey. Int. J. Cancer, *29*: 631–635, 1982.

16. Gallo, R. C. and Wang-Staal, F. Retroviruses as etiologic agents in some animal and human leukemias and lymphomas and as tools in elucidating the molecular mechanisms of leukemogenesis. Blood, *60*: 545–547, 1982.

17. Hidano, A., Kawakani, M., and Yago, A. Hypersensitivity to mosquito bite and malignant histiocytosis. Jpn. J. Exp. Med., *52*: 303–308, 1982.

18. Krikorian, J. G., Portlock, C. S., Cooney, P., and Rosenberg, S. A. Spontaneous regression of non-Hodgkin's lymphoma: a report of nine cases. Cancer, *46*: 2093–2099, 1980.

19. Strauchen, J. A., Moran, C., Goldsmith, M., and Greenberg, M. Spontaneous regression of gastric lymphoma. Cancer, *60*: 1872–1875, 1987.

20. Ziegler, J. L. Spontaneous remission in Burkitt's lymphoma. NCI Monogr., *44*: 61–65, 1976.

21. Grem, J. L., Hafez, G. R., Brandenburg, J. H., and Carbone, P. P. Spontaneous remission in diffuse large cell lymphoma. Cancer, *57*: 2042–2044, 1986.

Carcinoma of the Urinary Bladder Associated with Schistosomiasis in Egypt: The Possible Causal Relationship

Hassan Nabil TAWFIK

Department of Pathology, National Cancer Institute, Cairo University, Egypt

Abstract: Carcinoma of the urinary bladder is the most common malignancy in Egyptians. At the National Cancer Institute in Cairo, it accounts for 27.6% of all cancers—38.5% of cancers in the male and 11.3% in the female. This very high frequency is attributed to underlying schistosomiasis. The infection can lead to malignancy through local tissue damage, mechanical irritation, bilharzial toxins or through secondary bacterial infection. Bacterial products include nitrate reductase capable of synthesizing nitrosoamines and β glucuronidase enzymes, active at pH 7. Through liver involvement and dysfunction, tryptophan metabolism is disturbed, with the excretion of carcinogenic metabolites. Vitamin A deficiency is responsible for the squamous metaplasia and the high frequency of squamous cell carcinoma observed in the bladder.

The characteristic clinico-pathological features of cancer of the urinary bladder are outlined, mainly the occurrence at a young age, the male predominance, especially farmers, and the high association with schistosomiasis. The tumors are often first seen in an advanced stage, arising from the posterior bladder wall and vault. The trigone is only affected in 8.5% of the cases. Histologically, squamous cell carcinomas of low grade are the most frequent cell type. Lymph node involvement is low in spite of the advanced stage of the tumor. Therefore, the results of radical surgery are encouraging.

The results of a special study correlating the above parameters with the intensity of ova deposition are presented. Patients with heavy infection at a slightly earlier age but other tumor parameters the same are similar to those of egg-negative cases. This study indicates that other factors also play a role in the induction of tumors that are enhanced by the schistosomal infection. In Fayoum Province, schistosomiasis is decreasing while bladder cancer is increasing.

Urine cytology as a screening tool is effective in detecting early bladder cancer. Studies are now in progress to detect tumor associated antigens in sera and urine of patients.

The striking association between urinary schistosomiasis and bladder cancer in

Egypt was first noted by Goebel in 1905 (*1*). Ferguson in 1911 presented convincing evidence of the association (*2*).

Carcinoma of the urinary bladder is the commonest malignancy in Egyptians. It usually affects male farmers who suffer from chronic schistosomiasis. Bladder cancer develops insidiuously, being masked by preexisting cystitis; most sufferers, therefore, are discovered in a late stage (*3*).

Schistosomiasis resides in infected canals where the water current is weak and man is infected as he uses water for his daily needs or during irrigation of the fields. Thus, there is daily exposure, and the infection is severe and repeated. In most cases, the infection starts during childhood and reaches a peak at between 10 and 20 years of age (*4*).

Historical Review

Schistosomiasis probably existed in the Nile valley even before the existence of man himself. All medical papyri that were written about 1500 B.C. mentioned hematuria; it was referred to as "A-aa" disease. The information in these papyri had probably cumulated from the first dynasty many years earlier (3400 years B.C.). Hematuria or "A-aa" disease was cited in the Ebers papyrus 28 times, in the Berlin papyrus 12 times, in the Hearst papyrus 9 times, and in the London papyrus once. Thus it was mentioned 50 times reflecting the wide spread of the disease. The erect phallus was used as a symbol of the word (*5*).

In these old papyri not only was the symptomatology described but it was also stated that "A-aa" disease produced abdominal worms called "hrrw". Antimony sulphide (stibium) by mouth was mentioned among the several agents used in its treatment; however, it was stated that the disease was incurable. Such knowledge was probably obtained by the ancient Egyptians through the examination of viscera removed during embalmment. The kidneys were called "depti" (Edwin Smith papyrus) (*6*) while the ureters were described as two vessels secreting urine (Ebers papyrus). The bladder was called "sheptit". Schistosoma eggs were found in the kidneys of mummies of the 20th Dynasty (1200–1090 B.C.) (*7*).

Herodite and medieval Arabs described the high frequency of hematuria "that men of Egypt menstruate like women". During the Napoleonic expedition to Egypt several celebrated physicians commented on the severity and prevalence of Egyptian hematuria (*8*).

However, it was not until 1851 that Theodore Bilharze, the German Assistant Professor of Medicine in Cairo Medical School described the worm in the mesenteric veins (*9*). The worm was classified as schistosoma by Weinland 1858 (*10*).

Epidemiology of Schistosomiasis

The worms of *Schistosoma hematobium* are responsible for the involvement of the urogenital organs. The worms leave the liver before full maturity and migrate against the stream of blood in the portal tributaries to reach the vesico-prostatic plexus of veins. Here the female worms leave the males and pass into the smallest venules in the mucosa of the bladder, ureter, and other sites where they lay their eggs. A toxic substance secreted by the viable miracidium in the eggs helps their penetration of the mucosa and excites a cellular reaction in the tissues if eggs are entrapped.

In Africa, *S. hematobium* extends from central Africa where the Great Lakes are along the river Nile to the delta. It also extends west to the Gold Coast, Nigeria, and to south and east Africa. Several species are present in Iraq, Palestine, Saudi Arabia, Yemen, and India (*11*).

The disease varies in severity depending on the irrigation system used and exposure to infected water. Thus when canals are used for irrigation the disease is severe and infection is repeated (*e.g.*, Egypt and Iraq), while in areas depending on rainfall as in other parts of Africa and the Middle East the disease is less severe.

In Egypt *S. hematobium* infection is widespread in the Nile delta and valley. In 1980, the prevalence was 12.8–17.3% in the delta region, 27.1–33.6% in middle Egypt, and 17–37% in upper Egypt (*12*). This represents a considerable change from the figures of 1935 when 60% of the people in the delta, 80–90% in middle Egypt, and only 5% in upper Egypt were infected (*13*). Thus the disease is increasing in upper Egypt due to the broad introduction of perennial irrigation throughout the year. There are several campaign programs to combat the disease, but the persistence of infection reflects the various technical, medical, and social problems involved.

Schistosomiasis and Bladder Cancer

The main factors that suggest that carcinomas are caused either directly or indirectly by the parasite are:

1.   The high association between carcinomas and schistosomal cystitis.

2.   The high frequency of carcinoma of the urinary bladder in areas infested by schistosomiasis.

3.   The disease occurrence in farmers exposed to severe and repeated infestations. However, owing to internal migration bladder cancer is seen also in cities. The majority of Egyptians should actually be considered potentially infested unless otherwise proved. However, the severity of infestation does according to individual occupation. In a screening program conducted in Dakahilya province in the Delta region, bladder cancer was detected only in farmers.

4.   Bladder cancer in Egypt as a clinico-pathological entity quite different from that seen in the western world.

5.   Immunologic studies that suggest the presence of schistosomal antigens among specific tumor antigens.

In almost all Egyptian bladder cancer studies schistosoma eggs were found in a high percentage of cases. In early series reported from Egypt, schistosoma ova were present in 100% of the cases (*14*). With the advent of wide antibilharzial campaigns we can now separate two entities of bladder cancer in Egypt, a large one in which schistosoma eggs are present in tissues and another in which eggs are either not detectable or are absent. The frequency of egg positive cases in recent series is 83.1% (*15*).

In other countries where *S. hematobium* is endemic, bladder cancer is also frequent. In Egypt, there is no population-based incidence rate yet. The statistics of most hospitals and the Cairo NCI show that cancer of the urinary bladder is the most

TABLE 1. Comparison between Egg-positive and Egg-negative Cases

Trait[a]	Egg-positive (81.2%)		Egg-negative (18.2%)
	Heavy	Light	
Mean age (yrs.)	47.1	49.1	49.1
Less than 40 yrs.	25.9%	19.7%	8.5%
Sex ratio	8.7:1	4:1	2:1
Trigone involved	8.2%	9.0%	10.4%
Squamous cell carcinoma	82.7%	75.8%	76.0%
Verrucous carcinoma	9.3%	4.5%	6.3%

[a] Other parameters such as site, stage, and size as well as nodal involvement did not differ by infestation category.

frequent type of cancer in Egyptians, especially among males. In NCI Cairo records bladder cancer forms 38.5% of all malignancies in males and 11.3% of those in females, coming after breast cancer, thus accounting for 27.6% of all cancers encountered (16). The high figure in the NCI series reflects a selective referral of cases due to a special interest in the disease. In the Cairo metropolitan cancer registry which gathers its material from five main hospitals in Cairo including the NCI, bladder cancer was 15.8% of all cancers (17).

Cancer of the urinary bladder is also frequent in other areas of the Middle East and Africa where schistosomiasis is endemic. There is a high frequency in Iraq (18), Gold Coast (19), Nigeria (20), Mozambique (21), and South African Bantu (22). However, the relative frequency is less than that reported in Egypt due to the less severe nature of schistosomal infestation.

Salient Features of Bladder Cancer in Egypt

During the 5 years from 1982–1986, 1,302 specimens from radical cystectomies were examined at the pathology department of the NCI, Cairo. A separate study was done on 264 cases to quantitate the intensity of egg deposition. The cases were to three groups: 150 cases having heavy egg deposition, 66 cases having slight ova deposition, and 48 cases egg-negative cases (Table 1).

The average age in the whole group was 47.5 years and, for heavily infected patients, 47.1 years. Cases mildly infected or egg-negative had an average age of 49.1 years. Although no statistical difference was present, more heavily infected patients were below 40 years of age (25.9%), as compared to 19.7 and 8.5% in lightly infected and egg-negative patients, respectively.

There was a marked sex predilection in heavily infected patients. The male-female ratio was 8.7:1 compared to 4:1 in the lightly infected group and 2:1 in the egg-negative group.

→Fig. 1. a: nodular carcinoma of the posterior wall. The rest of the bladder is trabeculated due to bladder neck obstruction. b: sessile cauliflower tumor. The rest of the mucosa is rusty (sandy patch). c: whitish tumor and surrounding leukoplakia. d: verrucous carcinoma extending to bladder neck.

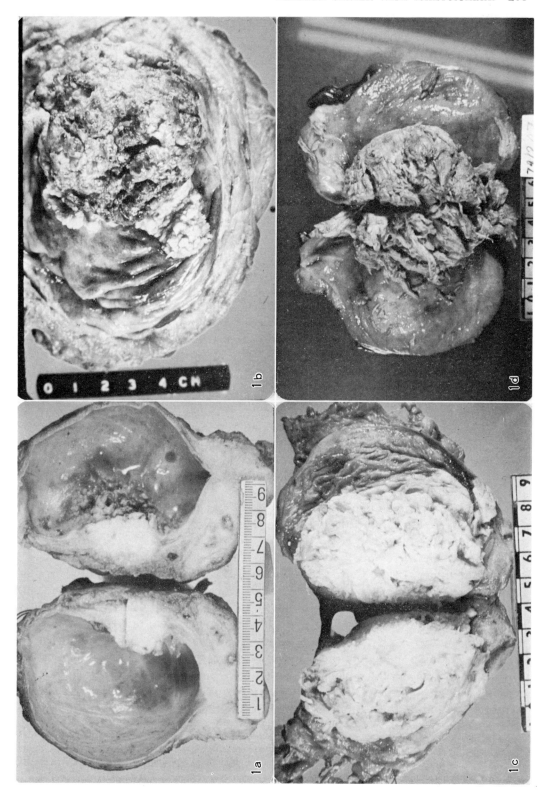

TABLE 2.   Histopathologic Types and Grades of Bladder Cancer

Type	No.	%	Grade %	
			Low	High
Squamous cell ca.	916	70.3	79.2	20.8
Verrucous ca.	86	6.6	100.0	—
Transitional cell ca.	190	14.6	55.0	45.0
Adenocarcinoma	66	5.1	9.0	91.0
Undifferentiated	44	3.4	—	100.0
Total	1,302	100.0	70.8	29.2

Most bladder cancers were seen as a raised sessile nodular masses (Fig. 1). In the present series, 61.4% of the tumors were nodular, 23.2% ulcerative, 6.6% verrucous, 6.9% papillary, and 1.9% diffuse. Verrucous carcinoma is a peculiar tumor seen where thick white filamentous masses of keratin project into the bladder lumen (Fig. 1). It has a broad pushing margin and does not involve lymph nodes although it might reach a large size (Fig. 2). Few cases of verrucous carcinoma are seen in egg-negative cases. In this study, there was no effect of intensity of ova deposition on the gross appearance of tumors.

The majority of tumors (64%) were large, between 5–10 cm, only a few cases (0.8%) were smaller than 2 cm. No difference in tumor size was seen between egg-positive and negative cases.

Most of the cases showed an advanced pathologic stage, P3: 61.5% and P4: 31.4%. The presence or the absence of eggs had no effect on the stage.

The trigone is usually spared in schistosoma associated cancers. In this study it was involved in 8.1% of the cases. The most common sites of tumor development were (in order of frequency) the posterior wall (30.5%), vault (27.3%), and the anterior wall (17.1%). Also, there was no difference in the site of tumors in egg-positive and negative cases.

Squamous cell carcinoma of the low grade variety was the commonest tumor (Table 2). There was no statistical difference between egg-positive and negative cases as far as tumor histology.

Lymph nodes were only involved in 18.5% of the cases in spite of the advanced stage of the tumor. In the Cairo NCI series, extensive pelvic clearance of nodes was usually done at the time of cystectomy. The low frequency of nodal involvement might reflect the low grades of most of these tumors as well as the obstruction of the pelvic lymphatics by schistosomal fibrosis. In other words, one effect of the parasite (fibrosis) may block another effect (progression of the neoplasia).

The remaining mucosa of the bladder was never healthy. Squamous metaplasia was seen in 51% of the cases, being more frequent with heavy egg deposits. Glandular cystitis was seen in 13% of the cases. Severe dysplasia and carcinoma *in situ* were seen in 5.1% and 8.2% of the bladders, especially in those severely infected.

→Fig. 2.   a: verrucous carcinoma, elongated keratinized processes with club-shaped invading processes. b: keratinized tadpole cells in urine. c: malignant transitional cells in urine. d: tubular adenocarcinoma with bilharzial ova.

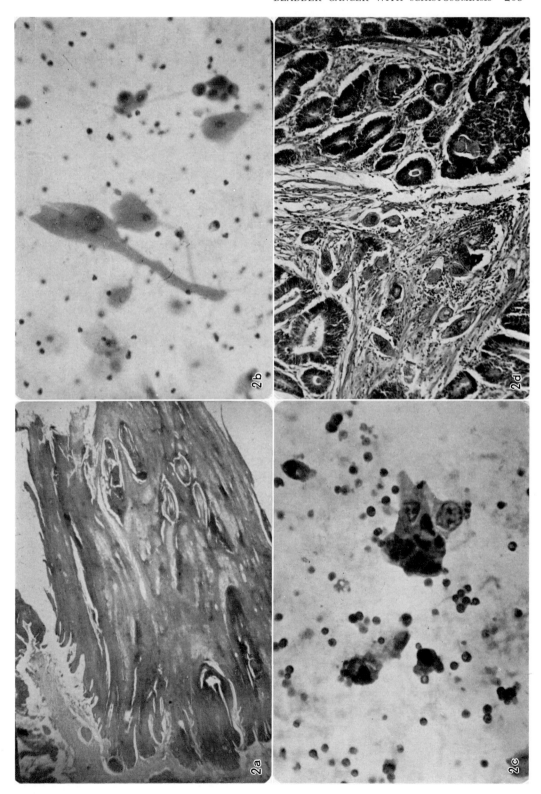

Multiple tumors were present in 15% of the cases with no statistical difference between egg-positive and-negative cases.

The above figures are in agreement with other reports on the frequency and pathological features of bladder cancer in Egypt (23, 24). However, there is no evidence that egg deposition has any effect on tumor pathology as previously suggested (25).

Early Detection of Schistosomal Bladder Cancer

Most cases of bladder cancer are first seen in the late stage when radical cystectomy is the only possible treatment. An attempt to discover early cases was carried out using urine cytology as a screening procedure. Urine cytology offers a technically feasible method applicable to the field, and acceptable to the population. Its sensitivity has been previously tested. The lapse time between schistosomal infection and bladder cancer allows ample time for the detection of these neoplasms.

A special field study was done in the Delta region where 8,744 inhabitants of the villages were screened. Ten bladder cancers were discovered in a high risk group of 4,769 patients; these were defined as farmers above the age of 20. No tumors were observed in non-farmers or individuals below 20 years of age (26). Therefore, a yield of 2:1,000 of high risk people was obtained. Seven of these tumors were superficial PIS-P2 tumors, which indicates the effectiveness of the screening.

Immunopathology of Schistosoma Associated Bladder Cancer

Schistosoma infected individuals are under constant immunological stress, either local or systemic (27, 28), so that immune mechanisms might be either protective or may contribute to tissue injury (29). Our studies showed that schistosoma infested bladder cancer patients have a significantly lower number of T lymphocytes and reduced delayed sensitivity (skin tests) to a purified protein derivatives of tuberculin and streptokinase-streptodornase (30). Immunoglobulins are deposited around hyperplastic schistosomal lesions in the bladder wall and in tumor tissue (31). Tumor specific bladder antigens were detected some of which cross reacted with schistosoma infected tissue or the mucosa of bladders not affected by the tumor (32). These antigens were present in the patients' sera; their isolation from the urine is underway. They might serve as a detection tool for cancer.

Possible Role of Schistosomiasis as Vesical Carcinogen(s)

The exact role played by schistosomiasis in the induction of bladder tumors is unknown; probably multiple factors act together. The parasite induces severe local damage on the vesical mucosa with secondary bacterial infection. Liver damage caused by the parasite results in derangement of the liver detoxication function and impairment of the tryptophan metabolism. Severe injury of the mucosa by the passage of egg and fibrocellular reaction in the lamina propria result in mucosal shedding, degeneration and attempts at regeneration with terminal metaplasia, mostly of the squamous type; but glandular and columnar metaplasias are also frequently encountered (*33*). The mucosal damage helps the absorption of free carcinogens in the bladder (*34*). This process is furthered by the stagnation of urine as a result of bladder neck obstruction in these cases (*35*). The eggs calcified by continuously irritating the mucosa might lead to carcinoma development (*36*). A chemical factor secreted by Miracidia has been suggested to have carcinogenic properties (*37*); the laboratory proof, however, is lacking. It is known that chronic mucosal irritation by stones, diverticulae or exostrophy, or paralytic sepsis can lead to carcinomas of the bladder.

Chronic bacterial infection in a schistosomal bladder is often intractable as a result of urine stasis and tissue injury. Most invaders are gram negative bacilli (55.1%); others are gram positive cocci (8%), anaerobic *Bacteroides* (4%), fungi (8.7%), and mixed infections (24.2%) (*38*). Bacterial products incriminated in the development of bladder cancers include β glucoronidase and nitrate reductase enzymes. The former liberates conjugated carcinogens in the bladder and is active at pH 7 (*39*). Nitrate reductase reduces nitrates to nitrosamines. A positive nitrite test correlated with the severity of urinary bacterial infection and with dysplastic changes in urinary sediments (*40*). The level of urinary nitrosodimethylamine is raised in bilharzial cystitis and bladder cancer (*41*).

Hicks *et al.* have found greater amounts of total N-nitroso compounds in the urine of patients infected with bacteria or schistosoma hematobium than in non-infected patients, and the highest values were for patients with both the parasite and nitrate-reducing bacteria (*41a*). However, no convincing evidence of mutagenic substances could be found in the urine through the use of the Ames *Salmonella* plate assay (*41b*). Newer methods, such as the detection of DNA adducts may be a promising approach to understanding the pathogenesis of these bladder cancers.

The liver is the habitat of the schistosoma worm which seldom induces a reaction unless they die. Most liver injury is caused by eggs carried back to the liver where they induce fibrosis in the large or fine portal tracts. Liver injury in infected patients leads to impairment of the metabolism of tryptophan with increased secretion of carcinogenic metabolites (*42*). Moreover, liver and tissue derived glucoronidase excretion is increased (*43*). Liver damage often results in a reduced level of vitamin A (*44*) which might be a factor in the induction of squamous metaplasia and squamous carcinoma. *In vitro*, it was shown that vitamin A inhibits keratinization of urinary bladder tumors (*45*).

Egyptian farmers consume a diet rich in nitrate from the fertilizers used. Their diet is deficient in vitamins A and B and they drink a lot of dark tea. They are exposed to a wide variety of chemicals used as pesticides and insecticides. These factors play a role in enhancing all the above mentioned factors. The possibility that drugs used in the treatment of bilharziasis play a role should also be considered because some are mutagenic (*46*).

Factors Against the Schistosomal Theory

There is no universal agreement on the exact role played by schistosomiasis in the induction of bladder tumors. Several investigators even doubt this role and stress other environmental factors such as dietary or chemical exposure of farmers. The problem of incriminating schistosomiasis is complicated by the absence of a good animal model. In rodents, *S. hematobium* is short-lived and usually suffers stunted growth, but if the animals mature, the eggs do not reach the genito-urinary system in a regular manner (*47*).

In non-human primates, the eggs are often deposited in the urinary system. Heavy infestation by *S. hematobium* induced only proliferative lesions morphologically similar to transitional cell carcinomas in a Talopoin monkey and in a Capuchin monkey (*48*). However, they lacked cellular atypia, mitosis or metastatic potentiality. Squamous metaplasia was present in other parts of the bladder mucosa. In another experiment, these lesions were found to regress and could not be transplanted (*49*).

Eggs are not deposited in the urinary bladder of small animals, mucosal changes in the form of squamous metaplasia and hyperplastic lesions have been described, and even a tumor-like mass was noted (*50*). However, such tumors are very few and need an added carcinogenic agent to develop. In areas of low endemicity, the association between the parasite and bladder cancer is less evident (*51*). In South African Bantu (*52*), Uganda (*53*), and southern Rhodesia (*54*) the association between schistosomiasis and cancer is less evident and in many cases the ova were not seen in the bladder tumors which have a higher percentage of the transitional type.

In Egypt, several factors should be considered. In particular, the high frequency of bladder cancer and the absolute number of cases have persisted in spite of vigorous antischistosomal and sanitary measures that were successful in reducing the intensity and frequency of schistosomiasis, especially in the Delta region. In Fayoum Province, which is an oasis situated south of Cairo, an active antischistosomal campaign since 1968 reduced schistosomal infestation from 60% to 10%, but carcinoma of the bladder is still the commonest cancer, accounting for about 50% of all malignancies in this area now (*55*). It may be that 20 years are not long enough for cancer reduction since there is a long latent period between the start of infection and the development of bladder cancer.

Certain trends in cancer incidence should be considered. There is a tendency towards higher age occurrence along with an increase in average survival time. In earlier series the average age was 40.2 years (*56*), while in more recent studies it was 47.5 years (*57*). Some studies in Egypt are beginning to show a rise in the frequency of transitional cell tumors (M. A. Ghoneim, personal communication).

In the previous study correlating tumor parameters with the intensity of egg deposition in tissues, it was evident that schistosoma associated cancers occur in slightly younger individuals, particularly males who, more than females, are heavily exposed to schistosomal infection. However, other tumor parameters, such as size, shape, site, stage, and histology were the same in both sexes. Even the verrucous type, thought to develop only in bilharzial bladder, has been found in egg-negative patients. Therefore, schistosoma-associated cancer is in no way different from cases of egg-negative individuals. Schistosoma may play only an enhancing role in the development of tumors which are possibly caused by other factors previously outlined.

REFERENCES

1. Goebel, G. Uber die bei bilharziakrankheit vorkommenden Blasentumoron mit besonderer beruchsichtigung des Karzinomas. Z. Krebsforsch., *3*: 369–513, 1905.
2. Ferguson, A. R. Associated bilharziasis and primary malignant disease of the urinary bladder, with observations in a series of forty cases. J. Path. Bact., *16*: 76–94, 1911.
3. El-Sebai, I. Clinical aspects, staging and management of cancer of the bilharzial bladder. *In;* I. El-Sebai (ed.), Cancer Bladder, Vol. 2, pp. 2–30, CRC Press, Boca Raton, Florida, 1983.
4. Higashi, G. I. and Aboul-Enein, M. I. Diagnosis and epidemiology of *Schistosoma hematobium* infections in Egypt. *In;* M. N. El-Bolkainy and E. Chu (eds.), Detection of Bladder Cancer Associated with Schistosomiasis, pp. 47–69, Al-Ahram Press, Cairo, 1981.
5. Kamal, H. Historical account of bilharziasis. Proc. 1st Int. Symp. Bilharziasis, Ministry of Science Res., Egypt, pp. 161–170, 1962.
6. Breasted, S. H. The Edwin Smith Papyrus. University of Chicago Press, 1930.
7. Ruffer, M. A. Studies on the paleopathology of Egypt. R. L. Monnie (ed.), University of Chicago Press, 1911.
8. Makar, N. Urological Aspects of Bilharziasis in Egypt. p. 1, Societe Orientale de Publicite Press, Cairo, 1955.
9. Bilharze, T. Fernere über das die pfortader des menschen bewohnende Distomun Haematobium und sein verhaltnis zu gewissen pathologischen bildungen. Ztschr Wissenschaft Zool., *4*: 72–76, 1852.
10. Weinland. Quoted by Kamed Mansour. The history of nomenclature of the bilharzia worm. Proc. 1st Int. Symp. Bilh., Ministry of Science Research, Egypt, pp. 239–242, 1962.
11. WHO. International work on Bilharziasis 1948–1958. WHO Chronicle, *1*: 1–9, 1959.
12. Mobarak, M. B. Report on the prevalence and control of schistosomiasis in Egypt. Ministry of Health, Cairo, 1980.
13. Scott, J. A. The incidence and distribution of the human schistosome in Egypt. Am. J. Hyg., *25*: 566–572, 1937.
14. Makar, U. Urological Aspects of Bilharziasis in Egypt. Societe Oriental de Publicite Press, Cairo 1955.
15. Aboul Nasr, A. L., Gazayerli, M. E., Fawzi, R. M., and El-Sebai, I. Epidemiology and pathology of cancer bladder in Egypt. Acta Unio. Int. Contra Cancrum, *18*: 528–537, 1962.
16. El-Sebai, I., El-Bolkainy, M. N., and Hussein, M. H. Cancer Institute Registry. Med. J. Cairo Univ., *41*: 175–181, 1973.
17. Aboul Nasr, A. L., Boutros, S. G., and Hussein, M. H. The cancer registry for the metropolitan Cairo area. Cancer Registration in 1977. Progress Report 5, Cairo Univ. Publ., p. 41, 1979.
18. Shamma, A. H. Schistosomiasis and cancer in Iraq. Am. J. Clin. Pathol., *25*: 1283–1287, 1955.
19. Edington, G. M. Malignant disease in the Gold Coast. Br. J. Cancer, *10*: 595–601, 1956.
20. Duncan, J. J. Cancer problems in Lagos. West African Med. J., *17*: 96–103, 1968.
21. Prates, M. D. and Gillman, J. Carcinoma of the urinary bladder in the Portuguese East African with special reference to bilharzial cystitis and preneoplastic reactions. S. Afr. J. Med. Sci., *24*: 13–40, 1959.
22. Hinder, R. A. and Schmaman, A. Bilharziasis and squamous carcinoma of the bladder.

S. Afr. Med. J., *43*: 617, 1969.

23. El-Bolkainy, M. N., Ghoneim, M. A., and Mansour M. A. Carcinoma of the bilharzial bladder in Egypt. Clinical and pathological features. Br. J. Urol., *44*: 561–570, 1972.

24. El-Bolkainy, M. N., Tawfik, H. N., and Kemel, I. A. Histopathologic classification of carcinomas in the Schistosomal bladder. *In;* M. N. El-Bolkainy and E. Chu (eds.), Detection of Bladder Cancer Associated with Schistosomiasis, pp. 107–123, Al-Ahram Press, Cairo, 1981.

25. Tawfik, H. N., Abull Ela, F., Anwer, N., and Ibrahim, A. S. Effect of severity of *Shistosoma* egg deposition on the pathology of cancer bladder. J. Cancer Inst., in press.

26. El-Bolkainy, M. N., Chu, E. W., Ghoneim, M. A., and Ibrahim, A. S. Cytologic detection of bladder cancer in a rural Egyptian population infested with schistosomiasis. Acta Cytol., *25*: 303–310, 1982.

27. Warren, K. S. Pathophysiology and pathogenesis of hepatosplenic schistosomiasis mansoni. Bull. N. Y. Acad. Sci., *44*: 280–294, 1968.

28. Warren, K. S. The secret of the immunopathogenesis of schistosomiasis. *In vivo* models. Immun. Rev., *61*: 189–213, 1982.

29. WHO. Report of an informal consultation on the immunopathological manifestations of schistosomiasis. Geneva, 1970.

30. El-Asfahani, A., Higashi, G. I., Sherif, M., Tawfik, H. N., Omar, S., Ibrahim, A. S., and Geith, H. Impaired immunologic reactivity in patients with urinary bladder cancer associated with bilharziasis. Proc. Int. Conf. Bilh. MPH, Cairo, 1978.

31. Tawfik, H. N., El-Maghraby, M., El-Asfahani, A., Daw, M., and Torky, H. The distribution of tissue bound immunoglobulins in bilharzial lesions and carcinoma of urinary bladder. Al-Azhar Med. J., *5*: 659–666, 1976.

32. Assaf, M.I.E. Immune labeling of carcinoma of the bilharzial bladder by anti tumor antibodies. Ph. D. Thesis, Zagazig Univ., Egypt, 1984.

33. Khafagy, M. M., El-Bolkainy, M. N., and Mansour, M. A. Carcinoma of the bilharzial urinary bladder. A study of the associated lesions in 86 cases. Cancer, *30*: 150–159, 1972.

34. Young, S. W., Farid, Z., and Bassily, S. Urinary Schistosomiasis. A 5-year clinical, radiological and functional evaluation. Trans. R. Soc. Trop. Med. Hyg., *67*: 379–383, 1973.

35. Badr, M., Zaher, M., and Fawzy, R. Further experience with bilharzial bladder neck obstruction. J. Egypt Med. Assoc., *41*: 624–629, 1958.

36. El-Aaser, A. A., Hassanein, S. M., El-Bolkainy, M. N., Omar, S., and El-Sebai, I. Bladder carcinogenesis using bilharzia infested Swiss Albino mice. Eur. J. Cancer, *14*: 645–649, 1979.

37. Makar, N. Cancer of the Bilharzial bladder. *In;* N. Makar (ed.), Urological Aspects of Bilharziasis in Egypt, S.O.P. Press, Cairo, 1955.

38. Isa, S.A.A., Aboul-Enein, M., and Abdel-Aziz, A. Bacteriologic and mycologic infection patterns in bilharzial bladder cancer. Proc. WHO Conf. Bladder Cancer, NCI, Cairo, 1985.

39. Abdel-Tawab, G. A., El-Zoghby, S. M., and Abdel-Samie, Y. M. Studies on the aetiology of bilharzial carcinoma of the urinary bladder VI. Beta-glucoronidase in urine. Int. J. Cancer, *1*: 383–389, 1966.

40. El-Aaser, A. A., El-Merzabani, M. M., El-Bolkainy, M. N., Ibrahim, A. S., Zakhary, N. I., and El-Morsi, B. A study on the aetiological factors of bilharzial bladder cancer in Egypt. 5. Urinary nitrite in rural population. Tumori, *66*: 409–412, 1980.

41. El-Merzabani, M. M., El-Aaser, A. A., and Zakhary, N. I. A study on the aetiological factors of bilharzial bladder cancer in Egypt. 1. Nitrosamines and their precursors in

urine. Eur. J. Cancer, *15*: 287–291, 1979.

41a. Hicks, R. M. Nitrosamines as possible etiologic agents in bilharzial bladder cancer. *In;* P. N. Magee (ed.), Banbury Report 12, Nitrosamines and Human Cancer, pp. 455–469, Cold Spring Harbor Laboratory, New York, 1982.

41b. Everson, R. B., Gad-el-Mawla, N. M., Attia, M.A.M., Chevlin, E. M., Thorgeirsson, S. S., Alexander, L. A., Flack, P. M., Staiano, N., and Ziegler, J. L. Analysis of human urine for mutagens associated with carcinoma of the bilharzial bladder by the Ames Salmonella plate assay: interpretation employing quantitation of viable lawn bacteria. Cancer, *51*: 371–377, 1983.

42. Abdel-Tawab, G. A., Kelda, F. S., and Kelda, N. L. Studies on the aetiology of bilharzial carcinoma of the urinary bladder. V. Excretion of tryptophan metabolites in urine. Int. J. Cancer, *1*: 377–382, 1966.

43. Fripp, P. J. The origin of urinary β-glucoronidase activity. Br. J. Cancer, *19*: 330–333, 1965.

44. Olson, J. A. Metabolism and function of vitamin A. Fed. Proc., *28*: 1670–1674, 1969.

45. Toyoshima, K. and Leighton, J. Vitamin A inhibition of keratinization in rat urinary bladder cancer cell line. Nara bladder tumor No. 2 in meniscus gradient culture. Cancer Res., *35*: 1873, 1876, 1975.

46. Bulay, O., Urman, M., Clayson, C. N., and Shubik, P. Carcinogenic effects of niridazol on rodents infected with schistosoma mansoni. J. Natl. Cancer Inst., *59*: 1625–1631, 1977.

47. Moore, D. V. and Meleney, H. E. Comparative susceptibility of common laboratory animals to experimental infection with *Schistosoma hematobium*. J. Parasit., *40*: 392–397, 1954.

48. Kuntz, R. E., Cheever, A. W., and Myers, B. J. Proliferative epithelial lesions of the urinary bladder of non human primates infected with schistosoma hematobium. J. Natl. Cancer Inst., *48*: 223–235, 1972.

49. Kuntz, R. E., Cheever, A. W., G. T., Moore, J. A., and Huang, T. Natural history of papillary lesions of the urinary bladder in Schistosomiasis. Cancer Res., *38*: 3836–3839, 1978.

50. Hashem, M. The aetiology and pathogenesis of the bilharzial bladder cancer. J. Egypt Med. Assoc., *44*: 857–966, 1961.

51. Gelfand, M., Weinberg, R. W., and Castle, W. M. Relation between carcinoma of the bladder and infestation with *Schistosoma hematobium*. Lancet, *1*: 1249–1251, 1967.

52. Higginson, J. and Oettle, A. G. Cancer of the bladder in the South African Bantu. Acta Unio. Int. Contra Cancrum, *18*: 579–584, 1962.

53. Dodge, O. G. Tumors of the bladder in Uganda Africans. Acta Unio. Int. Contra Cancrum, *18*: 548–552, 1962.

54. Houston, W. Carcinoma of the bladder in Southern Rhodesia. Br. J. Urol., *36*: 71–76, 1964.

55. Sherif, M., Ibrahim, A. S., Foad, A. M., and Guirguis, S. The Fayoum cancer registry. Cairo Univ. Natl. Cancer Inst., 1987.

56. Hashem, M. The aetiology and pathogenesis of bilharzial bladder cancer. Proc. 1st Int. Symp. Bilh. Ministry of Scientific Res. Egypt, pp. 697–700, 1962.

57. El-Bolkainy, M. N., Mokhtar, N. M., Ghoneim, M. A., and Hussein, M. H. The impact of Schistosomiasis on the pathology of bladder carcinoma. Cancer, *48*: 2643–2648, 1981.

Liver Cancer in an Endemic Area of Schistosomiasis Japonica in Yamanashi Prefecture, Japan

Yutaka INABA

Department of Hygiene, Juntendo University School of Medicine, Tokyo 113, Japan

Abstract: In Yamanashi Prefecture, schistosomiasis japonica has been endemic since the 16th century. Control of the disease has been very successful and no new case has been reported since 1977. Research has been conducted on the relationship between schistosomiasis and liver cancer, but no definite conclusion has been reached. We carried out several studies on this subject from the viewpoint of epidemiology.

A descriptive study showed a higher mortality rate for liver cancer in the endemic area of schistosomiasis than in the country as a whole, but not much difference from the mortality rate in the non-endemic area. A case-control study showed a high odds-ratio for cases with a history of schistosomiasis; however, the value is almost the same as for cases which had hepatitis B (HB) antigen. This study suggested a multiplicative effect of HB antigen, history of schistosomiasis and history of alcohol intake.

A retrospective cohort study showed a significantly high mortality rate for liver cancer in male inhabitants of the endemic area.

These results confirm that schistosomiasis was closely related to liver cancer. However, the follow-up study of liver cirrhosis showed no difference in the survival curve and death rate from liver cancer between schistosoma positive cases and negative cases. A cross-sectional study of the prevalence of HB virus showed a higher rate in inhabitants with a history of schistosomiasis than those without such a history. Although the above two studies were carried out in small samples, it is considered now that schistosomiasis is one of the co-factors of liver cancer and indirectly associated with it.

In Yamanashi Prefecture, which is located in the middle of Japan, a specific endemic disease with suspected ascites has been noticed since the 16th century. In the first decade of the 20th century, the disease, schistosomiasis japonica, was confirmed by many Japanese doctors. There were three main endemic areas of this disease in the country: the northern Kyushu district, the interprefectural area between Hiroshima and Okayama, and Yamanashi Prefecture (Fig. 1). Among these three areas,

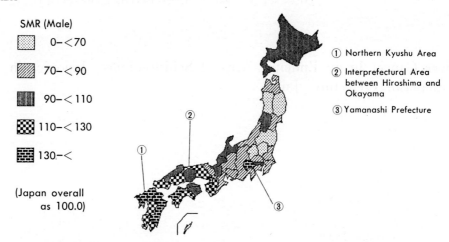

SMR (Male)

☐ 0–<70

▨ 70–<90

▥ 90–<110

▩ 110–<130

▦ 130–<

(Japan overall
as 100.0)

① Northern Kyushu Area

② Interprefectural Area
between Hiroshima and
Okayama

③ Yamanashi Prefecture

Fig. 1. Standardized mortality ratios (SMRs) of liver cancer (1975) and endemic areas of schistosomiasis in Japan.

Yamanashi Prefecture covered the largest region and had the most affected population.

In 1926, Katada described the mortality from malignant neoplasms by major sites from 1915 to 1924 in Yamanashi Prefecture (*1*). He indicated that the number of deaths from liver cancer was relatively higher in the endemic area of schistosomiasis than in the non-endemic area: 72 or 15.5% of 1,344 total malignant neoplasms in the endemic area, whereas 72 or 9.8% of 2,757 total malignant neoplasms in the non-endemic area. However, in other endemic areas of schistosomiasis in Asia, researchers have reported no relationship between liver cancer and schistosomiasis (*2, 3*). As the control of schistosomiasis has been very successful, there has been no case of the disease since 1977, but there are still many patients with other liver diseases in the endemic area. Recently, Japanese researchers reported a positive relationship between liver cancer and schistosomiasis and suggested a multiplicative association with hepatitis B (HB) virus infection (*4, 5*). With this background, we carried out several epidemiological studies in Yamanashi Prefecture.

Descriptive Epidemiology of Mortality Rates

The trend in mortality rates from liver cancer and liver cirrhosis in Yamanashi Prefecture is shown in Table 1. This table reveals a higher mortality rate from liver diseases in the prefecture than in Japan as a whole, but the difference has become less recently. Figure 1 shows the geographical distribution of the male liver cancer by the standardized mortality ratio (SMR) in Japan by prefecture. (The female distribution is similar). It indicates that the Yamanashi Prefecture area sustained particularly high mortality in the eastern part of Japan.

A correlation study of liver cancer mortality and HB antigen-positive rate in blood donors was carried out by municipality, but no positive relationship could be elucidated (*6*). In Yamanashi Prefecture, the HB antigen-positive rate in blood

TABLE 1.   Trends of Mortality for Liver Diseases in S-Town (per 100,000 population)

	Japan		Yamanashi Prefecture		SMR[a] of Yamanashi Prefecture	
	M	F	M	F	M	F
Liver cancer						
1970	11.7	6.9	20.8	11.4	—	—
1975	12.4	6.7	21.4	10.2	137.5	124.9
1980	17.6	7.6	31.4	9.2	151.9	96.0
1985	24.2	9.1	34.9	11.6	—	—
Liver cirrhosis						
1970	17.5	7.7	33.1	12.9	156.0	142.9
1975	19.9	7.5	30.3	12.6	123.1	114.8
1980	20.9	7.7	24.0	10.2	101.3	103.8
1985	20.4	8.4	21.4	11.6	—	—

[a] Standardized mortality ratio calculated with the mortality in Japan as 100.0.
—, not calculated. S-town is one of the highest districts shown in Fig. 2.

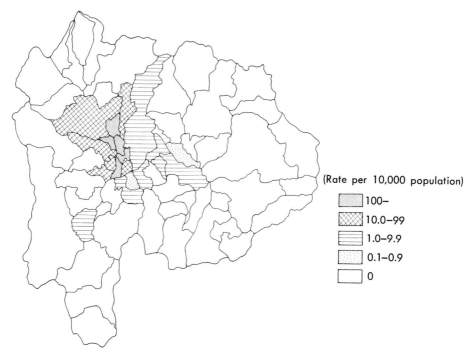

(Rate per 10,000 population)

100–
10.0–99
1.0–9.9
0.1–0.9
0

Fig. 2.   Prevalence rate of schistosomiasis japonica in Yamanashi Prefecture (1958–1962).

donors was about 2.0% in 1975, which was almost the same as the average in Japan as a whole.

Among 64 municipalities in Yamanashi Prefecture, 20 were endemic areas of schistosomiasis in 1958–1962 (Fig. 2); the population size in that area was about 400,000, almost the same as in the non-endemic area. Using the 1975 national population in Japan as the standard population, the SMR for liver cancer and liver

TABLE 2. Standardized Mortality Ratio (SMR) for Liver Cancer and Liver Cirrhosis in Yamanashi Prefecture (1973–1977)

Cause of death	Sex	Endemic area[a]				Non-endemic area[b]			
		Obs.	Exp.	SMR[c]	CI[d]	Obs.	Exp.	SMR[c]	CI[d]
Liver cancer	M	203	128.8	158.2	21.8	188	159.9	117.6	16.8
	F	109	73.2	148.9	28.0	130	91.8	141.6	24.3
Liver cirrhosis	M	315	200.0	157.5	17.4	228	243.1	93.8	12.2
	F	168	81.4	206.4	31.2	123	101.7	120.9	21.4

[a] 20 municipalities which were endemic areas of schistosomiasis in 1958–1962. [b] 44 other municipalities which were non-endemic areas. [c] Using the 1975 national population in Japan as the standard population. [d] 95% confidence interval.

cirrhosis in the endemic area and non-endemic area was calculated (7) (Table 2). The SMR for liver cirrhosis in the endemic area was about twice as high as in the non-endemic area; however, the SMR for liver cancer was only a little higher in the endemic area.

As is well known, the differential diagnosis between liver cirrhosis and liver cancer is very difficult; moreover, in the endemic area of schistosomiasis, there might be underdiagnosis of liver cancer because many clinical doctors have thought until recently that the end-point of schistosomiasis was liver cirrhosis. We will elucidate this hypothesis in the near future. Therefore, a problem in diagnosis may be unavoidable.

Case Control Study of Liver Cancer

From 1977 to 1979, in collaboration with seven hospitals in the endemic area a case-control study was carried out (8). The control group was selected from the same hospital as the cases matching sex and age, and excluding liver disease patients. The results of interviews of 62 pairs who were inpatients in the hospitals revealed that hepatoma was significantly correlated with HBs antigen, history of schistosomiasis and daily intake of alcohol, and that the odds ratios were 10.0, 9.5, and 3.2, respectively (Table 3). This study also suggested that these factors were multiplicatively related to hepatoma rather than additive. However, this study had the possibility of interviewer bias and recall bias because the information was obtained from attendant doctors, and so the odds ratios seemed to be overestimated.

TABLE 3. Matched Pair Analysis for Hospital Controls

Item	Case(+) control(−)	Case(−) control(+)	Odds ratio	Chi square
HBsAg	20	2	10.0	13.1**
Schisto.	19	2	9.5	12.2**
Alcohol	19	6	3.2	5.8*

HbsAg, HBs antigen; Schisto., history of schistosomiasis; alcohol, daily intake of alcoholic beverages.
** Significant at $p=0.01$ level. * Significant at $p=0.05$ level.

Retrospective Cohort Study in the Endemic Area of Schistosomiasis

This study was based on the inhabitants of a village in the endemic area in 1958. The mortality experience of 2,371 inhabitants was followed up for more than 20 years (*9*). The observed-expected ratio (O/E) was significantly high for liver cirrhosis (3.54 for males, 5.24 for females), liver cancer (males only, 2.59) and colorectal cancer (females only, 1.78). These O/E values were higher in agricultural households than in non-agricultural households, in those residing before 20 years of age than in those after 20 years of age, and in those having over 30 years of residence before 1958 than in those having under 30 years (Table 4).

These three studies revealed that schistosomiasis was closely related to liver cancer; however, its relative risk varied from 1.5 to 9.5. A retrospective study showed that, from among the above studies, the most reliable value was 2.0 to 3.0 in males.

Follow-up Study of Liver Cirrhosis Cases with Schistosomiasis

In order to verify that schistosomiasis promoted liver cirrhosis to liver cancer, 225 cases of liver cirrhosis were followed for about 6 years. These cases were selected

TABLE 4.   SMR by Sub-population

		Cancer of liver (male)	Liver cirrhosis	
			Male	Female
Agricultural household	O.	20	36	23
	E.	7.23	8.27	4.28
	O/E	2.77**	4.35**	5.37**
		(1.69–4.27)	(3.05–6.03)	(3.41–8.06)
Non-agricultural household	O.	7	6	8
	E.	3.21	3.63	1.64
	O/E	2.18	1.65	4.88**
		(0.87–4.49)	(0.60–3.60)	(2.10–9.61)
Age at residence				
<20	O.	18	29	11
	E.	6.09	7.03	1.55
	O/E	2.96**	4.13**	7.10**
		(1.75–4.67)	(2.76–5.92)	(3.54–12.70)
≥20	O.	9	13	20
	E.	4.30	4.83	4.36
	O/E	2.09	2.69**	4.59**
		(0.96–3.97)	(1.43–4.60)	(2.80–7.08)
Duration of residence				
<30	O.	9	10	7
	E.	4.09	4.89	2.88
	O/E	2.20*	2.05	2.43
		(1.00–4.18)	(0.98–3.76)	(0.97–5.01)
≥30	O.	18	32	24
	E.	6.31	6.97	3.04
	O/E	2.85**	4.59**	7.90**
		(1.69–4.51)	(3.12–6.48)	(5.06–11.75)

** Significant at 5% level.   * Significant at 1% level.   ( ) 95% confidence interval.

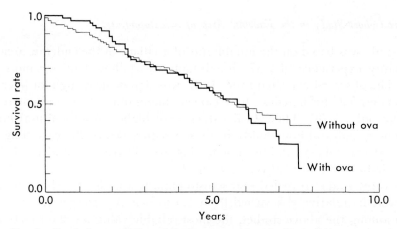

FIG. 3.   Survival curve of liver cirrhosis causes with and without *Schistosoma japonicum*.

TABLE 5.   Causes of Death, Liver Cirrhosis Cases with or without *Schistosoma japonicum*

Cause of death	*Schistosoma japonicum*				Total	(%)
	(+)	(%)	(−)	(%)		
Liver cancer	27	(39.7)	27	(61.4)	54	(48.2)
Others	41	(60.3)	17	(38.6)	58	(51.8)
Total	68	(100.0)	44	(100.0)	112	(100.0)

from a hospital in the endemic area for schistosomiasis and Juntendo Hospital in Tokyo. All cases were diagnosed by histological examination between 1976 and 1978. There was no difference in the survival curve between those with and without schistosomiasis (Fig. 3). Among 112 deaths during the observation period, there was no significant difference in the liver cancer rate between those with and without schistosomiasis (Table 5). Although the promoting effect of schistosomiasis to liver cancer has been reported in animal experiments (*10*), the result of our study did not support this hypothesis.

Cross-sectional Study on the Prevalence of HB Virus in Inhabitants of the Schistosomiasis Endemic Area

In a schistosomiasis endemic area, 122 inhabitants were studied for HB virus markers (*11*). Table 6 shows that HB virus markers in persons with a history of schistosomiasis were significantly higher than in those without such history. This suggested that needles contaminated by hepatitis virus (B or non-A non-B) may contribute to liver disease, because sodium antimony tartrate had often been used intravenously over a long period for the therapy of schistosomiasis.

The Role of Schistosomiasis Japonica in the Pathogenesis of Liver Cancer

As the carcinogenicity of *Schistosoma japonicum* has not been verified experimentally, schistosomiasis is considered a so-called "co-factor" in carcinogenesis. The

TABLE 6. HB Virus Markers in Inhabitants of the Schistosomiasis Endemic Area

History of schistosomiasis	HB virus markers			Positive (%)	Negative (%)	Total (%)
	HBsAg	HBsAb	HBcAb			
Positive	4	26	41	45 (66.2)	17 (31.5)	62 (50.8)
Negative	1	16	19	23 (33.8)	37 (68.5)	60 (49.2)
Total	5	42	60	68 (100.0)	54 (100.0)	122 (100.0)

mechanism of the co-factor has been suggested by several researchers. Pathological and clinical studies have led researchers to suspect that schistosoma was a promoting factor and HB virus was an initiating factor (4, 5). This theory seemed to be confirmed by experimental study (10). However, in our recent studies, although the results were based on small samples, we could not elucidate the promoting effect of the schistosomiasis, and we found evidence of the old HB virus infection, that is, non-A non-B liver virus infection. As the relationship between schistosomiasis and liver cancer is not so clear in other countries, in the present situation I consider that schistosomiasis might be indirectly associated with liver cancer. In China, a report (12) was presented recently which suggested that there is a close association between schistosomiasis japonica and mortality from colon cancer. Further study is required on the relationship between schistosomiasis and malignant neoplasms.

ACKNOWLEDGMENTS

The author thanks the administrative staff and his many co-workers in Yamanashi Prefecture for assistance in this research.

REFERENCES

1. Katada, B. A geo-statistical study on malignant neoplasms in Yamanashi Prefecture. Byourigaku Kiyou (Bull. Pathol.) 3: 777–933, 1926 (in Japanese).
2. Hartz, P. H. Role of schistosomiasis in the etiology of cancer of the liver in Chinese. Arch. Pathol., 39: 1–2, 1945.
3. Bonne, C. Cancer in Java and Sumatra. Am. J. Cancer, 25: 811–821, 1935.
4. Iuchi, M., Hayakawa, M., Kitani, K., Yamada, H., Iio, M., Sasaki, Y., and Kameda, H. Primary liver cancer in chronic schistosomiasis, second report. Acta Hepatol. Jpn., 14: 249–252, 1973 (in Japanese).
5. Nakashima, T., Okuda, K., Kojiro, M., Sakamoto, K., Kubo, Y., and Shimokawa, Y. Primary liver cancer coincident with schistosomiasis japonica. Cancer, 36: 1483–1489, 1975.
6. Inaba, Y., Yamamoto, S., Takahashi, L. E., Nakamura, K., Ono, T., and Nagahashi, M. The relationship of death from liver cancer and liver cirrhosis to the environmental factors in Yamanashi Prefecture, Japan. Jpn. J. Public Health, 24: 465–473, 1977 (in Japanese).
7. Inaba, Y. A statistical study on the mortality in the endemic area of schistosomiasis Japonica in Yamanashi Prefecture—with special emphasis on the malignant neoplasms of the digestive tract. Jpn. J. Public Health, 29: 585–590, 1982 (in Japanese).

8. Inaba, Y., Maruchi, N., Matsuda, M., Yoshihara, N., and Yamamoto, S. A case-control study on liver cancer with special emphasis on the possible aetiological role of schistosomiasis. Int. J. Epidemiol., *13*: 408–412, 1984.

9. Inaba, Y. A cohort study on the causes of death in an endemic area of schistosomiasis japonica in Japan. Ann. Acad. Med. Singapore, *13*: 142–148, 1984.

10. Miyasato, M. Experimental study of the influence of *Schistosoma japonicum* infection on carcinogenesis of mouse liver treated with 2-FAA. Jpn. J. Parasit., *33*: 41–48, 1984 (in Japanese).

11. Inaba, Y., Yoshihara, N., and Horimi, T. Cross-sectional study on HB virus infection rate among inhabitants in the endemic area of schistosomiasis japonica. J. Yamanashi Med. Assoc., *13*: 11–15, 1985 (in Japanese).

12. Zhong, Xu. and De-Long, Su. *Schistosoma japonicum* and colorectal cancer; An epidemiological study in the People's Republic of China, Int. J. Cancer, *34*: 315–318, 1984.

GENETIC AND OTHER
HOST FACTORS

UNUSUAL OCCURRENCES AS CLUES TO CANCER ETIOLOGY, R. W. MILLER ET AL. (EDS.),
JAPAN SCI. SOC. PRESS, TOKYO/TAYLOR & FRANCIS, LTD., PP. 221–231, 1988

PRINCE TAKAMATSU MEMORIAL LECTURE

Rare Cancers: Clues to Genetic Mechanisms

Alfred G. Knudson, Jr.

Institute for Cancer Research, Fox Chase Cancer Center, Philadelphia, Pennsylvania, 19111, U.S.A.

Abstract: Virtually every kind of cancer can occur in hereditary form. Such hereditary cancers are rare, but have been informative out of proportion to their frequencies because some of them have illuminated mechanisms important in the genesis of cancer generally. The prototypes of hereditary cancer have been two uncommon tumors, retinoblastoma and Wilms' tumor. Genetic epidemiologic analysis of these tumors led to the formulation of a model for their origin following two events. According to this model the first event could already be present in the germline, thereby giving rise to the heritable forms of these diseases; the second event would occur somatically in one or more cells of the relevant organ. Both events would occur somatically in the non-hereditary form. It was proposed that the two events involved mutation or loss of both copies of a particular gene; *i.e.*, these genes are recessive in oncogenesis.

Cytogenetic analyses of rare deletion cases of retinoblastoma permitted the localization of the retinoblastoma gene to chromosomal band 13q14. Deletion was also proposed as the mechanism for the rare conjunction of Wilms' tumor and aniridia; deletions of chromosomal band 11p13 were subsequently found. Deletions were also found in tumor cells of some patients with the non-hereditary forms of these two tumors, lending support to the idea that the same loci were involved in the two forms.

The application of molecular genetic techniques led to verification of the recessive hypothesis for both retinoblastoma and Wilms' tumor and to the cloning of the gene of the former. These accomplishments are leading to a new understanding of mechanisms of oncogenesis and their involvement even in the common cancers of adults.

I am greatly honored to present the Prince Takamatsu Memorial Lecture at this symposium. I am only one of many foreigners who have greatly admired and appreciated the interest and personal involvement of so many members of the Imperial Family of Japan in biology and medicine. In particular, the efforts of Her

Imperial Highness, Princess Takamatsu, and of His Imperial Highness, the late Prince Takamatsu, have not gone unnoticed; the Princess Takamatsu Symposia are internationally acclaimed.

The problem of cancer, to which the resources of the Princess Takamatsu Cancer Research Fund are dedicated, is still a great one for all nations. Yet there is excitement in the circles of cancer research, owing primarily to knowledge of genetic changes in cancer cells that are shedding light on mechanisms of carcinogenesis and suggesting new approaches to reversal of the malignant state.

Last year at this symposium the subject was that of viral oncogenes and their putative parents, host proto-oncogenes. The study of rare events was critical to that body of research, the rare events involving the incorporation of modified proto-oncogenes into the genomes of certain retroviruses. Today I would like to discuss another group of rare events, the hereditary cancers of man, whose study has revealed a second class of cancer genes. Both classes of genes appear to have roles in the origin not only of the rare cancers that were first studied, but also of the common cancers generally.

The first cancer genes, oncogenes, were discovered because of their dominant genetic activity; their continued presence and activity is essential for the elicitation and maintenance of the malignant state. In contrast, the newer class of cancer gene is recessive in oncogenesis; the mutation or loss of both copies of a gene is essential for oncogenesis. Such genes have been referred to as recessive oncogenes, or, because their normal alleles are antioncogenic, as antioncogenes.

The discovery and characterization of recessive oncogenes, or antioncogenes, has depended upon research at three different levels: patient, chromosome, and DNA. Patients and their families have provided epidemiologic genetic clues; their chromosomes, cytogenetic clues; their DNAs, molecular genetic clues. Here I plan to review these clues, indicate the present state of our knowledge of antioncogenes, and suggest some implications for the future.

Epidemiologic Genetic Clues

Epidemiologic genetic clues to the existence of antioncogenes came primarily from the study of two uncommon tumors, retinoblastoma and Wilms' tumor. Retinoblastoma has been the prototypic tumor and the key to the discovery of recessive cancer genes. This has been so because its heritability is high and because rare cases with constitutional deletion permitted chromosomal localization of the gene.

With an incidence of about five per 10^5 births in most countries, retinoblastoma accounts for only about three percent of the burden of cancer in children. However, it accounts for a much higher fraction of *heritable* cancer in children. For retinoblastoma some 25–30 percent or so of cases are affected with tumors in both eyes. Fifty percent of the offspring of these bilateral cases are at high risk of the disease, as expected for dominant inheritance, whether the previous family history is positive or not, so all should be thought of as germline mutations. In addition, 10–15 percent of unilaterally affected persons pass on a high risk of tumor to 50 percent of their children, so it can be concluded that about 40 percent of cases are heritable and 60 percent are not (*1*).

If some heritable cases are unilaterally affected, and some bilaterally affected, the inherited mutation is clearly not sufficient to cause tumor. The very large number (about 10^8) of cells in each eye that are derived from retinoblasts suggests that the formation of a tumor is an exceedingly rare cellular event. I calculated that the mean number of tumors per gene carrier was three (1), and that the distribution of tumors among cases followed closely the Poisson function, indicating the chance occurrence of these events at a regular frequency. I concluded that tumor develops in heritable cases as the result of two events, one a heritable mutation and one a postzygotic event in a somatic (retinal) cell. This latter event would have a frequency of the order of 10^{-7} per cell division, a frequency compatible with that of somatic mutation.

If heritable cases were caused by two mutations, one germinal and one somatic, what might be the mechanism in the 60 percent of cases that are not heritable? A hypothesis was that two mutations might be operating in these cases too, but both would be somatic, occurring post-zygotically. This hypothesis led to a prediction regarding the ages of appearance of the tumors in heritable and non-heritable cases. I noted the age at diagnosis for each case, and then plotted the fraction of cases not yet diagnosed *vs.* age. The curve for heritable cases followed the expectation for a single somatic event, that for non-heritable cases followed the expectation for two somatic events. From this it was concluded that the two forms of retinoblastoma are caused in the same way, the only difference being that in one the first mutation is germinal, in the other, somatic.

If two mutations are necessary, what might be their relationship, if any? A simple hypothesis is that they affect the two copies of some autosomal genetic locus; *i.e.*, the mutation would be recessive at the cellular level in causing cancer. This presents a confusion in terminology, because the inheritance of retinoblastoma is dominant. One must therefore specify whether the term is being applied at the level of the individual or at the level of the cell; inheritance of *predisposition* to retinoblastoma is *dominant*, while the *mechanism* of carcinogenesis is *recessive*.

This notion of a recessive mechanism was supported by an observation on the hereditary human disease, Bloom's syndrome. Chromosomes from patients with this rare recessively inherited disorder show an increased incidence of breakage and rearrangement. A particularly striking finding is the quadriradial figure, similar to that observed in meiotic chromosomes, indicative of pairing of homologous chromosomes. There is a high rate of sister chromatid exchanges (2) and even occasional exchanges between paired homologous chromosomes. Anna Meadows and her colleagues observed a child with Bloom's syndrome who provided still further evidence for recombination (3). He was afflicted with leukemia, as often happens in this syndrome; in fact, such patients are at risk for a range of cancers, with a virtual certainty of some malignancy by the age of 30 years. This child was black, actually with intermediate pigmentation. However, his skin revealed numerous darker areas of pigmentation adjacent to very pale areas. They were reminded of "twin spotting" in *Drosophila*, a phenomenon in which cells on a background of intermediate phenotype segregate into cells of polarized phenotypes. They concluded that this child was heterozygous for a pigment gene and that somatic recombination had produced homozygous dark and light daughter cells that had grown into clones. They further concluded that the high incidence of cancer in the syndrome might be the result of such recombination. If cancer can be caused by mutations in recessive cancer genes, then the second event could be either a new mutation (including point mutation, deletion, and monosomy) or somatic recombination with segregation of a homozygous daughter cell. The site of a particular cancer in the syndrome would depend upon the site of a first somatic mutation, while the high incidence of cancer could be explained by the high frequency of one kind of second event (recombination). A corollary of this idea is that recombination also occurs in normal persons and can be a mechanism for the second event in them. The first event would necessarily entail mutation (in the broad sense), whereas the second event could be caused by either mutation or recombination.

Louise Strong and I applied the notion of two events to two other tumors of children, Wilms' tumor and neuroblastoma (4, 5). Like retinoblastoma both of these tumors affect paired organs, which aids in the assessment of multiple origin. In addition, heritable forms of each were known. As anticipated, we found that bilateral tumors were more common among hereditary cases than among all cases combined. We also found that the age distribution of cases paralleled that of retinoblastoma; for both Wilms' tumor and neuroblastoma the heritable cases were distributed as expected for a single somatic event, the non-heritable cases, as for two somatic events. The same conclusion was reached: two events were always necessary, the first being a germline mutation in hereditary cases, a somatic mutation in non-hereditary cases.

Notice was taken of a condition that is occasionally associated with Wilms' tumor, *viz.*, aniridia. Robert Miller and his colleagues had assembled convincing epidemiologic evidence of an association between sporadic congenital aniridia and Wilms' tumor; the hereditary form of aniridia was not so associated (6). We found that the distribution of ages at diagnosis of tumor was similar to that for hereditary cases of Wilms' tumor. We proposed that, if the genes for hereditary Wilms' tumor and aniridia are near each other in the same chromosome, then a chromosomal deletion could include both genes, leading to aniridia and predisposition to Wilms' tumor (4). The aniridia would be sporadic because affected persons would be so severely affected by gene loss as to cause reduced viability and/or infertility; nearly all cases would be expected to represent new germline mutations. Discovery of such a deletion would point to the location of the Wilms' tumor gene.

Epidemiologic genetic clues led us to the conclusion that two events were necessary for the development of certain cancers in children, and possibly of a broad spectrum of tumors, since virtually every kind of cancer appears in hereditary form (7). We further supposed that the mechanism of oncogenesis was recessive at the cellular level. Evidence bearing on that mechanism came from the study of tumor cells themselves.

Cytogenetic Clues

Greatest progress in providing such evidence has been made with retinoblastoma and Wilms' tumor, because for each of these tumors there is a small fraction (about 3–5 percent) of cases whose somatic cells all show a specific deletion in one chromosome. The first such patients were reported before the advent of chromosomal banding techniques, so specification of the site, or even the precise chromosome, was not possible, although the deleted chromosome was clearly in the 13–15 group. Anna Meadows observed such a patient, suspecting deletion because of mild mental retardation, which is not usually a feature associated with retinoblastoma. Chromosomal banding of peripheral blood cells revealed heterozygosity for a deletion in the long arm of chromosome 13. Comparison of this banded karyotype with those of four previously reported cases pointed to band 13q14 as the critical site common to all (8). This was subsequently corroborated in a patient with a deletion within this band (9). We proposed that hereditary cases of retinoblastoma without deletion involve a submicroscopic mutation, and that non-hereditary cases involve a somatic mutation, microscopic or submicroscopic, at the same locus.

As noted earlier, we had suggested that aniridia with Wilms' tumor might be associated with a germline deletion (4). This has proven to be correct. The first cytogenetic analysis of a case showed a translocation between chromosomes 8 and 11 (10). Subsequent analyses of that case and other cases revealed that chromosomal band 11p13 was deleted in all (11). Again, the supposition was that hereditary cases without a constitutional deletion involve a submicroscopic mutation at the same site.

The original hypothesis called for somatic mutation in non-hereditary cases as a first event at the same site affected by germline mutation in the hereditary cases. One way to check this hypothesis would be to look for chromosome 13 aberrations in tumor cells in patients with the non-hereditary form of retinoblastoma. Although only 3–5 percent of patients have a constitutional deletion at 13q14, it might be expected that deletion would be better tolerated in a specialized somatic cell than in a germ cell and developing organism. On the other hand, karyotypes of tumor cells are not as clear as those of blood cells, so small deletions that are apparent in the latter might not be noticed in tumor cells. Several investigators have reported on this problem, and the consensus is that about 15 percent or so of tumors reveal monosomy or deletion of chromosome 13, the deletion site always including 13q14. Similar studies have been performed on Wilms' tumor, with similar results too, except that monosomy 11 has not been reported in tumors.

The deletion cases of retinoblastoma and Wilms' tumor pointed to chromosomal bands 13q14 and 11p13, respectively, as sites of mutation for all cases of those tumors. However, other kinds of evidence were necessary to demonstrate the correctness of this hypothesis. Such evidence was supplied by biochemical studies on deletion and hereditary cases.

Robert Sparkes made the happy discovery that the only gene then known to be located on chromosome 13, the gene for the enzyme esterase D, was affected by 13q14 deletion (12). Cases with this constitutional deletion were hemizygous for esterase D; the deletion included the esterase D locus on the deleted chromosome, reducing the mean level of esterase D activity in blood to 50 percent of normal. Since even the smallest identifiable deletion demonstrated this behavior, Sparkes concluded that the two genes were very closely linked.

This information was then used by Sparkes to show that the heritable form of retinoblastoma not associated with deletion also involved chromosome 13q14

(*13*). This was possible because of a polymorphism of the enzyme in human populations. This polymorphism consists of a two allele system that affects electrophoretic mobility of the enzyme. All individuals are types 1-1, 1-2, or 2-2. Families suitable for study include those in which a parent who had survived retinoblastoma and was type 1-2, married a person of type 1-1 or 2-2, and had both affected and unaffected children. If the genes are not linked, the esterase D alleles should segregate randomly without regard to tumor status. If they are very closely linked, the affected children in a pedigree should all be of one type and the unaffected children of another type, indicating no genetic recombination. Sparkes found no recombination.

The esterase D gene could also be used in an examination of retinoblastoma tumors, whether hereditary or not hereditary. I had proposed that retinoblastoma was the prototype of a recessive cancer mutation, and that the second somatic event, which converted a heterozygous cell into a homozygous or hemizygous mutant cell, could be accomplished by any of several mechanisms, namely, loss of chromosome 13, deletion of that chromosome in the 13q14 region, a small submicroscopic mutation at that site, or somatic recombination, with segregation of a cell homozygous for the mutation on the homologous chromosome (*14*). The proposed mechanisms for the development of the second event were in some cases local, as with point mutation, and sometimes gross, as with monosomy, deletion, and recombination. Events in the latter category have implications for associated markers. If we consider a hereditary case of retinoblastoma with esterase D type 1-2 in which the acquired mutation in the tumor affects only the retinoblastoma locus, then the esterase D locus would retain heterozygosity. On the other hand, if a hereditary case with esterase D type 1-2 developed a tumor on the basis of a gross event, then only one esterase D allele should be found in the tumor. Indeed, both results were found in different cases (*15*). The first report that *both* copies of esterase D were abnormal was made by William Benedict and his colleagues (*16*), who examined a patient whose blood level of esterase D was 50 percent of normal, despite absence of a demonstrable deletion. The authors proposed that this case involved an occult deletion. The tumor, on the other hand, had just one chromosome 13 and no measurable esterase D activity, from which it was concluded that the normal 13 had been lost during tumorigenesis. These findings implied loss of both copies of the linked retinoblastoma gene as well.

Studies of both retinoblastoma and Wilms' tumor were severely limited by the lack of availability of polymorphic genetic markers on chromosomes 11 and 13. This has been a common problem for linkage studies generally. A new tool was required to pursue the investigations further; that tool was molecular genetics, which has provided an abundance of polymorphic DNA markers.

Molecular Genetic Clues

Molecular analysis of these mechanisms depended upon widespread variations among individuals with respect to specific DNA sequences, especially those that do not code for the gene product. When genomic DNA is digested by a restriction endonuclease at one of the variant sites but not the other, this polymorphism can be detected by the technique of Southern blotting. Hybridization of the DNAs with a

DNA probe that recognizes both of the digested sequences permits detection of fragments of different sizes. If the larger fragment is designated as 1 for a given probe, and the smaller by 2, then different individuals could have 1-1, 1-2, or 2-2 genotypes. Such polymorphic DNA fragments are called restriction fragment length polymorphisms, or RFLP's. RFLP's have been found for DNAs of known genes, such as insulin and H-ras oncogene, although most of the hundreds of available RFLP's have not been identified with known genes.

These RFLP's can then be used just as esterase D was used, to test for linkage or for loss of heterozygosity in tumors. Webster Cavenee was the first to use such DNA probes in a search for loss of heterozygosity. He and his colleagues first studied retinoblastoma, using a panel of probes known to hybridize with unique sequences located on chromosome 13 (17). Informative persons were those who were heterozygous for one or more of these probes. Comparison of Southern blots from normal cells and tumor cells from the same person permitted analysis of mechanism in some cases. Particularly interesting are cases in which a tumor that has two intact chromosomes 13 has retained heterozygosity for a DNA fragment that lies between the centromere and band 13q14, but has lost heterozygosity for more distal markers. This finding indicates that somatic recombination occurred, with the tumor cells acquiring one mutant chromosome and one chromosome whose proximal long arm is derived from the non-mutant chromosome and whose distal long arm is derived from the mutant chromosome. Such an exchange evidently occurs following pairing of homologous chromosomes, with crossing-over between two chromatids of different homologues. In other cases all of the markers had lost heterozygosity in tumor cells, a finding compatible with either recombination between the centromere and the proximal DNA marker or with loss of one chromosome and duplication of the remaining one by successive non-disjunctions. In still other instances loss of heterozygosity has resulted from monosomy or deletion.

In some instances heterozygosity has been retained in the tumor for all possible markers. This is the result one would expect with a local mutational second event, such as a point mutation or an intragenic deletion. Such a result has been found in about 40 percent of retinoblastomas.

Similar findings have been reported for Wilms' tumor, using markers on chromosome 11. The insulin, beta globin, and H-ras genes are located near the end of chromosome 11, and DNA from all show polymorphisms. Recombination or chromosomal loss or deletion should lead to loss of heterozygosity, a result noted in about 60 percent of tumors (18).

Each of the originally proposed mechanisms for second events apparently operates for the tumors studied. There is even a variation on one of the mechanisms, with a second non-disjunction leading to two identical mutant chromosomes.

The availability of linked DNA markers was then used to search for the "retinoblastoma gene" and for abnormalities in it in tumors. One such marker was localized to the immediate region of the retinoblastoma gene, and further found to be abnormal in a few tumors. Stephen Friend, working in Robert Weinberg's laboratory, discovered that this probe had two further properties of interest: (1) it hybridized with DNA of the mouse, indicating a level of evolutionary conservation associated with the transcribed portions of genes, and (2) it hybridized with a messenger RNA from immortalized fetal retinoblasts (*19*). This probe was therefore used to study DNA from normal and tumor cells, the latter from persons with re- tinoblastoma or osteosarcoma, a tumor sometimes found in patients with retino- blastoma. Deletions of all or part of the tumor DNA were found in about 30 per- cent of cases. In one case only an internal portion of the detectable DNA was deleted, indicating that this probe was indeed detecting the retinoblastoma gene. This dis- covery was quickly verified and extended by two other groups of investigators (*20*, *21*).

The retinoblastoma gene is very large, of the order of magnitude of 200,000 base pairs of DNA. However, its messenger RNA is only 4,700 base pairs, so the coding sequences are a minor part of the whole. A complementary DNA has been sequenced by Wen-Hwa Lee and his colleagues (*22*), and this sequence has been used to predict the amino acid sequence of the corresponding protein. A portion of this protein has been synthesized and used as an antigen to produce an antibody against the authentic protein. This antibody reveals that the cellular protein is nu- clear. Furthermore, fractionated cellular protein, identified by antibody, has DNA binding activity, as was predicted from the putative amino acid sequence. It may therefore be that the normal product of the retinoblastoma gene is a protein that regulates the activity of other genes by combining with their regulatory domains.

Consequences

There is now no doubt of the existence of two classes of genes that qualify as cancer genes in the sense that abnormalities in their function lead to cancer. These genes are commonly called proto-oncogenes, or oncogenes, and recessive oncogenes, or anti-oncogenes. An understanding of their roles in some human cancers came about through the investigation of two uncommon cancers of children, Burkitt's lymphoma and retinoblastoma. Now other, more common, tumors seem to involve one or the other of these mechanisms. Oncogene abnormality associated with chro- mosomal translocation operates in a number of hematopoietic malignancies, in- cluding chronic myelocytic leukemia. Anti-oncogene abnormality has been invoked for colon cancer, breast cancer, small cell cancer of the lung, and renal carcinoma.

The clearest evidence on the latter cancers is for colon cancer. Walter Bodmer and his colleagues (*23*) have recently shown, by linkage with an RFLP, that the gene for polyposis coli is located on chromosome arm 5q. With linked DNA probes they then investigated non-hereditary colon cancer, testing the hypothesis that hereditary and non-hereditary forms of this cancer involve the same genetic mech- anism. They found that more than 20 percent of non-heritable colon cancers showed loss of heterozygosity for at least one linked marker, a finding consistent with a first event of somatic mutation at one of the copies of the polyposis coli gene, and a second gross event causing loss of the other copy (*24*). This percentage could be as high as 40 percent, but is still lower than the 60 percent observed for retinoblastoma and Wilms' tumor. This discrepancy is not surprising, because colon cancer is probably a heterogeneous category of tumors. For example, there are two separate hereditary predispositions to colon cancer, one associated with polyps and one not. If non-he- reditary colon cancer sometimes involves one of these loci and sometimes the other, then loss of heterozygosity for either alone could well be in the range of 20–40 percent.

The importance of oncogenes and anti-oncogenes goes beyond carcinogenesis. Both classes of genes are clearly important in normal development and physiology, and may even be associated with other diseases than cancer, notably embryologic defects. This possibility emerges from my own study of hereditary renal carcinoma in rats, a phenomenon originally described by Eker (25). Susceptibility to this tumor is dominantly inherited, as with so many human tumors. We believe that tumor formation requires a second somatic event, effecting loss of the normal gene copy. The gene seems to be a recessive lethal in the whole animal, since presumptive homozygotes die at a fetal age of 9–10 days (unpublished results). Evidently the normal allele of the renal carcinoma gene is important in development.

Another example of developmental abnormality associated with a cancer gene is provided by a mutant called lethal giant larva in *Drosophila*. In homozygotes for this mutation the putative optic center of the adult fly behaves abnormally, failing to undergo normal differentiation and giving rise to a neuroblastoma-like tumor that is lethal to the larva (26). The cloned gene is able to correct the defect in mutant cells (27). It will now be of interest to see if the DNA of the normal retinoblastoma gene can be transfected into tumor cells to reverse their oncogenicity. Hope that this may be possible stems from the observation of Eric Stanbridge and his colleagues that a normal chromosome 11p segment can reverse the tumorigenicity of Wilms' tumor (28). Such a finding would provide final proof of the recessiveness of oncogenic mutations of the gene, and raise the possibility of a new approach to the treatment of tumors caused by the recessive mechanism.

ACKNOWLEDGMENTS

Preparation of this manuscript was supported by Grants CA-06927 and CA-43211 from the United States Public Health Service and by an appropriation from the Commonwealth of Pennsylvania.

REFERENCES

1. Knudson, A. G. Mutation and cancer: statistical study of retinoblastoma. Proc. Natl. Acad. Sci. U.S.A., *68*: 820–823, 1971.
2. Chaganti, R. S., Schonberg, S., and German, J. A manyfold increase in sister chromatid exchanges in Bloom's syndrome lymphocytes. Proc. Natl. Acad. Sci. U.S.A., *71*: 4508–4512, 1974.
3. Festa, R. S., Meadows, A. T., and Boshes, R. A. Leukemia in a black child with Bloom's syndrome. Cancer, *44*: 1507–1510, 1979.
4. Knudson, A. G., Strong, L. C. Mutation and cancer: a model for Wilms' tumor of the kidney. J. Natl. Cancer Inst., *48*: 313–324, 1972.
5. Knudson, A. G. and Strong, L. C. Mutation and cancer: neuroblastoma and pheochromocytoma. Am. J. Hum. Genet., *24*: 514–532, 1972.
6. Miller, R. W., Fraumeni, J. F., and Manning, M. D. Association of Wilms' tumor with aniridia, hemihypertrophy and other congenital malformations. N. Engl. J. Med., *270*: 922–927, 1964.
7. Knudson, A. G., Strong, L. C., Anderson, D. E. Heredity and cancer in man. Prog.

Med. Genet., *9*: 113–158, 1973.

8. Knudson, A. G., Meadows, A. T., Nichols, W. W., and Hill, R. Chromosomal deletion and retinoblastoma. N. Engl. J. Med., *295*: 1120–1123, 1976.

9. Yunis, J. J. and Ramsay, N.K.C. Retinoblastoma and subband deletion of chromosome 13. Am. J. Dis. Child., *132*: 161–163, 1978.

10. Ladda, R., Atkins, L., Littlefield, J., Neurath, P., and Marimuthu, K. M. Computer-assisted analysis of chromosomal abnormalities: detection of a deletion in aniridia/Wilms' tumor syndrome. Science, *185*: 784–787, 1974.

11. Francke, U., Holmes, L. B., Atkins, L., and Riccardi, V. M. Aniridia-Wilms' tumor association: evidence for specific deletion of 11p13. Cytogenet. Cell Genet., *24*: 185–192, 1979.

12. Sparkes, R. S., Sparkes, M. C., Wilson, M. G., Towner, J. W., Benedict, W., Murphree, A. L., and Yunis, J. J. Regional assignment of genes for human esterase D and retinoblastoma to chromosome band 13q14. Science, *208*: 1042–1044, 1980.

13. Sparkes, R. S., Murphree, A. L., Lingua, R. W., Sparkes, M. C., Field, L. L., Funderburk, S. J., and Benedict, W. F. Gene for hereditary retinoblastoma assigned to human chromosome 13 by linkage to esterase D. Science, *219*: 971–973, 1983.

14. Knudson, A. G. Retinoblastoma: a prototypic hereditary neoplasm. Semin. Oncol., *5*: 57–60, 1978.

15. Godbout, R., Dryja, T. P., Squire, J., Gallie, B. L., and Phillips, R. A. Somatic inactivation of genes on chromosome 13 is a common event in retinoblastoma. Nature, *304*: 451–453, 1983.

16. Benedict, W. F., Murphree, A. L., Banerjee, A., Spina, C. A., Sparkes, M. D., and Sparkes, R. S. Patient with 13 chromosome deletion: evidence that the retinoblastoma gene is a recessive cancer gene. Science, *219*: 973–975, 1983.

17. Cavenee, W. K., Dryja, T. P., Phillips, R. A., Benedict, W. F., Godbout, R., Gallie, B. L., Murphree, A. L., Strong, L. C., and White, R. L. Expression of recessive alleles by chromosomal mechanisms in retinoblastoma. Nature, *305*: 779–784, 1983.

18. Koufos, A., Hansen, M. F., Lampkin, D. B., Workman, M. L., Copeland, N. G., Jenkins, N. A., and Cavenee, W. K. Loss of alleles at loci on human chromosome 11 during genesis of Wilms' tumour. Nature, *309*: 170–172, 1984.

19. Friend, S. H., Bernards, R., Rogelj, S., Weinberg, R. A., Rapaport, J. M., Albert, D. M., and Dryja, T. P. A human DNA segment with properties of the gene that predisposes to retinoblastoma and osteosarcoma. Nature, *323*: 643–646, 1986.

20. Lee, W-H., Bookstein, R., Hong, F., Young, L-J., Shew, J-Y., and Lee, E. Y-H. P. Human retinoblastoma susceptibility gene: cloning, identification, and sequence. Science, *235*: 1394–1399, 1987.

21. Fung, Y-K. T., Murphree, A. L., T'Ang, A., Qian, J., Hinrichs, S. H., and Benedict, W. F. Structural evidence for the authenticity of the human retinoblastoma gene. Science, *236*: 1657–1661, 1987.

22. Lee, W-H., Shew, J-Y., Hong, F. D., Sery, T. W., Donoso, L. A., Young, L-J., Bookstein, R., and Lee, E. Y-H. P. The retinoblastoma susceptibility gene encodes a nuclear phosphoprotein associated with DNA binding activity. Nature, *329*: 642–645, 1987.

23. Bodmer, W. F., Bailey, C. J., Bodmer, J., Bussey, H.J.R., Ellis, A., Gorman, P., Lucibello, F. C., Murday, V. A., Rider, S. H., Scambler, P., Sheer, D., Solomon, E., and Spurr, N. K. Localization of the gene for familial adenomatous polyposis on chromosome 5. Nature, *328*: 614–616, 1987.

24. Solomon, E., Voss, R., Hall, V., Bodmer, W. F., Jass, J. R., Jeffreys, A. J., Lucibello, F. C., Patel, I., and Rider, S. H. Chromosome 5 allele loss in human colorectal car-

cinomas. Nature, *328*: 616–619, 1987.

25. Eker, R., Mossige, J., Johannessen, J. V., and Aars, H. Hereditary renal adenomas and adenocarcinomas in rats. Diag. Histopathol., *4*: 99–110, 1981.

26. Gateff, E. Malignant neoplasms of genetic origin in *Drosophila melanogaster*. Science, *200*: 1448–1459, 1978.

27. Jacob, L., Opper, M., Metzroth, B., Phannavong, B., and Mechler, B. M. Structure of the 1(2) gl gene of *Drosophila* and delimitation of its tumor suppressor domain. Cell, *50*: 215–225, 1987.

28. Weissman, B. E., Saxon, P. J., Pasquale, S. R., Jones, G. R., Geiser, A. G., and Stanbridge, E. J. Introduction of a normal human chromosome 11 into a Wilms' tumor cell line controls its tumorigenic expression. Science, *236*: 175–180, 1987.

UNUSUAL OCCURRENCES AS CLUES TO CANCER ETIOLOGY, R. W. MILLER ET AL. (EDS.),
JAPAN SCI. SOC. PRESS, TOKYO/TAYLOR & FRANCIS, LTD., PP. 233–242, 1988

Chromosomes and Cancer Families

D. G. HARNDEN

Paterson Institute for Cancer Research, Christie Hospital and Holt Radium Institute, Manchester, M20 9BX, England, UK

Abstract: At the beginning of this century Theodor Boveri predicted that specific chromosome changes would be found to have a causal role in neoplasia. We are now beginning to acquire the evidence to substantiate this hypothesis. The evidence comes from two particular sources, (i) genetic environmental interactions and (ii) specific constitutional chromosome aberrations. Cancer incidence varies throughout the world. This is often due to the interaction of an environmental agent with a genetically varied population. Using UV and ionising radiation as examples it is argued that some individuals are more susceptible to genetic damage by these agents. Moreover, the genetic lesions which are caused by these agents are now being shown to be relevant to cancer. In the radiosensitive syndrome ataxia-telangiectasia for example, specific chromosome rearrangements have been defined which seem likely to be directly involved in the development of leukaemia in these patients. The second line of evidence comes from the study of patients who have constitutional chromosome abnormalities associated with susceptibility to specific cancers. It has now been shown that these chromosome changes mark the location of genes which are involved in the development of cancer and that these same loci are also important in the non-familial forms of these diseases. Thus we are beginning to understand for the first time the mechanistic pathway that leads from environmental agents, through chromosome damage, to the alteration of specific genes which control the neoplastic process.

Chromosome abnormalities are found in many tumour cells and there has been much discussion as to whether the aberrations are causal, or whether they are secondary but important, or perhaps even epiphenomena of no particular importance. It is interesting to look back at the work of Theodor Boveri who observed the orderly separation of chromosomes in normal cells and in his monograph of 1914 (*1*) made certain predictions about the relationships of chromosome abnormalities to the development of cancer, which look quite remarkable in view of recent developments in this field (Table 1).

TABLE 1. Predictions by Boveri

1)	Genomic rearrangements are causal.
2)	Monoclonal origin
3)	Specific aberrations associated with particular neoplasms
4)	Defect on one chromosome, compensated in diploid state, is manifest on loss of the homologous chromosome.
5)	State of differentiation of tissue will be critical.
6)	Genomic changes caused by exogenous agents
7)	Some apparently normal cancers will prove to be pseudo-diploid.
8)	Leukaemias will be similar to solid cancers.

Derived from Wolf (2)

It is now clear that some of the chromosome changes found in cancer and leukaemia involve alterations in genes which are of great importance in the development of neoplasia. Moreover, for the first time it seems possible that the mechanisms which link damage caused by environmental agents to the neoplastic process may be amenable to investigation. Our new understanding has come from a number of different sources but only two of these will be considered in this presentation (a) genetic environmental interactions and (b) constitutional chromosome aberrations.

Genetic Environmental Interactions

While it is clear that environmental factors play a crucial role in determining the occurrence of cancer, it is equally important to recognise that these environmental agencies are acting upon a very varied human population. The pattern of cancer incidence in the population will therefore be determined by both factors. Individual variation in response may be due to physiological variations in the way in which the environmental stimulus is handled by the individual, or to genetic differences between individuals. There is now much evidence to show that this latter is an important mechanism in carcinogenesis.

1. UV radiation

Let us first consider a rather obvious example to establish the principle. The ultra violet radiation in sunlight has a large potential for causing damage to the DNA in the nuclei of human skin cells but the actual amount of damage will depend upon the length and intensity of the exposure, the ability of the light to reach the skin cell nuclei and the capacity of these cells for repair. Table 2 shows the incidence of skin cancers in different populations in different parts of the world. It can be deduced that skin cancer is dependent upon the amount of sunlight exposure (white males in El Paso, Texas have six times more cancer than white males in Birmingham, England) but also upon the degree of skin pigmentation (white males in Birmingham have 20 times more skin cancer than black males in Ibadan). This is, therefore, a well documented but often overlooked, example of interaction between an environmental carcinogen and a genetically determined predisposing factor.

This particular example can be taken a little further since in several genetic diseases the reduced capacity of the cells to repair UV induced DNA damage, also

TABLE 2. Incidence of Skin Carcinoma (ICD 173)

	Male	Female
Ibadan, Nigeria	2.6	2.9
El Paso, Texas (Spanish)	35.2	36.1
(other White)	278.5	137.6
England, Birmingham	49.4	30.8
Liverpool	45.8	30.1
Japan, Miyagi	1.4	1.2
Okayama	1.7	4.8
Osaka	1.1	0.4

From Waterhouse et al. (3)

Age standardised rates/10^5-population (Based on truncated world population)

determines susceptibility to skin cancer. For example, patients with xeroderma pigmentosum (XP) vary in their capacity to carry out excision repair of DNA damage and this variation is correlated with severity of the symptoms of the disease including the induction of skin cancers. It is interesting to note that these two genetic factors can interact with each other so that patients with XP who also have strongly pigmented skin are less severely affected than XP patients with poorly pigmented skin.

The precise mechanism by which the sensitivity to UV light leads on to the development of cancer is still not clear even after intensive investigation but clearly DNA damage is implicated. The frequency of mutations is increased in XP cells compared to normals after UV exposure (4) but these mutations per se have not been linked directly to cellular transformation and tumour induction.

2. Ionising radiation

There have been a number of attempts to demonstrate variation in sensitivity to ionising radiation. Weichselbaum et al. (5) have studied the sensitivity to killing by ionising radiation of cells taken from patients who have shown an unusual sensitivity to radiation as measured by skin erythema. No correlation was detected. Similarly Smith et al. (6) have studied a group of patients showing an unusually severe skin reaction to radiotherapy. They observed that all 6 of the patients studied had either a reduced D_0 value or a low extrapolation number and the two most severely affected patients had low values for both measures. However, they had only 2 'normal' controls and it is not clear that the observed variation was statistically outside normal variation.

It is quite clear that there is substantial variation between 'normal individuals' in measurements of cellular radiosensitivity. Arlett and Harcourt (7) described radiosensitivity of a large number of human cell strains and define the normal range of D_0 values to lie between 97 and 180 rads, but this cellular variation was not correlated with any clinical measure of radiosensitivity. In a later paper, however, Arlett (8) reports a degree of hypersensitivity at the cellular level and a reduced capacity for repair of potential lethal damage in four individuals judged to be radiosensitive following radiotherapy using a range of clinical criteria. There is thus some evidence that 'normal' individuals vary in cellular radiosensitivity though the differences are not large and it is not always clear that this variation correlates with the variation in radiosensitivity which is noted in clinical practice.

Ataxia Telangiectasia (A-T)

A-T is a rare recessively inherited syndrome involving progressive cerebellar degeneration, and distinguished from other forms of ataxia by the striking telangiectases on the eyes, face and ears.

1.   Radiosensitivity

It is now well known that A-T patients are sensitive to ionising radiation and to a limited range of radiomimetic drugs. In view of the theme of this meeting it may be of interest to outline briefly how this was recognised. In 1966, Hecht and his colleagues (*9*) drew attention to the association of A-T with leukaemia and chromosome abnormalities in peripheral blood cells. For this reason my colleagues and I were studying a number of patient with A-T (*10, 11*). One of these patients developed a lymphoma and following a course of radiotherapy died after a severe adverse reaction to the radiation. Discussions between Dr. Gillian Mann and Dr. R. W. Miller who knew of 2 other similar cases led to the publication of a case report (*12*) which drew general attention to the problem of clinical radiosensitivity in A-T. With this knowledge and the example of XP before us Dr. Malcolm Taylor, Professor Bryn Bridges and I planned a series of experiments on cells from A-T patients including banked cells from the patient referred to above which led to the publication of the first report identifying cellular radiosensitivity in A-T patients (*13*). It is now well documented that all A-T patients are sensitive to ionising radiation though recently it has been shown that the syndrome is perhaps not as clearly defined as had been thought. Taylor *et al.* (*14*) report 3 patients with some of the features of A-T who show levels of chromosomal and cellular radiosensitivity intermediate between normal individuals and classical A-T.

Some aspects of the sensitivity to ionising radiation are now clear. There is a defect in repair of radiation induced DNA lesions best illustrated by the absence of potential lethal damage repair of lesions induced by low LET radiation (*15*). Further, whereas normal cells respond to exposure to ionising radiation by rapidly reducing the rate of DNA replication synthesis, A-T cells do not do so (*16*). Cox *et al.* (*17*) have reported that A-T cells show a lack of fidelity in the repair of specific DNA lesions in transfected plasmids. However, Green and Lowe (*18*) using a different plasmid failed to find any DNA repair related defect. The precise nature of the defect at the molecular level is thus still undefined.

The important question of how these abnormalities of DNA repair and DNA replication relate to the susceptibility to leukaemia, lymphoma and other cancers in A-T is also not yet answered. However, important clues are emerging from a study of the chromosomes of these patients.

2.   Chromosome Aberrations

Not only are A-T cells unusually sensitive to the induction of chromosome damage by ionising radiation (*19*) but also the occurrence of spontaneous chromo-

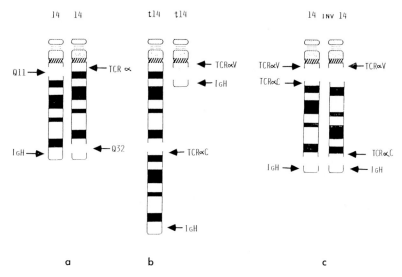

FIG. 1. Chromosome rearrangements in ataxia-telangiectasia. (a) two normal chromosomes 14 showing the breakpoints at q11 and q32, and the location of the TCRα and IgH genes (b) *t*(14; 14) (q11; q32) showing that the breakpoint at q11 splits the TCRα gene separating the variable (V) and constant (c) regions. (C) inv (14) (q11 q32) showing the same breakpoints as in (b).

some abnormalities in peripheral blood lymphocytes and other cells is a major feature of A-T patients. Clones of lymphocytes carrying specific chromosome abnormalities are found in a high proportion of these patients. Many of these clones involve specific chromosomal breakpoints, particularly at 14q11 and at 14q32 (*20*). Indeed, the commonest rearrangements are the reciprocal translocation *t*(14;14) (q11; q32) and the inversion *t*(14) (q11q32). It is becoming clear that these breakpoints are at or close to specific gene loci which are involved in the development and differentiation of T cells (Fig. 1). Kennaugh *et al.* (*21*) have shown, using *in situ* hybridisation techniques, that DNA probes for the α chain of the T cell receptor (TCRα) and for the immunoglobulin heavy chain gene (IgH) that, in a patient with a *t*(14; 14), the break point at 14q11 falls within the α chain locus of the T cell receptor and that the breakpoint at 14q32 is proximal to the IgH locus.

On several occasions clones of cells have been studied both before and after the emergence of leukaemia. In some cases, at least, the clonal karyotype is closely associated with the occurrence of leukaemia. For example Taylor and Butterworth (*22*) followed a patient with a complex karyotype including an inversion of chromosome 14 during the evolution of a T cell leukaemia. Detailed analysis of the breakpoints in this clone shows that the breakpoint at 14q11 occurs at the J region of the TCRα gene while the 14q32 breakpoint is downstream, *i.e.*, proximal to the IgHCμ locus (*23*). The authors conclude that there is an as yet undiscovered gene downstream from the IgH locus which is important in leukaemogenesis.

It seems possible therefore that in A-T we are close to making the link between the induction of genetic lesions by an environmental agent and the initiation of neoplasia.

Constitutional Chromosome Rearrangements and Neoplasia

While A-T is a good example of the involvement of chromosome abnormalities in familial cancer and also a good example of how chance happenings at the clinical level can lead on to a deeper understanding of neoplasia, it is by no means unique. There are now many other examples of specific chromosome abnormalities associated with familial neoplasia. These differ from A-T in being constitutional abnormalities and in several of these cases the initial clue to the association came from clinical observation on a single case (Fig. 2, Table 3).

1.   Retinoblastoma

Lele *et al.* (*24*) described the first case of deletion of a 'D group' chromosome in a child with retinoblastoma. This patient was entirely normal at birth and although development was slow she seemed quite healthy till bilateral retinoblastoma was recognised at 10 months of age. There was no family history of retinoblastoma. A large deletion of a D group chromosome was clearly identified in both tumour and normal somatic cells. It was thought at the time that this was chromosome 15

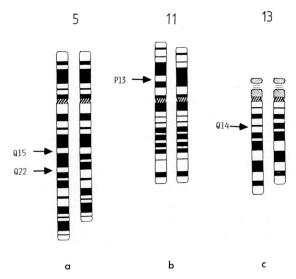

FIG. 2.   Chromosome deletions in hereditary cancer susceptibility. In each case the normal chromosome is on the left. (a) del (5) (q15 q22) in familial adenomatous polyposis. (b) del (11) (p13) in Wilms' AGR syndrome. (c) del (13) (q14) in retinoblastoma.

TABLE 3.   Constitutional Chromosome Abnormalities Associated with Cancer Susceptibility

Chromosome abnormality	Syndrome	Cancer susceptibility	Reference
del 13 (q 14)	Multiple congenital abnormalities (MCA)	Retinoblastoma	Lele *et al.* (*24*)
del 11 (p 13)	Aniridia-genitourinary retardation syndrome (AGR)	Wilms' tumour	Riccardi *et al.* (*29*)
del 5 (q 15-q22)	Familial adenomatous polyposis & MCA	Carcinoma of the colon	Herrera *et al.* (*31*)

(using non-banded chromosomes). Five other cases of retinoblastoma examined at the same time were chromosomally normal. However, the authors clearly were aware of the significance of their finding—"the possibility remains that deletion of a part of this chromosome removed a normal allele which would have allowed the (abnormal) gene to become active in its hemizygous form".

Since this early description it has taken nearly 20 years to approach an understanding of the significance of the deletion. Briefly, this visible chromosome deletion at 13q14 is found in around 5% of cases of retinoblastoma. It is also clear that sub-microscopic deletions are present in a small number of cases as measured by the deletion of the closely linked esterase D gene or of linked anonymous DNA probes. More important, however, deletion of all or part of chromosome 13 or a translocation involving 13q14 is found in a substantial proportion of retinoblastoma tumours (25). In appropriate families this can be measured by loss of heterozygosity for polymorphic markers in this region, even in the absence of overt chromosome change. The pattern that has emerged is consistent with the hypothesis of Knudson (26) that two hits are required for the initiation of the neoplastic process in retinoblastoma and that in hereditary retinoblastoma one of these hits is inherited. There is now the further implication that the retinoblastoma gene is at this locus and moreover that, at the cellular level it behaves in a recessive manner. The nature of this locus is now the subject of intense investigation. Friend et al. (27) described the isolation of a fragment of DNA from this region which they put forward as a candidate for the retinoblastoma gene. Characterisation of the gene product suggests that this protein, which is present in many normal cells but not in retinoblastoma cells, is a phosphoprotein with DNA binding properties suggesting that it may be a gene with a regulatory function (28).

2.   Wilms' tumour

In 1978 Riccardi and his colleagues (29) described 3 cases of a syndrome comprising aniridia, genito-urinary abnormalities and mental retardation (AGR) all of whom had deletions of the short arm of chromosome 11. One of these patients had a Wilms' tumour.

It has subsequently been shown that there is a close association between Wilms' tumour, the AGR triad and an interstitial deletion at 11p13. As with retinoblastoma it has been possible to demonstrate loss of heterozygosity at this locus using linked genes and DNA probes not only in Wilms' tumour but also in rhabdomyosarcoma and hepatoblastoma (30).

3.   Familial adenomatous polyposis (FAP)

With the models of retinoblastoma and Wilms' tumour already well known the exploitation of a single case of polyposis coli described by Herrera et al. (31) has been both rapid and dramatic. This patient is a 42 year old white male with mental retardation, colon carcinoma, horseshoe kidney, absence of left lobe of the liver, agenesis of the gall bladder and multiple colonic polyps (possible Gardner's syndrome). He has a deletion of chromosome 5 defined as either del (5) (q13q15) or del (5) (q15q22). The authors state that he is the first case of polyposis coli with a deletion of chromosome 5.

Bodmer *et al.* (*32*), realising the significance of this case, used a series of DNA probes known to be on chromosome 5 to study linkage with polyposis coli in 124 members of 13 different families. One probe showed a close linkage to FAP and subsequent *in situ* hybridisation showed the probe to localise at 5q21–q22 consistent with the findings of Herrera *et al.*. This study was taken a stage further by Solomon *et al.* (*33*) who showed that in the tumour cells from non-familial cases of carcinoma of the colon there was a loss of heterozygosity at this locus in at least 20% of the cases studied. Ten out of 40 cases studied showed loss of one allele of a highly polymorphic, locus specific mini-satellite probe which maps at 5q34-q ter. This finding is most consistent with loss of the whole of the long arm of chromosome 5 and possibly of the whole chromosome.

The extension of the observation of an abnormality in a single case, through a familial situation, to the recognition of a consistent abnormality in a common cancer is remarkable. In this instance, the link was made in just over one year largely because the technology for exploitation of such situations is now available.

Conclusions

From this brief survey I want to draw two conclusions. First, we are now beginning to understand the importance of genetic change in neoplasia. We have 3 elements. (i) Environmental agents which cause cancer often also cause DNA and/ or chromosome damage. (ii) Visible chromosome changes and other genetic lesions are found in cancer cells. (iii) Some cancers have an inherited basis. Till recently it has not been possible to link these three approaches and even now our knowledge of the association is imperfect. However, from the studies described in this report it can be postulated that chromosome and DNA damage induced by radiation is an integral part of the neoplastic process (A-T and XP); that this may well act by the selection of specific rearrangements which affect critical loci (clones in A-T); that constitutional chromosome abnormalities affecting the same or similar loci are critical in the development of neoplasia (retinoblastoma, Wilms' tumour and familial adenomatous polyposis); and that some at least of the chromosome abnormalities seen in cancers are the same as, or are similar in nature to these highly specific inherited or induced abnormalities and play a vital part in the development of cancer.

Thus, we are at last getting some answers to the questions raised so long ago by Boveri.

Second, in keeping with the theme of this symposium, it is clear that the recognition of unusual clinical features in patients can be exploited and lead to an understanding of disease processes at the cellular and molecular level. The recognition of clinical radiosensitivity in an A-T patient has led to the identification of a DNA repair defect and may also help us to understand how DNA damage leads on to highly specific chromosome abnormalities associated with neoplasia. The observation in 3 separate instances of congenital malformations associated with chromosome deletion and neoplasia is leading towards the identification of the genes responsible for these cancers. It may therefore be possible to exploit similar observations in the future.

REFERENCES

1. Boveri, T. Zur Frage der Entstehung maligner Tumoren, Gustave Fischer, Jena, 1914.
2. Wolf, U. T. Boveri and his book "On the Problem of the Origin of Malignant Tumours." *In;* J. German (ed.), Chromosomes and Cancer, pp. 3–20, Wiley, New York, 1974.
3. Waterhouse, J.A.H., Muir, C., Correa, P., and Powell, J. Cancer Incidence in Five Continents, Vol. III, International Agency for Research on Cancer, Lyon, 1976.
4. Maher, V. M. and McCormick, J. J. Effect of DNA repair on the cytotoxicity and mutagenicity of UV irradiation and of chemical carcinogens in normal and xeroderma pigmentosum cells. *In;* J. M. Yuhas, R. W. Tennant, and I. D. Regan (eds.), Biology of Radiation Carcinogenesis, pp. 129–145, Raven Press, New York, 1976.
5. Weichselbaum, R. R., Epstein, J., and Little, J. B. *In vitro* radiosensitivity of human diploid fibroblasts derived from patients with unusual clinical responses to radiation. Radiology, *121*: 479–482, 1976.
6. Smith, K. C., Haln, R. T., Hoppe, R. T., and Earle, J. D. Radiosensitivity *in vitro* of human fibroblasts derived from patients with a severe skin reaction to radiotherapy. Int. J. Rad. Onc. Biol. Phys., *6*: 1573–1575, 1980.
7. Arlett, C. F. and Harcourt, S. A. Survey of radiosensitivity in a variety of human cell strains. Cancer Res. *40*: 926–932, 1980.
8. Arlett, C. *In;* E. M. Fielden, J. F. Fowler, J. H. Hendry, and D. Scott (eds.), Proceedings of the 8th International Congress of Radiation Research. Vol. 2. The Radiosensitivity of Cultured Human Cells, pp. 424–430, Taylor & Francis Ltd., London, 1987.
9. Hecht, F., Koler, R. D., Rigas, D. A., Dahnke, G. S., Case, M. P., Tisdale, V., and Miller, R. W. Leukaemia and lymphocytes in ataxia telangiectasia. Lancet, *ii*: 1193, 1966.
10. Harnden, D. G. Ataxia telangiectasia syndrome: cytogenetic and cancer aspects. *In;* J. German (ed.), Chromosomes and Cancer, pp. 620–636, John Wiley & Sons Inc., New York, 1974.
11. Oxford, J. M., Harnden, D. G., Parrington, M., and Delhanty, J.D.A. Specific chromosome aberrations in ataxia telangiectasia. J. Med. Genet., *12*: 251–262, 1975.
12. Cunliffe, P. N., Mann, J. R., Cameron, A. H., Roberts, K. D., and Ward, H.W.C. Radiosensitivity in ataxia telangiectasia. Br. J. Radiology, *48*: 374–376, 1974.
13. Taylor, A.M.R., Harnden, D. G., Arlett, C. F., Harcourt, S. A. Lehmann, A. R., Stevens, S., and Bridges, B. A. Ataxia-telangiectasia: a human mutation with abnormal radiation sensitivity. Nature, *258*: 427–429, 1975.
14. Taylor, A.M.R., Flude, E., Laher, B., Stacey, M., McKay, E., Watt, J., Green, S. H., and Harding, A. E. Variant forms of ataxia telangiectasia. J. Med. Genet., *24*: 669–677, 1987.
15. Cox, R. A cellular description of the repair defect in ataxia telangiectasia. *In;* B. A. Bridges and D. G. Harnden (eds.), Ataxia Telangiectasia—a cellular and molecular link between cancer, neuropathology and immune deficiency, pp. 141–153, John Wiley, Chichester, 1982.
16. Lavin, M. F., Ford, M. D., and Houldsworth, J. DNA replication in ataxia telangiectasia cells after exposure to ionising radiation. *In;* B. A. Bridges and D. G. Harnden (eds.), Ataxia Telangiectasia—a cellular and molecular link between cancer, neuropathology and immune deficiency, pp. 319–326, John Wiley, Chichester, 1982.
17. Cox, R., Debenham, P., Masson, W. K., and Webb, M.B.T. Ataxia telangiectasia: a human mutation giving high frequency misrepair of DNA double-stranded scissions. Mol. Biol. Med., *3*: 229–244, 1986.

18. Green, M.H.L. and Lowe, J. E. Failure to detect a DNA repair-related defect in the transfection of ataxia telangiectasia cells by enzymatically restricted plasmid. Int. J. Rad. Biol., *52*: 3, 437–446, 1987.

19. Taylor, A.M.R. Cytogenetics of ataxia telangiectasia. *In;* B. A. Bridges, D. G. Harnden (eds.), Ataxia telangiectasia: a cellular and molecular link between cancer, neuropathology, and immune deficiency, pp. 53–82, John Wiley, Chichester, 1982.

20. McCaw, B. K., Hecht, F., Harnden, D. G., and Teplitz, K. L. Somatic rearrangement of chromosome 14 in human lymphocytes. Proc. Natl. Acad. Sci. U.S.A., *72*: 2071–2075, 1975.

21. Kennaugh, A., Butterworth, S., Hollis, R., Baer, P., Rabbits, T. H., and Taylor, A.M.R. The chromosome breakpoint at 14q32 in an ataxia telangiectasia *t* (14; 14) T cell clone is different from the 14q32 breakpoint in Burkitt's and an inversion T cell lymphoma. Human Genet., *73*: 254–259, 1986.

22. Taylor, A.M.R. and Butterworth, S. V. Clonal evolution of T-cell chronic lymphocytic leukaemia in a patient with ataxia telangiectasia. Int. J. Cancer, *37*: 4, 511–516, 1986.

23. Baer, R., Heppell, A., Taylor, A.M.R., Rabbits, P. H., Boullier, B., and Rabbits, T. H. The breakpoint of an inversion in a T cell leukaemia, sequences downstream of the immunoglobulin heavy chain locus implicated in tumorigenesis. Proc. Natl. Acad. Sci. U.S.A., *84*: 9069–9073, 1987.

24. Lele, K. P., Penrose, L. S., and Stallard, H. B. Chromosome deletion in a case of retinoblastoma. Ann. Haem. Genet., *27*: 171–174, 1963.

25. Cavanee, W. K., Dryja, T. P., Philips, R. A., Benedict, W. F., Godbout, R., Gallie, B. L., Murphree, A. L., Strong, L. C., and White, R. L. Expression of recessive alleles by chromosomal mechanisms in retinoblastoma. Nature, *305*: 779–784, 1983.

26. Knudson, A. G. Mutation and cancer: Statistical study of retinoblastoma. Proc. Natl. Acad. Sci. U.S.A., *68*: 820–823, 1971.

27. Friend, S. H., Bernard, S. R., Rogelj, S., Weinberg, R. A., Rapaport, J. M., Albert, D. M., and Dryja, T. P. A human DNA segment with properties of the gene which predisposes to retinoblastoma and osteosarcoma. Nature, *323*: 643–646, 1986.

28. Lee, W-H., Shew, J-Y., Hong, F. D., Sery, T. W., Donoso, L. A., Young, L. J., Brookstein, R., and Lee, E. Y-H. The retinoblastoma susceptibility gene encodes a nuclear phosphoprotein associated with DNA binding activity. Nature, *329*: 642–645, 1987.

29. Riccardi, V. M., Suhansky, E., Smith, A. C., and Francke, U. Chromosomal imbalance in the aniridia—Wilms' tumour association: 11p interstitial deletion. Pediatrics, *61*: 604–610, 1978.

30. Koufos, A., Hansen, M. F., Copeland, N. G., Jenkins, N. A., Lampkin, B. C., and Cavenee, W. K. Loss of heterozygosity in three embryonal tumours suggests a common pathogenic mechanism. Nature, *316*: 330–334, 1985.

31. Herrera, L., Kakati, S., Gibas, L., Pietrzak, E., and Sandberg, A. A. Gardner's syndrome in a man with an interstitial deletion of 5q. Am. J. Med. Genet., *25*: 473–476, 1986.

32. Bodmer, W. F., Bailey, C. J., Bodmer, J., Bussey, H.J.R., Ellis, A., Gorman, P., Lucibello, F. C., Murday, V. A., Rider, S. H., Scambler, P., Sheer, D., Solomon, D., and Spurr, N. K. Localisation of the gene for familial adenomatous polyposis on chromosome 5. Nature, *328*: 614–616, 1987.

33. Solomon, E., Voss, R., Hall, V., Bodmer, W. F., Jass, J. R., Jeffreys, A. J., Lucibello, F. C., Patel, L., and Rider, S. H. Chromosome 5 allele loss in human colorectal carcinomas. Nature, *328*: 617–619, 1987.

KEYNOTE LECTURE

The Familial Syndrome of Sarcomas and Other Neoplasms

Frederick P. Lı

Clinical Studies Section, Clinical Epidemiology Branch, National Cancer Institute, Boston, Massachusetts 02115, U.S.A.

Abstract: Observation of one kindred with sarcoma, breast cancer and other neoplasms has led to the recognition of a familial cancer syndrome in young patients.
To date, 24 affected families have been enrolled in the Cancer Family Registry of
the National Cancer Institute, and 21 others have been reported in the literature.
The major feature of the syndrome is an autosomal dominant pattern of breast
cancers and sarcomas of bone and soft tissue at unusually early ages. Additional
components of the syndrome appear to be brain tumors, leukemia, and adrenocortical carcinoma in children and adolescents. Family members are prone to develop
multiple primary cancer. In addition to descriptive reports, the syndrome has been
detected in segregation analysis of a consecutive series of children with soft tissue
sarcomas; in studies of breast cancer among mothers of unselected children with
sarcomas; and in prospective observation for new cancers in our previously reported
families. Laboratory studies are in progress to seek the gene(s) associated with this
syndrome of diverse cancers. Studies of this rare disorder may provide new insights
into the pathogenesis of the 5 component tumors, particularly breast cancer, the
commonest cancer among women in the United States and elsewhere.

A Clinical Observation

Studies of this cancer syndrome began with the observation of one affected
family. My introduction to the family occurred in 1967, soon after I joined Dr.
Robert W. Miller and Dr. Joseph F. Fraumeni, Jr. at the National Cancer Institute.
I heard about the family during a social conversation, was intrigued by the cancer
cluster, and arranged to see the proband. The family pedigree revealed that 3 young
patients had developed a soft tissue sarcoma, a rare neoplasm with an incidence
rate of approximately 1 per 100,000 persons in the general population (*1*). Cancer
of the breast and other sites had also developed among family members (Fig. 1).
A search of the literature revealed only isolated families with this constellation of
neoplasms.

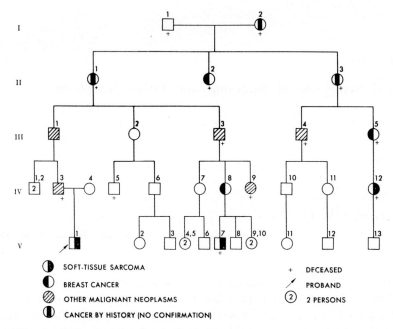

FIG. 1. Pedigree of the first family in the series.

Epidemiological Studies

Descriptive studies: To find similarly affected families, Dr. Miller suggested a review of death certificates and medical charts of children with soft tissue sarcomas. He had employed this approach to identify associations between birth defects and childhood cancers, such as aniridia and Wilms' tumor (*2*). Dr. Fraumeni and I visited 17 hospitals in 11 cities in the U.S. to abstract 280 medical charts of children with rhabdomyosarcoma. In addition we examined all death certificates for children with this neoplasm in the United States, 1960–64 (*3*). Three sib-pairs with childhood soft tissue sarcoma were found, when 0.06 sib-pair was expected on a chance basis (*1*). The 4 kindreds combined had 26 cancers, including 11 sarcomas, 7 breast cancers and 8 other tumors. Four of the breast cancers were in young mothers of sarcoma cases. Other young family members had diverse cancers, including leukemia and brain tumor. No environmental carcinogens were found to account for these familial cancer clusters. Fraumeni and I speculated that soft tissue sarcomas, breast cancer, and other neoplasms in young patients may represent a hereditary cancer syndrome.

To date, we have collected a total of 24 affected kindreds (8 previously reported) in the Cancer Family Registry of the National Cancer Institute, and have identified 21 other affected families in the literature (Table 1) (*1*, *4–18*). In our 24 families, each proband developed a sarcoma at age 45 or earlier, and at least 2 other relatives had cancer within this age-period. There were a total of 151 cancer patients in the 24 affected blood lines. Cancer in 119 of these patients (79%) was diagnosed before age 45, when only 10 percent of all cancers develop in the general population (*19*). The pattern of cancer in our families was consistent with autosomal dominant in-

TABLE 1. Cancers in Our 24 Families and in 21 Other Families in the Literature

Tumor[a]	No. of patients, (percent)[b]	
	NCI series (24 families)	Literature series[c] (21 families)
Sarcoma:	56 (37%)	44 (25%)
Soft tissue	35 (23%)	17 (10%)
Bone	21 (14%)	18 (10%)
Unknown site		9 (5%)
Breast	35 (23%)	46 (26%)
Brain	14 (9%)	25 (14%)
Leukemia	9 (6%)	10 (6%)
Adrenocortical	4 (3%)	9 (5%)
Other	33 (22%)	41 (23%)
All cancers	151 (100%)	175 (99%)

[a] Only first cancers are considered among those with multiple primaries.   [b] Cancer in 231 of the 325 patients in the combined series was diagnosed before age 45.   [c] See refs. *4–14*.

TABLE 2. Multiple Primary Cancers in 39 Members of 45 Families with the Syndrome

First cancer	Second cancer			
	Breast	Sarcoma	Brain, adrenal, leukemia	Other
Breast[a]	—	1	2	2
Sarcoma	1	14	3	4
Brain, adrenal, leukemia	0	1	2	0
Other	0	2	2	5

[a] Bilateral breast cancer is considered one neoplasm.

heritance. Sarcomas and breast cancer accounted for 91 (60 percent) of the neoplasms. The 56 sarcomas originated in both soft tissues and bone. The soft tissue sarcomas arose at a wide range of ages and anatomic regions, and were diverse in histology. Nearly all bone cancers were osteosarcoma that arose in the lower limbs between ages 5 and 28 years. Among the 35 breast cancer patients, 8 had bilateral neoplasms that often occurred at early ages (median, 33 years; range 22–47). Additional components of the syndrome, accounting for 18 percent of the cancers, occurred in 14 patients with brain tumors, 8 with leukemia, and 4 with adrenocortical carcinoma before age 45. The pattern of cancers in the 21 families in the literature is similar to that in our series (Table 1) (*4–14*). In particular, sarcoma and breast cancer comprised one-half of the cancers in these families, and brain tumors, leukemia, and adrenocortical carcinoma comprised another 25 percent. Also, both series show the tendency of family members to develop multiple primary cancers, often at early ages. Among the 39 patients with multiple cancers, 24 had 2 of the neoplasms featured in the syndrome, 10 had one component, and only 5 had none (Table 2). Second cancers in 6 of the 15 patients in our series occurred in the field of radiotherapy and appear to be due in part to the exposure.

Analytical studies: Familial clusters of cancer can be due to chance association. Therefore, we have followed the 4 families in our original report for the develop-

TABLE 3. Cancers in 4 Families, pre-1969 and 1969–80[a]

Tumor	Number of cancers[b]	
	pre-1969	1969–80[c]
Sarcoma	12	4
Breast cancer	11	5
Other	13	7
Total	36	16

[a] See ref. *20*. [b] Ages at diagnosis of cancer: 0–14 years, 12 cases; 15–34 years, 18 cases; ≥ 35 years, 22 cases. [c] Cancers expected between 1969 and 1980: 0.5 case; $p < 0.01$ when compared with 16 observed cases.

ment of additional cancers. If cancer aggregation in these families were due to chance, surviving family members would not be expected to develop an excess of new cancers. If, on the other hand, the families have a cancer syndrome, an excess of breast cancers, sarcomas and other neoplasms might occur on prospective observation. Between 1969 and 1980, we found that 10 of 31 surviving blood relatives developed a total of 16 additional cancers (*20*). The number exceeds the 0.5 cancers expected in these families by chance ($p < 0.01$). There were 4 soft tissue sarcomas, 5 breast cancers, and 7 other neoplasms (Table 3). Thus the 4 families are prone to develop these cancers, and work is in progress to extend the follow-up to all 24 families in our Registry.

The familial association between sarcoma and breast cancer has also been examined in other analytical studies. Williams and Strong performed segregation analysis of 159 families with probands who were 3-year survivors of a childhood soft tissue sarcoma (*21*). In 9 familial clusters, an autosomal dominant pattern of cancers was detected. One-half of the presumed gene carriers were affected by age 30 years, and 90 percent by age 60. A high frequency of multiple primary cancers was observed. The abnormal allele appears to have a low population frequency (0.00002). In a segregation analysis of 18 high-risk families with breast cancer and associated cancers, Go *et al.* (*22*) have identified 2 kindreds with an autosomal dominant pattern of breast cancer, sarcoma, and other neoplasms. Other studies by Birch and associates have examined the occurrence of cancer among the mothers of a population-based series of children with soft tissue and bone sarcomas (osteosarcoma and chondrosarcoma) (*23*, *24*). These mothers had a 3-fold increase of breast cancer, often at young ages, but not an excess of other cancers.

Laboratory Studies

We have conducted laboratory studies to seek the gene(s) involved in this cancer syndrome. The initial studies employed laboratory assays available in the late 1960's and early 1970's. These investigations examined unbanded and banded chromosomes of peripheral lymphocytes, titers of antibodies to Epstein-Barr virus and oncofetal antigens (carcinoembryonic antigen, alpha-fetoprotein, and human chorionic gonadotropin), immunoglobulin levels and lymphocyte blastogenic response to several mitogens, and fibroblast transformation *in vitro* by SV-40 virus and its T-antigen (*25*). The first decade of study of serology and somatic tissues yielded little definitive data. Recent reports on one affected family indicated that the cultured fibroblasts from several members are relatively resistant to killing by ionizing radiation, and that one fibroblast line has an activated oncogene (c-*raf-1*) detected in transfection experiments (*26, 27*). However, other families with this cancer syndrome did not manifest this radioresistance phenomenon, and additional studies of the role of oncogenes are in progress (*11*).

Our attention has now shifted from studies of fibroblasts to tumor tissues, particularly sarcoma cells. However, fresh tumor tissue from families with the syndrome is rarely available. Consequently we have studied, based on Knudson's postulate, sporadic (non-familial) sarcomas for genes that may predispose to this familial sarcoma syndrome (*28*). Non-random cytogenetic changes have been found in several histological subtypes of sarcoma: translocation between chromosomes 12 and 16 (*t*(12; 16)) in liposarcoma; *t*(X; 18) in synovial sarcoma; *t*(11; 22) in Ewing's sarcoma; *t*(3; 12) in lipoma; *t*(2; 13) in alveolar rhabdomyosarcoma; and 3p rearrangements in other rhabdomyosarcomas (*29, 30*). Molecular studies of childhood rhabdomyosarcoma by Koufos *et al.* have revealed loss of heterozygosity in the short arm of chromosome 11 (*31*). In addition, we have recently detected homozygous deletion in 3 of 16 soft tissue sarcomas examined with the retinoblastoma (Rb) gene probe that was isolated from chromosome 13q14 (*32*). Loss of genes in this region has been found in breast cancer, and the involvement of chromosome 13q in this familial syndrome merits additional investigation (*33*).

Comment

Why have we pursued studies of this rare syndrome for nearly 2 decades? The disorder affects only a few families and has almost no public health impact. The reason is that several major forms of childhood cancer are involved and that another component, breast cancer, is the commonest neoplasm among women in many parts of the world. The etiology and pathogenesis of breast cancer remain poorly understood despite intense study with conventional methods. Our approach is to study the rare, but hopefully informative, families with this cancer syndrome to gain new insights into genetic mechanisms involved in breast cancer and childhood neoplasms in general. This strategy is exemplified by the recent studies of the rare families with adenomatous polyposis to localize a gene involved in carcinoma of the colon (*34*). The same genetic abnormality has been found in fresh tumor tissue from sporadic (non-familial) cancer of the colon (*35*).

REFERENCES

1. Li, F. P. and Fraumeni, J. F., Jr. Soft-tissue sarcomas, breast cancer, and other neoplasms: A familial syndrome? Ann. Intern. Med., *71*: 747–752, 1969.
2. Miller, R. W., Fraumeni, J. F., Jr., and Manning, M. D. Association of Wilms's tumor with aniridia, hemihypertrophy and other congenital malformations. N. Engl. J. Med., *270*: 922–927, 1964.
3. Li, F. P. and Fraumeni, J. F., Jr. Rhabdomyosarcoma in children: Epidemiologic

study and identification of a familial cancer syndrome. J. Natl. Cancer Inst., *43*: 1365–1373, 1969.

4. Pearson, A.D.J., Craft, A. W., Ratcliffe, J. M., Birch, J. M., Morris-Jones, P., and Roberts, D. F. Two families with the Li-Fraumeni cancer family syndrome. J. Med. Genet., *19*: 362–365, 1982.

5. Epstein, L. I., Bixler, D., and Bennett, J. E. An incident of familial cancer. Cancer, *25*: 889–891, 1970.

6. Duncan, M. H. and Miller, R. W. Another family with the Li-Fraumeni cancer syndrome. JAMA, *249*: 195, 1983.

7. Meisner, L. F., Gilbert, E., Ris, H. W., and Haverty, G. Genetic mechanisms in cancer predisposition. Report of a cancer family. Cancer, *43*: 679–689, 1979.

8. Bottomly, R. H., Trainer, A. L., and Condit, P. T. Chromosome studies in a "Cancer Family". Cancer, *28*: 519–528, 1971.

9. Lynch, H. T., Mulcahy, G. M., Harris, R. E., Gurgis, H. A., and Lynch, J. F. Genetic and pathologic findings in a kindred with hereditary sarcoma breast cancer, brain tumors, leukemia, lung, laryngeal, and adrenal cortical carcinoma. Cancer, *41*: 2055–2064, 1978.

10. Lynch, H. T., Krush, A. J., Harlan, W. L., and Sharp, E. A. Association of soft tissue sarcoma, leukemia, and brain tumors in families affected with breast cancer. Am. Surg., *39*: 199–206, 1973.

11. Little, J. B., Nove, J., Dahlberg, W. K., Troilo, P., Nichols, W. W., and Strong, L. C. Normal cytotoxic response of skin fibroblasts from patients with Li-Fraumeni familial cancer syndrome to DNA-damaging agents *in vitro*. Cancer Res., *47*: 4229–4234, 1987.

12. Miller, C. W. and McLaughlin, R. B. Osteosarcoma in siblings. Report of two cases. J. Bone Joint Surg., *59*-A: 261–262, 1977.

13. Lynch, H. T., and Gurgis, H. A. Childhood cancer and the SBLA syndrome. Med. Hypotheses, *5*: 15–22, 1979.

14. Smith, J. W., Ali, K., Caces, J. N., Coburn, T. P., Kumar, A.P.M., and Mauer, A. M. Familial cancer: The occurrence of bone cancer in male members of a family in multiple generations. Clin. Res., *28*: 869–A, 1980.

15. Fraumeni, J. F., Jr., Vogel, C. L., and Easton, J. M. Sarcomas and multiple polyposis in a kindred. Arch. Intern. Med., *121*: 57–61, 1968.

16. Li, F. P., Tucker, M. A., and Fraumeni, J. F., Jr. Childhood cancer in sibs. J. Pediatr., *88*: 419–423, 1976.

17. Blattner, W. A., McGuire, D. B., Mulvihill, J. J., Lampkin, B. C., Hananian, J., and Fraumeni, J. F., Jr. Genealogy of cancer in a family. JAMA, *241*: 259–261, 1979.

18. Mulvihill, J. J., Gralnick, H. R., Whang-Peng, J., and Leventhal, B. G. Multiple childhood osteosarcomas in an American Indian family with erythroid macrocytosis and skeletal anomalies. Cancer, *40*: 3115–3122, 1977.

19. Young, J. L., Perry, C. L., and Asire, A. J. (eds.), Surveillance, Epidemiology, and End Results: Incidence and Mortality Data, 1973–1977. Nat. Cancer Inst. Monogr., *57*: 70–73, 1977.

20. Li, F. P. and Fraumeni, J. F., Jr. Prospective study of a family cancer syndrome. JAMA, *247*: 2692–2694, 1982.

21. Williams, W. R., and Strong, L. C. Genetic epidemiology of soft tissue sarcomas of children. *In;* H. J. Muller, and W. Weber, (eds.), Familial Cancer. 1st Int. Res. Conf., pp. 151–153, Karger, Basel, 1985.

22. Go, R.C.P., King, M. C., Bailey-Wilson, J., Elston, R. C., and Lynch, H. T. Genetic epidemiology of breast cancer and associated cancers in high-risk families. I. Segrega-

tion analysis. J. Natl. Cancer Inst., *71*: 455–461, 1983.

23. Hartley, A. L., Birch, J. M., Marsden, H. B., and Harris, M. Breast cancer risk in mothers of children with osteosarcoma and chondrosarcoma. Br. J. Cancer, *54*: 819–823, 1986.

24. Birch, J. M., Hartley, A. L., Marsden, H. B., Harris, M., and Swindel, R. Excess risk of breast cancer in the mothers of children with soft tissue sarcomas. Br. J. Cancer, *49*: 325–331, 1984.

25. Li, F. P. and Fraumeni, J. F., Jr. Familial breast cancer, soft-tissue sarcomas, and other neoplasms. Ann. Intern. Med., *83*: 833–834, 1975.

26. Bech-Hansen, N. T., Blattner, W. A., Sell, B. M., McKeen, E. A., Lampkin, B. C., Fraumeni, J. F., Jr., and Patterson, M. C. Transmission of *in-vitro* radioresistance in a cancer-prone family. Lancet, *1*: 1335–1337, 1981.

27. Chang, E. H., Pirollo, K. F., Qiang Zou, Z., Cheung, H. Y., Lawler, E. L., Garner, R., White, E., Bernstein, W. B., Fraumeni, J. F., Jr., and Blattner, W. A. Oncogenes in radioresistant, non-cancerous skin fibroblasts from a cancer prone family. Science, *237*: 1036–1039, 1987.

28. Knudson, A. G., Jr. Retinoblastoma: A prototypic hereditary neoplasm. Semin. Oncol., *5*: 57–60, 1978.

29. Van Den Berghe, H. Chromosome anomalies in solid tumors and their significance. Cancer Genet. Cytogenet., *28*: 49–54, 1987.

30. Turc-Carel, C., Dal Cin, P., Limon, J., Rao, U., Li, F. P., Corson, J. M., Zimmerman, R., Parry, D. M., Cowan, J. M., and Sandberg, A. A. Involvement of chromosome X in primary cytogenetic change in human neoplasia: Nonrandom translocation in synovial sarcoma. Proc. Natl. Acad. Sci U.S.A., *84*: 1981–1985, 1987.

31. Koufos, A., Hansen, M. F., Copeland, N. G., Jenkins, N. A., Lampkin, B. C., and Cavenee, W. K. Loss of heterozygosity in three embryonal tumours suggests a common pathogenic mechanism. Nature, *316*: 330–334, 1985.

32. Friend, S. H., Horowitz, J. M., Gerber, M. R., Wang, X. F., Bogeman, E., Li, F. P., and Weinberg, R. A. Deletion of a DNA sequence in retinoblastomas and mesenchymal tumors. Proc. Natl. Acad. Sci. U.S.A., in press.

33. Lundberg, C., Skoog, L., Cavenee, W. K., and Nordenskjold, M. Loss of heterozygosity in human ductal breast tumors indicates a recessive mutation on chromosome 13. Proc. Natl. Acad. Sci. U.S.A., *84*: 2372–2376, 1987.

34. Bodmer, W. F., Bailey, C. F., Bodmer, J., Bussey, H.J.R., Ellis, A., Gorman, P., Lucibello, F. C., Murday, V. A., Rider, S. H., Scambler, P., Sheer, D., Solomon, E., and Spurr, N. K. Localization of the gene for familial adenomatous polyposis on chromosome 5. Nature, *328*: 614–616, 1987.

35. Solomon, E., Voss, R., Hall, V., Bodmer, W. F., Jass, J. R., Jeffreys, A. J., Lucibello, F. C., Patel, I., and Rider, S. H. Chromosome 5 allele loss in human colorectal carcinomas. Nature, *328*: 616–619, 1987.

Where Have Dysplastic Nevi Led Us?

Margaret A. Tucker

Epidemiology and Biostatistics Program, Division of Cancer Etiology, National Cancer Institute, National Institutes of Health, Bethesda, Maryland 20892, U.S.A.

Abstract: In 1977, Dr. Mark Greene and Dr. Wallace Clark examined members of the B. and K. families, in which several individuals had developed cutaneous malignant melanoma. They recognized that both families had nevi that were unusual in morphology, pattern, distribution, size, and number. These dysplastic nevi identify the individuals in melanoma-prone families who are at increased risk of melanoma; the cumulative risk of melanoma approaches 100% in affected members. Formal genetic analyses have revealed that the dysplastic nevus and melanoma traits appear to be pleiotropic effects of a single, highly penetrant, autosomal dominant gene. Linkage studies have revealed weak linkage with Rh on the short arm of chromosome 1 (1p), and excluded linkage with the HLA region on chromosome 6p, transferrin on 3q, H-ras on 11p, and Gm on 14q. The most promising location for the melanoma/dysplastic nevus susceptibility locus remains chromosome 1p. Future studies will focus on the localization of the melanoma gene, and then the characterization of the gene product to elucidate the etiology of melanoma.

The story of dysplastic nevi began in late 1975. After giving a lecture at Fox Chase, Philadelphia, Dr. Robert W. Miller made ward rounds with Dr. Michael Mastrangelo, who had been caring for many patients with melanoma. In response to a question, Dr. Mastrangelo said that several families had been affected. Dr. Miller suggested to Dr. Mark Greene, who had recently joined his staff, that he look into the family cases as a possible research project.

On a Sunday in April of 1976, Drs. Mark Greene, Wallace Clark, Michael Mastrangelo, John Mulvihill, and Richard Cohen (a dermatologist caring for the K. family) met 25 members of the K. family in the outpatient clinic of the St. Francis Hospital in Trenton, New Jersey. They drew blood, obtained skin biopsies for fibroblasts, examined the family's skin, and took clinical photographs. They noticed that the family had numerous, extremely unusual pigmented lesions, predominantly on the back. On the back of one family member was an intact melanoma, Clark's Level II, 0.51 mm thick. Dr. Clark returned to his office and reviewed all of the pathology slides from members of the K. family again. He realized that the histology of the lesions in the K. family was similar to the histology of lesions from another patient he had seen, Mrs. B. Dr. Clark asked her to return to his clinic. When he reexamined her, he took a detailed family history, and discovered that her mother had had a melanoma. Dr. Clark and Greene then examined the members of the B. family and discovered that they had very similar lesions to those in the K. family. Numerous members of both families had large, irregular, flat nevi, with variable pigmentation and unusual distribution. The nevi occurred not only on the sun-exposed areas, as is the pattern for common acquired nevi, but also on doubly-covered areas, such as the buttocks, female breast, and perineum. Recognizing that they did not yet understand the natural history or pathobiology of these distinctive lesions, Drs. Greene and Clark decided to give them a deliberately nondescriptive name, and named the lesions B-K moles, in recognition of the contributions of these first two families (1).

Dr. Greene then took a year to complete his medical oncology training at the National Cancer Institute. During his clinical year, he identified other individuals with familial melanoma and B-K moles. Upon his return to the Epidemiology Branch, he and Dr. Clark began contacting additional families from the registry of cancer-prone families maintained by the Family Studies Section of the NCI. Families with two or more living members with melanoma were invited to be involved in a fairly complicated clinical and laboratory study of familial melanoma. The design of the study included a physical examination, total body photography, phlebotomy, skin biopsy for fibroblasts, and multiple nevus biopsies to pathologically confirm the diagnosis of B-K moles. Fourteen families with melanoma were willing to participate. The Hereditary Cutaneous Malignant Melanoma Project was started as a collaboration which still continues between the NCI and the Pigmented Lesion Group of the University of Pennsylvania.

When I arrived at the NCI after my residency training, Dr. Greene asked if I would be interested in working on the melanoma project with him. The first families were coming in for the clinical and laboratory evaluations. Over the next two years, we examined 401 members of the 14 families, which are the base of the Hereditary Cutaneous Malignant Melanoma Project. These 401 individuals included 69 melanoma patients, 195 adult blood relatives, 91 spouses, and 46 children.

This project has had a major impact on the knowledge of the biology and etiology of melanoma. In studying the families, it became obvious that the cardinal features of the B-K moles were disorderly growth and cytologic atypia of the melanocytes (2). In other systems, this pattern is called dysplasia, so that the name of these lesions was changed from B-K moles to dysplastic nevi (3). Drs. Clark and Elder have characterized the unique histopathology of these lesions, and established diagnostic criteria (4). After reviewing the histologic slides from this study, and from similar patients seen in the Pigmented Lesion Clinic, Dr. Clark has developed a model of tumor progression based on the evolution of dysplastic nevi to melanoma, similar to the tumor progression that leads from cervical dysplasia to carcinoma (4).

Over the years of this study, the natural history of these nevi has unfolded. The dysplastic nevi are not present at birth, but usually first appear as an increased number of morphologically normal nevi during midchildhood (5). The scalp may be the first place that morphologically atypical lesions appear. During puberty, the characteristic morphology of flat, large, variably pigmented, irregularly shaped nevi develops. New nevi continue to develop during adulthood, well into ages 50–60s, in contrast to normal nevi, which rarely appear after age 40. The nevi appear to go through cycles of activity, when new nevi develop and existing nevi enlarge or change (6). The triggers for this activity are not known, but the nevi frequently change during times of hormonal changes, such as puberty and pregnancy, and after intense sun exposure. We have followed several patients in whom we have photographically documented the progression of dysplastic nevi to melanoma (7). Dysplastic nevi are now accepted by most investigators to be clinically and histologically distinct precursors of malignant melanoma (8).

Dysplastic nevi identify those individuals in the families who are at high risk of melanoma (9). Almost all the melanomas have occurred in the family members who have dysplastic nevi. From the prospective followup data on these families, individuals with dysplastic nevi have a 148-fold increased risk of developing a melanoma compared to the general population; those family members who have already had one melanoma have a 500-fold increased risk of developing another melanoma. The cumulative probability of developing melanoma among family members with dysplastic nevi approaches 100% (9). During the study, 60 new melanomas have been diagnosed among 28 family members. Seven people have developed their first melanoma during our followup period. Eighteen melanomas were diagnosed during the intake examination of the project; 42 of the melanomas were diagnosed during followup. Many of the family members with melanoma develop multiple primary lesions, usually superficial spreading type (9). One young woman developed 15 separate primary melanomas by age 32.

Recognizing that individuals with dysplastic nevi in melanoma-prone families are at extremely high risk of melanoma, we have developed clinical guidelines to aid in early diagnosis or prevention of melanoma. We recommend that individuals: 1) examine their own skin monthly using clinical photographs for comparison; 2) undergo health care provider examinations every 3 to 6 months; 3) have early excisional biopsies of any changing nevi; 4) avoid sunburn at all cost; 5) if feasible, avoid exogenous hormones. To educate family members and health care providers about the recognition of dysplastic nevi, separate videotapes for family members, health care providers, and pathologists have been created and made widely available. In addition, we have more recently developed pamphlets and posters for physicians' offices. These guidelines have had an impact on the care of the family members. Most of the melanomas which have occurred during the followup period have been much thinner lesions, with a better prognosis (9). Almost twice as many histologically borderline lesions have been removed as melanomas.

The distribution of the melanomas on the skin of family members is not unusual compared to the distribution of melanomas in unselected groups of melanoma patients (9). The most common site for males is the back; for females, it is the lower leg, followed by back. The patients tend to be younger than those with sporadic melanoma, with a mean age of onset of 30 years for the first melanoma (9). The youngest family member to date was 11 years old when he developed his first melanoma. Affected family members, therefore, have multiple melanomas at an early age, similar to the patterns seen in other cancers with a familial component to their etiology (10, 11). Those affected members with the most nevi are at the highest risk of melanoma (6). The family members do not seem to be at significantly increased risk of other types of cancer, however (12). In the followup period of seven years, 32 cases of cancer were observed, compared to 7.4 expected, but the excess was attributable entirely to 22 excess cases of melanoma. Site-specific analyses revealed no significant risks at any site other than melanoma in affected or unaffected family members (12).

By inspection of the pedigrees, it appeared as though melanoma and dysplastic nevi might be autosomal dominant traits. The first attempt at segregation analysis could not confirm this, because of problems with the ascertainment of the families, and the frequency of dysplastic nevi in the general population (13). A novel analytic approach used by Dr. Sherri Bale, however, established that dysplastic nevi and melanoma are pleiotropic effects of a single, autosomal dominant gene, with approximately 90% penetrance (14).

Once it was established that the melanoma trait was controlled by a single gene, it seemed reasonable to try to establish the chromosomal location of the gene. Linkage analyses with available polymorphic markers excluded approximately 8% of the genome, and were consistent with weak linkage with the Rhesus blood group locus on chromosome 1p. A maximum lod score of 1.56 at 30% recombination was found between the melanoma/dysplastic nevus trait and Rh (13). Recent laboratory efforts have concentrated on developing DNA probes which might be more closely linked to the melanoma/dysplastic nevus gene. To date, about 20 markers on 1p have been developed. In addition, several areas of putative linkage suggested by other investigators have been definitively excluded by strongly negative lod scores less than −2. The regions around HLA on chromosome 6p (15), transferrin on 3q (16), Ha-ras-1 on 11p (17), and Gm on 14q (18) have been excluded. The most promising location for the melanoma / dysplastic nevus susceptibility locus remains chromosome 1p. This location also seems plausible because the most common chromosomes which are altered in melanoma tumors and cell lines derived from melanomas or melanoma metastases are 1, 6, and 7 (19).

Other laboratory studies have shown increased breaks, rearrangements and deletions in the chromosomes of lymphocytes among family members with the melanoma/ dysplastic nevus trait (20). The involved chromosomes tended to be those with putative fragile sites. We are in the process of trying to confirm this observation on a larger number of patients and family members. In addition to the routine cytogenetics, a fragile site analysis is also being conducted.

One of the variables associated with an increased number of chromosomal abnormalities in lymphocytes from individuals with the melanoma/dysplastic nevus trait was extensive sun exposure. The individuals with the most sun exposure also tended to have the most nevi and melanomas. To try to elucidate the mechanism of this melanoma susceptibility, *in vitro* assays of sensitivity to UV light have been done. Fibroblasts from affected individuals were found to have normal response to ionizing radiation. In contrast, the fibroblasts have increased sensitivity to UV irradiation. The rate of *de novo* DNA synthesis and DNA repair were normal. When the lines were exposed to 4-nitroquinoline-1-oxide, which is both ionizing and ultraviolet radiation mimetic, the cells again were sensitive, with normal *de novo* DNA synthesis and repair (21–23). Lymphoblastoid lines from affected individuals showed normal sensitivity to ultraviolet radiation, but a 2–4 fold increase in mutagenesis following UV exposure. This level of increased mutagenesis is intermediate between normal cells and those from patients with xeroderma pigmentosum (24). The mechanism of the UV sensitivity has not yet been completely elucidated. When the susceptibility gene is localized and characterized, the mechanism of UV sensitivity may be clarified.

The discovery and description of dysplastic nevi have not only led to the characterization of melanoma/dysplastic nevi as a single gene trait which accounts for at least 10% of cutaneous melanomas (25), but they have also led to an increased understanding about nonfamilial melanoma. Early on, Dr. David Elder and Dr. Wallace Clark of the Pigmented Lesion Clinic in Philadelphia recognized that similar dysplastic nevi occurred on individuals who had melanoma, but did not a positive family history of melanoma (26). Histologically, these lesions are indistinguishable from the dysplastic nevi occurring in the familial setting. Dysplastic nevi also occur in histologic continuity with nonfamilial melanomas (4). Other groups have confirmed this observation in different patient populations (27). The most current estimates are that between 30 and 50% of nonfamilial melanomas occur in individuals with dysplastic nevi (4, 27, 28). Several groups have examined patient populations to determine the prevalence of dysplastic nevi among the general population. It appears that approximately 2 to 9% of the general white population have dysplastic nevi (29–31). One recent estimate of dysplastic nevus prevalence was as high as 17% (32).

Dr. Ken Kraemer suggested a classification scheme for nonfamilial and familial dysplastic nevi. Type A refers to individuals or kindreds in which only one person has dysplastic nevi. Type B refers to individuals or kindreds where several individuals in the families have dysplastic nevi, but no melanoma. Type C individuals (or families) have dysplastic nevi and melanoma, with no other affected individuals in the family. Type D1 kindreds have familial dysplastic nevi with one individual with melanoma; type D2 have familial dysplastic nevi and several members who have had melanoma (33). The very high melanoma risks in our families reflect the risk in D2 families only.

We have used an average prevalence rate (5%) of dysplastic nevi to estimate the risk of melanoma among individuals with dysplastic nevi without a family history of melanoma (34). These individuals have about a 7-fold increased risk of melanoma, with a cumulative lifetime risk of about 6%. This is obviously much lower than the risk among gene carriers in melanoma-prone families. Quantifying the risk of melanoma in individuals with nonfamilial dysplastic nevi has major importance for the development of public health measures, since these individuals are a group at increased risk, in whom intervention may make a significant difference in melanoma incidence and mortality.

Analytic epidemiologic studies have confirmed the importance of dysplastic nevi as a risk factor for melanoma. Case-control studies where investigators have looked at nevi as a risk factor have demonstrated risks between 6–25 fold associated with the presence of increased number of nevi (35–41). Few of these studies have discriminated between dysplastic and common acquired nevi. Recent studies by Holly and Rousch have shown, however, that most of the risk associated with nevi is due to the presence of dysplastic nevi (32, 42). The risks associated with nondysplastic nevi have not been found to be significant.

In addition, individuals with dysplastic nevi who become immunosuppressed are at increased risk of melanoma. In a histologic review of melanoma following renal transplantation, Dr. Greene and Dr. Clark showed that 50% of the people who developed melanoma had evidence of a precursor dysplastic nevus in contiguity with the melanoma (43). While I was a medical oncology fellow at Stanford University Medical Center, I spent quite a bit of time in the lymphoma clinic and diagnosed 2 melanomas on Hodgkin's disease patients who also had dysplastic nevi. This led me to review all the patients with second primary melanomas following Hodgkin's disease who were treated at Stanford. This study revealed that individuals with Hodgkin's disease have an 8-fold increased risk of melanoma compared to the general population (44). Again, most of the patients who developed melanoma had documented dysplastic nevi, 2 histologically confirmed, and 3 based on clinical observation. There was one deceased patient for whom we could not document the presence of dysplastic nevi. He developed an advanced melanoma which may have obliterated the precursor lesion. The immunosuppression accompanying Hodgkin's disease or renal transplantation may provide the environment which allows the dysplastic nevi to transform to melanoma. The presence of dysplastic nevi appears to be a marker which identifies those individuals at increased risk of melanoma after immunosuppression.

In summary, the alert observation of Drs. Greene and Clark that members of a family with melanoma had abnormal appearing moles has transformed the field of melanoma pathology, genetics, biology, and epidemiology. We hope that we are on the verge of localizing the susceptibility locus, which will be invaluable in elucidating the etiology of melanoma. Once the gene is localized, we will be able to characterize the gene product which will then give us the mechanism of melanoma susceptibility. When the gene is identified, the differences in gene expression among different populations can then be explored. These differences in gene expression may particularly explain the ethnic differences in melanoma risk. Although speculative, one could envision that the gene might have something to do with ultraviolet sensitivity. Once the mechanism of susceptibility is understood, we may be better able to prevent melanoma.

ACKNOWLEDGMENTS
I would like to thank Dr. Joseph Fraumeni and Dr. Robert Miller for their continuous strong support of the melanoma project from its inception; Dr. Sherri Bale and Ms. Mary Fraser for their critical review of the manuscript; and Ms. Mildred Jacobus for her editorial assistance.

REFERENCES
1. Clark, W. H., Jr., Reimer, R., Greene, M. H., Ainsworth, A., and Mastrangelo, M. Origin of familial malignant melanoma from heritable melanocytic lesions. Arch. Dermatol. *114*: 732–738, 1978.
2. Elder, D. E., Greene, M. H., Bondi, E., and Clark, W. H. Acquired melanocytic nevi and melanoma: the dysplastic nevus syndrome. *In;* B. Ackerman (ed.), Pathology of Malignant Melanoma, pp. 185–215, Masson, New York, 1981.
3. Greene, M. H., Clark, W. H., Tucker, M. A., Elder, D. E., Kraemer, K. H., Fraser, M. C., Bondi, E. E., Guerry, D., Hamilton, R., and LaRossa, D. Precursor naevi and

cutaneous malignant melanoma. A proposed nomenclature. Lancet, *ii*: 1024, 1980.

4. Clark, W. H., Jr., Elder, D. E., Guerry, D., Epstein, M. H., Greene, M. H., and Van Horn, M. A study of tumor progression—the precursor lesions of superficial spreading and nodular melanoma. Hum. Pathol., *15*: 1147–1165, 1984.

5. Tucker, M. A., Greene, M. H., Clark, W. H., Jr., Kraemer, K. H., Fraser, M. C., and Elder, D. E. Dysplastic nevi on the scalp of prepubertal children from melanoma-prone families. J. Pediat., *103*: 65–69, 1983.

6. Kraemer, K. H. and Greene, M. H. Dysplastic nevus syndrome. Familial and sporadic precursors of cutaneous melanoma. Dermatol. Clin., *3*: 225–237, 1985.

7. Greene, M. H., Clark, W. H., Jr., Tucker, M. A., Elder, D. E., Kraemer, K. H., Guerry, D., IV, Witmer, W. K., Thompson, J., Matozzo, I., and Fraser, M. C. Acquired precursors of cutaneous malignant melanoma: the familial dysplastic nevus syndrome. N. Engl. J. Med., *312*: 91–97, 1985.

8. Consensus Conference: Precursors to malignant melanoma. J. Am. Med. Assoc., *251*: 1864–1866, 1984.

9. Greene, M. H., Clark, W. H., Jr., Tucker, M. A., Kraemer, K. H., Elder, D. E., and Fraser, M. C. High risk of malignant melanoma in melanoma-prone families with dysplastic nevi. Ann. Intern. Med. *102*: 458–465, 1985.

10. Knudsen, A. G., Jr. Mutation and cancer: Statistical study of retinoblastoma. Proc. Natl. Acad. Sci. U.S.A., *68*: 820–823, 1971.

11. Li, F. P. and Fraumeni, J. F., Jr. Soft-tissue sarcomas, breast cancer, and other neoplasms: A familial syndrome? Ann. Intern. Med., *71*: 747–752, 1969.

12. Greene, M. H., Tucker, M. A., Clark, W. H., Jr., Kraemer, K. H., Elder, D. E., and Fraser, M. C. Hereditary melanoma and the dysplastic nevus syndrome. The risk of cancers other than melanoma. J. Am. Acad. Dermatol., *16*: 792–797, 1987.

13. Greene, M. H., Goldin, L. R., Clark, W. H., Jr., Lovrien, E., Kraemer, K. H., Tucker, M. A., Elder, D. E., Fraser, M. C., and Rowe, S. Familial cutaneous malignant melanoma. Autosomal dominant trait possibly linked to the Rh locus. Proc. Natl. Acad. Sci. U.S.A., *80*: 6061–6075, 1983.

14. Bale, S. J., Chakravarti, A., and Greene, M. H. Cutaneous malignant melanoma and dysplastic nevi—evidence for autosomal dominance and pleiotropy. Am. J. Hum. Genet., *38*: 188–196, 1986.

15. Bale, S. J., Greene, M. H., Mann, D., Murray, C., Goldin, L., and Johnson, A. H. Familial melanoma is not linked to the HLA complex on chromosome 6. Int. J. Cancer, *36*: 439–443, 1985.

16. Bale, S. J., Greene, M. H., and Lovrien, E. Hereditary melanoma, the dysplastic nevus syndrome and transferrin. Cancer Genet. Cytogenet., *23*: 279–280, 1986.

17. Gerhard, D. S., Dracopli, N. C., Bale, S. J., Houghton, A. N., Watkins, P., Payne, C. E., Greene, M. H., and Housman, D. Evidence against H-*ras*-1 involvement in sporadic and familial melanoma. Nature, *325*: 73–75, 1987.

18. Buchmann, R. B., Bale, S. J., Greene, M. H., and Pandey, J. P. Immunoglobulin allotypes and familial cutaneous malignant melanoma (CMM)/dysplastic nevi (DN): A family study. Exp. Clin. Immunogenet., in press.

19. Herlyn, M., Thurin, J., Balaban, G., Bennicelli, J. L., Herlyn, D., Elder, D. E., Bondi, E., Guerry, D., Nowell, P., Clark, W. H., and Koprowski, H. Characteristics of cultured human melanocytes isolated from different stages of tumor progression. Cancer Res., *45*: 5670–5676, 1985.

20. Caporaso, N., Greene, M. H., Tsai, S., Pickle, L. W., and Mulvihill, J. J. Cytogenetics in hereditary malignant melanoma and dysplastic nevus syndrome. Is dysplastic nevus

syndrome a chromosome instability disorder? Cancer Genet. Cytogenet., *24*: 299–314, 1987.

21. Smith, P. J., Greene, M. H., Devlin, D. A., McKeen, E. A., and Paterson, M. C. Abnormal sensitivity to UV-radiation in cultured skin fibroblasts from patients with hereditary cutaneous malignant melanoma and dysplastic nevus syndrome. Int. J. Cancer, *30*: 39–445, 1982.

22. Smith, P. J., Greene, M. H., Adams, D., and Paterson, M. C. Abnormal responses to the carcinogen 4-nitroquinoline 1-oxide of cultured cells from patients with dysplastic nevus syndrome and hereditary cutaneous malignant melanoma. Carcinogenesis, *4*: 911–917, 1983.

23. Howell, J. W., Greene, M. H., Corner, R. C., Maher, V. M., and McCormick, J. J. Fibroblasts from patients with hereditary cutaneous malignant melanoma and abnormally sensitive to the mutagenic effect of simulated sunlight and 4-nitroquinoline 1-oxide. Proc. Natl. Acad. Sci. U.S.A., *81*: 1179–1183, 1984.

24. Perera, M.I.R., Um, K. I., Greene, M. H., Waters, H. L., Bredberg, A., and Kraemer, K. H. Hereditary dysplastic nevus syndrome. Lymphoid cell ultraviolet hypermutability in association with increased melanoma susceptibility. Cancer Res., *46*: 1005–1009, 1986.

25. Kopf, A. W., Hellman, L. J., Rogers, G. S., Gross, D. F., Rigel, D. S., Friedman, R. J., Levenstein, M., Brown, J., Golomb, F. M., Roses, D. F., Gumport, S. L., and Mintzis, M. M. Familial malignant melanoma. J. Am. Med. Assoc., *256*: 1915–1919, 1986.

26. Elder, D. E., Goldman, L. I., Goldman, S. C., Greene, M. H., and Clark, W. H., Jr. Dysplastic nevus syndrome. A phenotypic association of sporadic malignant melanoma. Cancer, *46*: 1787–1794, 1980.

27. Rhodes, A. R., Harrist, T. J., and Day, C. L. Dysplastic melanocytic nevi in histologic association with 234 primary cutaneous melanomas. J. Am. Acad. Dermatol., *9*: 563–574, 1983.

28. Taylor, M. R., Guerry, D., IV, Bondi, E. E., Shields, J. A., Augsburger, J. J., Lusk, E. J., Elder, D. E., Clark, W. H., Jr., and Van Horn, M. Lack of association between intraocular melanoma and cutaneous dysplastic nevi. Am. J. Ophthalmol., *98*: 478–482, 1984.

29. Rhodes, A. R., Sober, A. J., Mihm, M. C., and Fitzpatrick, T. B. Possible risk factors for primary cutaneous melanoma. Clin. Res., *28*: 232A, 1980.

30. Crutcher, W. A. and Sagebiel, R. W. Prevalence of dysplastic naevi in a community practice. Lancet, *i*: 729, 1984.

31. Cooke, K. R., Spears, G.F.S., and Elder, D. E. Dysplastic naevi identified in a cross-sectional survey, (submitted)

32. Holly, E. A., Kelly, J. W., Shpall, S. N., and Chiu, S-H. Number of melanocytic nevi as a major risk factor for malignant melanoma. J. Am. Acad. Dermatol., *17*: 459–468, 1987.

33. Kraemer, K. H., Greene, M. H., Tarone, R., Elder, D. E., Clark, W. H., Jr., and Guerry, D., IV. Dysplastic naevi and cutaneous melanoma risk. Lancet, *ii*: 1076–1077, 1983.

34. Kraemer, K. H., Tucker, M. A., Tarone, R., Elder, D. E., and Clark, W. H., Jr. Risk of cutaneous melanoma in dysplastic nevus syndrome types A and B. N. Engl. J. Med., *315*: 1615–1616, 1986.

35. Østerlind, A., Tucker, M. A., Hou-Jensen, K., Stone, B. J., Engholm, G., and Jensen, O. M. The Danish case-control study of cutaneous malignant melanoma. I. The im-

portance of host factors. Int. J. Cancer, in press.

36. Holman, C.D.J. and Armstrong, B. K. Pigmentary traits, ethnic origin, benign nevi, and family history as risk factors for cutaneous malignant melanoma. J. Natl. Cancer Inst., *72*: 257–266, 1984.

37. Nordlund, J. J., Kirkwood, J., Forget, B. M., Scheiber, A., Albert, D. M., Lerner, E., and Milton, G. W. Demographic study of clinically atypical (dysplastic) nevi in patients with melanoma and comparison subjects. Cancer Res., *45*: 1855–1861, 1985.

38. Green, A., MacLennan, R., and Siskind, V. Common acquired naevi and the risk of malignant melanoma. Int. J. Cancer, *35*: 297–300, 1985.

39. Swerdlow, A. J., English, J., Mackie, R. M., O'Doherty, C. J., Hunter, J.A.A., Clark, J., and Hole, D. J. Benign melanocytic naevi as a risk factor for malignant melanoma. Br. Med. J., *292*: 1555–1559, 1986.

40. Swerdlow, A. J., English, J., Mackie, R. M., O'Doherty, C. J., Hunter, J.A.A., and Clark, J. Benign naevi association with high risk of melanoma. Lancet, *ii*: 168, 1984.

41. Elwood, J. M., Williamson, C., and Stapleton, P. J. Malignant melanoma in relation to moles, pigmentation, and exposure to fluorescent and other lighting sources. Br. J. Cancer, *53*: 65–74, 1986.

42. Roush, G. C., McKay, L., Forget, B., Titus, L., and Kirkwood, J. Dependence of total nevi on dysplastic nevi in determining risk for melanoma. Prev. Med., *15*: 699, 1986.

43. Greene, M. H., Young, T. I., and Clark, W. H. Malignant melanoma in renal transplant patients. Lancet, *i*: 1196–1199, 1981.

44. Tucker, M. A., Misfeldt, D., Coleman, C. N., Clark, W. H., Jr., and Rosenberg, S. A. Cutaneous malignant melanoma after Hodgkin's disease. Ann Intern. Med., *102*: 37–41, 1985.

UNUSUAL OCCURRENCES AS CLUES TO CANCER ETIOLOGY, R. W. MILLER ET AL. (EDS.),
JAPAN SCI. SOC. PRESS, TOKYO/TAYLOR & FRANCIS, LTD., PP. 261–273, 1988

Genetic Models for Linkage Analysis of Ataxia-telangiectasia

Richard A. Gatti,*1 Daniel E. Weeks,*2 and Malcolm Paterson*3

*Departments of Pathology*1 *and Biomathematics,*2 *UCLA School of Medicine, Los Angeles, CA 90024, and the Molecular Genetics and Carcinogenesis Laboratory, Cross Cancer Institute, Edmonton, Canada T6G 1Z2*3

Abstract: Ataxia-telangiectasia (AT) is a multifaceted autosomal recessive disorder, inherited as a single gene in each family, presumably due to a defective DNA processing protein such as a recombinase, endonuclease or even a regulatory DNA-binding protein. We are attempting to identify the chromosomal location of the AT gene(s) by performing linkage analyses on a variety of genetic models.

At least five AT complementation groups have been defined. This genetic heterogeneity complicates linkage analysis. Model I assumes that the complementation genes are clustered into a single genomic region and, therefore, lod scores of linkage data from *all* families can be added. Model II assumes that the AT complementation genes are dispersed throughout the genome and the lod scores cannot be added. This model necessitates assigning the complementation group of every family that is included in the linkage analyses and reduces the number of families in each data base.

Model III utilizes heterozygote identification to follow the AT gene (in a Group A pedigree of 61 members) as a dominant trait, thereby increasing the amount of linkage information that can be derived from that family. Model IV will focus only on consanguineous offspring of first-cousin marriages, seeking to identify the location of the AT gene(s) by the increased degree of homozygosity of genetic markers in close proximity. This model has several advantages, including that much smaller numbers of patients are required. Model V assumes that a subset of our patients will carry deletions and can be used to confirm the relationship of a candidate gene to the AT phenotype.

Progress: Models I and II have been used to survey 7% and 2% of the genome, respectively. (An additional 5% of the genome can be added for exclusion of the X chromosome on clinical grounds.) Model III is intended to survey the entire genome. Our initial studies have surveyed approximately 30% of the genome. Several areas of increased lod scores have been identified and are under further investigation.

Historical Note

The frequent occurrence of cancer in patients with ataxia-telangiectasia (AT) was noted in early reports of the disorder (*1–3*). What seemed especially provocative was the preponderence of lymphoid malignancies, a class of neoplasms also noted in patients with other immunodeficiency disorders (*4*). These observations were pursued mainly by two groups: 1) researchers affiliated with the Minnesota Immunodeficiency Cancer Registry (*5, 6*) and 2) Swift and coworkers (*7–10*). The Registry evolved from data used in a 1971 world literature review by Gatti and Good (*4*) and remains to this day a worldwide data base. Swift *et al.* attempted to define the epidemiology of the disorder within the United States and this encompassed, naturally, information on the incidence and types of cancer (*8*). Recently, these same investigators have published a report on the cancer epidemiology of heterozygotes as well; this latter study revealed that, unlike in homozygotes, non-lymphoid cancers predominate (*10*). When the AT heterozygote frequency of approximately 2.8% is considered together with an estimated 7.6-fold increase in breast cancer in female AT heterozygotes, Swift theorizes that 18% of breast cancer patients may in fact be heterozygous carriers of the AT gene (*10*).

Another important clue to cancer etiology was gleaned from an AT patient by an astute clinician, Dr. Sam Gotoff, who noted "an untoward response to X-irradiation" in a child receiving conventional radiotherapy for a malignant tumor (*11*). This has been independently confirmed by others (*12–14*) and led to the laboratory observation that cultured AT fibroblasts are, without exception, hypersensitive to ionizing radiation (*15, 16*). Moreover, cultured cells from obligatory heterozygotes (*i.e.*, parents of AT patients) exhibit a radioresponse intermediate between that shown by cells from healthy donors and cells from patients. This intermediate radiation hypersensitivity forms the basis of several heterozygote detection assays; unfortunately, all are time-consuming and labor-intensive and none are 100% reliable (*17*). Several research groups also demonstrated that fusion of fibroblasts from some pairs of AT patients corrects the radiation hypersensitivity (*18–22*). This observation has been exploited to define, thus far, five distinct complementation groups in AT (A, C, D, E, and V1) and makes a strong argument for a genetic etiology of both the radiation hypersensitivity and the cancer susceptibility.

Immunologists have traditionally viewed AT as primarily an immunodeficiency disorder and as an Experiment of Nature in which cancer immunosurveillance is defective. Many immune defects have been reported in AT patients; however, these patients lacked any one uniform immunological defect that would act as a common denominator for the cancer etiology. One of us (R.A.G.) has tried to follow the segregation of some of these apparently random immune defects within families (*23*) and found that these defects do not segregate as Mendelian genetic traits. Realizing the importance of a single gene that if defective may concurrently predispose to cerebellar degeneration, cancer susceptibility, radiation hypersensitivity, chromosomal instability, elevated alphafetoprotein and premature aging, we elected to try to first determine its chromosomal location through genetic linkage analysis, with the long-term goal of defining its molecular structure, regulation of its expression and function of its protein product.

Requirements for Genetic Linkage Analysis

Genetic linkage analysis attempts to determine whether the alleles at one locus are inherited independently of alleles at another locus. If the alleles at the two loci are found to cosegregate, the loci are considered linked and in close physical proximity to each other in the genome. This implies that mapping the location of one locus will map the location of the other locus as well. Any Mendelian locus with sufficient allelic variation can serve as a genetic marker for linkage studies with a disease trait, the disease trait serving as the other locus.

To establish the statistical significance of linkage between any two markers requires data on a group of informative matings. At least one parent in an informative mating must be heterozygous at both loci. Significance is measured by comparing the expected number of crossover (recombination) events to the observed number. The major limitation to linkage analysis is lack of a sufficient number of informative matings. Until very recently, the common remedy to this problem was to increase the number of disease families tested. Regretably, this becomes difficult to do when studying a relatively uncommon disorder such as AT. Alternatively, one can increase the heterozygosity of the markers used. Within the past year a new category of genetic markers (DNA probes) has been developed which is called "variable number of tandem repeats" (VNTRs). VNTRs derive from genomic regions of great genetic variability (*24*). Many VNTR markers are so polymorphic that over 80% of the general population carry two different alleles, *i.e.*, are heterozygous for that marker. (The usefulness or informativeness of a marker can be expressed by either its frequency of heterozygosity in an outbred population or by its "polymorphic information content" or PIC (*25*).)

From the standpoint of linkage analysis, the human genome is extremely large. Even when the new highly informative markers are used on large nuclear families containing an aggregate of several hundred meioses, they can only distinguish linkage over recombination distances of approximately 15–20 centiMorgans (cM), *i.e.*, 15–20 million base pairs. The genome is estimated to be 3,300 cM. If the number of meioses in a linkage study is small, even highly informative markers can be expected to detect significant linkages over distances of only 1–10 cM. In fact, most markers being used to date are biallelic, not multiallelic and, in our experience, even when used on large numbers of segregants, can only distinguish linkage over distances of 1–5 cM. Obviously, the ideal linkage study would include large numbers of meioses and many highly informative markers spaced equidistantly so as to survey the entire genome. The number of such markers that would be necessary to survey the entire genome can be calculated: if one assumes an exclusion interval of 20 cM for each marker, 3,300 divided by 20=165 markers. In order to find these 165 equidistant markers, many more markers will have to be cloned and mapped. Having a complete panel of highly informative, equidistant markers minimizes the number of meioses needed for study and is the goal of linkage analysis scientists. To date, two extensive linkage maps with a combined total of approximately 900 markers have been developed, in a world-wide collaboration with the Center for Studying Human Polymorphisms (CEPH) in Paris. Together they cover over 95% of the genome (*26*, *27*).

When linkage analysis is applied to localization of disease genes, one additional requirement must be met. The disease gene must segregate as a single Mendelian factor, *i.e.*, the disease population must be genetically homogeneous. While it is possible to design linkage studies to detect linkage to multigene models, the amount of information necessary is forbidding and will not be addressed here.

Models for Localizing the AT Gene(s)

Our first requirement in performing linkage analysis of AT was to identify a homogeneous population large enough to generate significant lod scores. (The lod score is a statistic that represents the log base 10 of the odds in favor of linkage. A lod score of greater than 3 is taken as evidence for linkage.)

Ascertainment of the diagnosis of AT has not been a problem. We have used three diagnositic criteria: 1) progressive cerebellar ataxia with onset in early childhood, 2) elevated alphafetoprotein, and 3) radioresistant DNA synthesis of fibroblasts (*28*) (performed by Robert Painter). In addition, after making some minor adjustments in our cytogenetic techniques, we have been able to detect aberrations of chromosomes 7 and 14 in the lymphocytes of all subsequent patients examined (*29*). Fibroblasts have also been sent to N.G.J. Jaspers for complementation group assignments (*22*).

The genetic marker data were initially analyzed in accordance with two genetic models of AT:

Model I (clustered AT genes) assumes that the complementation genes cluster in a single region of the genome and, therefore, would all be linked to the same set of markers. Thus, under this model, the lod scores from all families can be added.

Model II (dispersed AT genes) assumes that the complementation genes are dispersed in the genome and each must be studied independently for linkage. Thus, only lod scores of families identified as belonging to a specific group can be combined. We have chosen to examine only families that have been assigned to complementation group A since this group is most common among our families.

Realizing that 1) we would not accumulate a sufficient number of families with multiple affected members under either of these models, and 2) it would be many months before assignments could be made on additional families, we developed another model:

Model III (heterozygote identifications) allows the segregation of the AT gene to be followed by heterozygote detection assays, thereby increasing the informativeness of the AT marker itself in a single large Group A pedigree. Blood and skin samples were taken from 61 members representing three generations and four branches of the family. Cultures were established for fibroblasts and lymphoblasts. DNA was isolated from peripheral blood lymphocytes and lymphoblasts.

At a WHO workshop in 1985 on "identification of AT heterozygotes", the reliability of various heterozygote assays was considered in depth and it was concluded that in the best laboratories, accuracy would approach 80–90% (*30*). In examining the pedigree used in Model III, all fibroblast cultures were coded as to their relationship to affected members and to one another. Of seven obligate heterozygotes tested, six were identified as heterozygotes by Paterson and coworkers

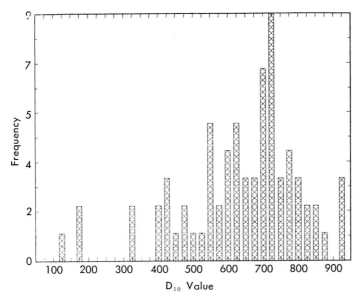

FIG. 1. Heterozygote assignments: distribution of D_{10} values for members of Amish pedigree used as Model III and controls. The three values below 200 are from AT homozygotes.

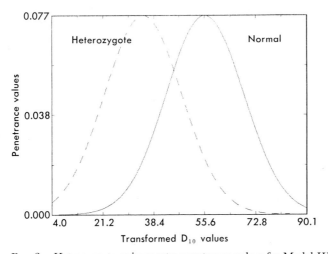

FIG. 2. Heterozygote assignments: penetrance values for Model III.

using a chronic low-dose gamma-irradiation method (*17*). Even with repeated testing of the discordant member's fibroblasts, the data were not compatible with clear heterozygote assignment. Better separation of these two populations is possible by transforming the raw D_{10} values displayed in Fig. 1. This permits a model where the "normal" and "heterozygote" populations come from two normal distributions with common variance and different means. We found that the two means differed by about 1.6 standard deviations (Fig. 2). In order to improve the discrimination between the two groups, additional coded heterozygotes and normals are being studied.

It is possible that the Model III data alone will not generate lod scores of greater than 3. We will then need to confirm and extend such potential linkages by pursuing them in the expanded Models I and II data. Simulations indicate that Model I or Model II may be adequate to establish tight linkage.

Two additional models are being developed:

Model IV (consanguineous affecteds) evaluates genomic regions for increased homozygosity in consanguineous affecteds. The underlying paradigm here is that an affected offspring of a first-cousin marriage will be homozygous for all markers in the region around the AT gene while the probability of homozygosity of any random marker unlinked to AT in the same first-cousin offspring is only:

$$1/16 + (15/16)(p)$$

where p is the probability that the marker is homozygous in a random population. Significant lod scores can be generated in this way using relatively small numbers of patients (*31, 32*). However, for logistical reasons, DNA is limited on these consanguineous patients and, therefore, Model IV will be used primarily to extend and confirm potential linkages identified by Model III. In addition to requiring only small numbers of patients, Model IV has two other advantages: 1) it is independent of heterozygote identification assays, which have a 10–20% error, and 2) it is not essential that all patients be assigned to specific complementation groups.

In order to examine the amount of information available in approximately forty consanguineous affecteds, let us assume a sequential sampling approach (*33, 34*). Under this approach, observations are taken one at a time, and one of three actions is taken after each observation: 1) accept the null hypothesis (H_0) of no linkage between the marker and the AT disease gene, 2) accept the alternative hypothesis (H_1) of linkage in a certain percentage of the affecteds, 3) continue sampling. We

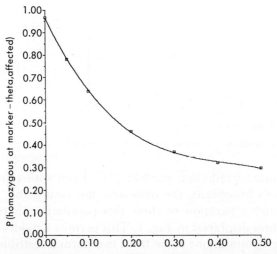

FIG. 3. Theoretical probability of marker homozygosity in an affected offspring of a first-cousin marriage where the marker is homozygous in 25% of a random population. Homozygosity increases as the marker approaches the AT gene.

wished to calculate the average number of observations needed to reach a decision. In order to make such calculations manageable, we assume the following: 1) let the probability of concluding there is linkage when in fact there is no linkage be 0.001. This corresponds to the traditional significance level of a lod score of 3. 2) Let the probability of concluding there is no linkage when in fact there is linkage be 0.01. This corresponds to a lod score of -2. 3) Let our marker have four alleles of equal frequency. This marker is heterozygous 75% of the time in a random sample of unrelated individuals. 4) Our alternative hypothesis must be very specific: let H_1 represent linkage in a fraction of the affecteds between the marker and the AT disease gene at a recombination fraction of theta, and no linkage in the remaining affecteds. 5) All the affecteds are offspring of first-cousin matings, so each affected has an inbreeding coefficient of 1/16.

Using the marker described above, the conditional probability of an affected being homozygous for the marker which is theta recombination units from the AT gene decreases from 0.968 to 0.296 as theta increases from 0 to 50% (Fig. 3). As can be seen, our ability to distinguish between H_0 and H_1 depends on the magnitude of the difference between the expected amounts of homozygosity under the two hypotheses. This intuitively implies that the marker must be closely linked to the AT disease gene in order for linkage to be detected.

In sequential analysis, we continue sampling only until we reach a decision. For any given experiment, the number of observations needed to reach a decision is random. But mathematical analysis permits us to calculate the average sample num-

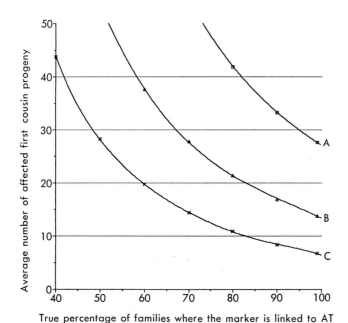

FIG. 4. Theoretical calculations estimating the number of first-cousin affecteds required in order to accept or exclude linkage as the genetic homogeneity among the tested affecteds increases (*i.e.*, when complementation groups are not known for all AT affecteds tested). This will also vary according to the distance of the given marker from the AT gene: Curve A is for theta= 0.10, Curve B is for theta=0.05, and Curve C is for theta=0.

ber (ASN) required to reach a decision. Note that this does not tell us which decision (H_0: no linkage or H_1: linkage) is made. Figure 4 shows the ASN as a function of the true percentage of affecteds in whom the marker is linked to AT. If we have about forty affecteds, and if the recombination fraction theta is 10%, then the proportion of affecteds linked to the AT gene must be greater than 80% in order for any decision at all to be reached. We presently are collecting samples on 25 consanguineous families and expect to have DNA on over 40 consanguineous affecteds available for testing soon.

Model V (deletional mutations) assumes that a subpopulation of AT patients will have deletions within their affected AT gene(s). Extrapolating from what is known about other disease genes, the proportion of this subpopulation can vary considerably. In alpha-thalassemia, almost all affecteds are due to deletions whereas in beta-thalassemia and most other diseases, the majority of defects are point mutations. We anticipate that at least a small subset of AT homozygotes will carry deletions in the region of their defective AT genes. Therefore, if a probe appears to be a good candidate for the AT gene, it can be hybridized to digested DNA from large numbers of affecteds with the expectation that some of these affecteds will show DNA fragments of abnormal size on Southern blots. If restriction enzymes are used which yield large fragments, these deletions are more likely to be detected. Enzymes such as NotI and SacII cut DNA at rare sequences and, by using pulsed field or inverted field gels, fragments of 100–1,000 kb can be visualized for this screening. The major limitation to these studies would be that deletions will probably be missed unless the probe used is actually part of the AT gene itself. Thus, Model V would be most useful in confirming that an AT gene has indeed been identified. It has the added advantage that a candidate gene does not need to be polymorphic in order to be tested since these studies do not depend upon genetic cosegregation or linkage.

Conclusion of Linkage Analyses

Thus far, we have used Models I and II for screening the blood protein markers (*35*) and we are just completing our first round of analyses of Model III data using approximately 110 markers. Model I data are meaningful for exclusion of linkage only if Model I is correct (*i.e.*, AT genes *are* clustered). In contrast, Model II exclusions should be meaningful for AT (Group A) even if Model I is correct. Whereas the data derived from Model I exclude 7% of the genome, the data base for Model II is smaller and the data exclude only about 2%. An additional 5% of the genome can be added for exclusion of most of the X chromosome on clinical grounds.

As we have recently published (*35*), the cumulative lod scores of sixteen families (Model I) for 23 informative markers revealed no linkage. Positive total lod scores appear in the data for RH, MNS, and PI. The maximum lod score (Z_{max}) for an RH/AT linkage was 0.77 at a recombination fraction theta=0.2. Z_{max} for MNS/AT was 0.65 at theta=0.13, and Z_{max} for PI/AT was 0.99 at theta=0. Lod scores below -2 for BF and GLO1 give exclusion intervals for thetas of [0, 0.14] and [0, 0.06], respectively, supporting our earlier report of non-linkage to HLA (*36*). The Model I data excluded approximately 236 cM or 7% of the autosomal genome (*37*).

The cumulative lod scores of eight Group A families (Model II) for 22 informative markers again showed no linkage. Positive total lod scores were found for RH, PI, ACP1, and MNS. The Z_{max} were: for RH/AT, 1.23 at theta=0.10; for PI/AT, 0.71 at theta=0; for ACP1/AT, 0.33 at theta=0.03; and for MNS/AT, 0.35 at theta=0.20. Altogether, these Model II data exclude approximately 72 cM or 2% of the genome.

Using Model II, the Z_{max} for the RH/AT combination was 1.51 when male and female thetas were allowed to differ. In this case, the maximum occurred when the female theta was zero and the male theta was 0.18. Thus, the Group A families showed no definite recombination events between RH and AT in mothers and at least one recombination in fathers.

The contribution of each family to the cumulative lod scores for RH/AT showed that one particular family (AT004) accounted for most of the positive evidence for linkage. Three families actually showed negative lod scores for thetas close to zero. On the other hand, among the families whose complementation groups have not yet been assigned, three families (AT006, AT007, and AT008) showed positive lod scores; one family (AT002) was not informative for linkage, and the remaining three families (AT009, AT017, and AT019) had negative lod scores. In any case, the data using either Model I or II are consistent with the conclusion that RH and AT are not *closely* linked.

While the relationship between RH (1p36.2–34) and AT is interesting, it is not convincing. As mentioned above, the elevated lod score reflects the evidence from mainly one family; other families negate the relationship. Further, data for other markers on chromosome 1, such as PGM1 (1p22.1), AMY2 (1p21), and Duffy (1p21–q23), show negative lod scores with exclusion intervals for PGM1, AMY2, and Duffy of 5 cM, 4 cM, and 1 cM, respectively. PGD (1p36.2–p36.13) was not informative in our families. On the other hand, taken together these data are still compatible with an assignment of AT Group A to the terminal end of chromosome 1p, and this possibility is being investigated.

An approximate exclusion interval of [0, 0.07] for BF excludes HLA-A and -B loci and again supports our earlier report of no linkage to HLA (*36*). We have additional preliminary data from Model III that also support this conclusion. This is of interest in view of the linkage of hereditary spinocerebellar ataxia to HLA (*38*).

A linkage of PI (*i.e.*, alpha-1-antitrypsin) to AT would tend to contradict our previous report of non-linkage to GM (*35*) since PI is located at 14q32.1, proximal to the IGH gene complex at 14q32.3 of which GM is a part. Two possible explanations for this apparent inconsistency are: 1) Model II is the correct model and the GM/AT linkage was masked in the earlier study by data from non-Group A families, or 2) the AT Group A gene is proximal to PI and thereby would be closer to PI than to GM. With regard to the earlier report, the two families with the most negative lod scores were later assigned to two different complementation groups (*i.e.*, Family 5, Group C; Family 6, Group A); thus, we still do not have sufficient information on complementation groups to definitively evaluate GM/AT linkage for Model II. The most likely interpretation of the data reported herein is that they do *not* support linkage of AT to the 14q31–32 region and are consistent with our earlier conclusion.

A linkage assignment around the MNS marker (4q28–31) would be interesting in view of the fact that AT homozygotes have elevated serum alphafetoprotein levels and the alphafetoprotein gene maps to 4q11–13 (*40*). However, we found no evidence of linkage of AT to GC, which maps to 4q12–13 (*41*).

We are now in a position, using the heterozygote assignments in Model III, to extend our observations regarding all of the above positive lod scores for the blood protein markers. In a collaboration with the Howard Hughes Medical Institute in Utah, another 80 markers have been tested on this pedigree. Preliminary assignment of quantitative variables for the probability that each unaffected member carries an AT gene were entered into the MENDEL genetic linkage program (*42*) for analysis of 110 genetic markers. Data analysis is still in progress at this writing. In addition, we are analyzing data on polymorphic candidate genes including thy-1 (*43*), alphafetoprotein (*40, 44*) and the T cell receptor alpha chain and beta chains (*45*).

We estimate that using 110 markers on Model III will independently survey approximately 15–30% of the genome. This estimate is based on preliminary analyses which show that a 0.58 PIC-marker excludes approximately 5 cM (in either direction). Conservatively estimating an average PIC for the 110 markers to be 0.4 and a conservative exclusion interval of 10 cM, we can multiply 110 by 10 cM = 1,100 cM (*i.e.*, 30% of the genome surveyed). However, because Models I, II, and III make different genetic assumptions and exclude some of the same regions, the percents of exclusion are not cumulative.

ACKNOWLEDGMENTS

This work was supported by USPHS National Research Service Awards GM-07104 and GM-08185, U.S. Department of Energy ER8760548, American Cancer Society CD 328, Ataxia-telangiectasia Medical Research Foundation, Alberta Heritage Foundation for Medical Research, National Cancer Institute (Canada), Concern Foundation, Drown Foundation, ELM Fund and Children's World. We thank Dr. Mark Leppert and Ken Lange for their comments in the preparation of this manuscript.

REFERENCES

1. Peterson, R.D.A., Kelly, W. D., and Good, R. A. Ataxia-telangiectasia. Its association with a defective thymus, immunological-deficiency disease, and malignancy. Lancet, *i*: 1189–1193, 1964.

2. Hecht, F., Koler, R. D., Rigas, D. A., Dahke, G. S., Case, M. P., Tisdale, V., and Miller, R. W. Leukemia and lymphocytes in ataxia-telangiectasia. Lancet, *ii*: 1193, 1966.

3. Sedgwick, R. P. and Boder, E. Ataxia-telangiectasia. *In;* P. J. Vinken and G. W. Bruyn (eds.), Handbook of Clinical Neurology, Vol. 14, pp. 267–339, North-Holland Publ. Co., Amsterdam, 1972.

4. Gatti, R. A. and Good, R. A. Occurrence of malignancy in immunodeficiency diseases. Cancer, *28*: 89–98, 1971.

5. Kersey, J. H., Spector, B. D., and Good, R. A. Primary immunodeficiency diseases and cancer: the Immunodeficiency Cancer Registry. Int. J. Cancer, *12*: 333–347, 1973.

6. Spector, B. D., Filipovich, A. H., Perry, G. S., and Kersey, J. H. Epidemiology of cancer in ataxia-telangiectasia. *In;* B. A. Bridges and D. G. Harnden (eds.), Ataxia-

telangiectasia—A Cellular and Molecular Link between Cancer, Neuropathology and Immune Deficiency, pp. 103–138, John Wiley and Sons, Publ., Chichester, 1982.

7. Swift, M., Sholman, L., Perry, M., and Chase, C. Malignant neoplasms in the families of patients with ataxia-telangiectasia. Cancer Res., *36*: 209–215, 1976.

8. Morrell, D., Cromartie, E., and Swift, M. Mortality and cancer incidence in 263 patients with ataxia-telangiectasia. J. Natl. Cancer Inst., *77*: 89–92, 1986.

9. Swift, M., Morrell, D., Cromartie, E., Chamberlin, A. R., Skolnick, M. H., and Bishop, D. T. The incidence and gene frequency of ataxia-telangiectasia in the United States. Am. J. Hum. Genet., *39*: 573–583, 1986.

10. Swift, M., Reitnauer, P. J., Morrell, D., and Chase, C. L. Breast and other cancers in families with ataxia-telangiectasia. N. Engl. J. Med., *316*: 1289–1294, 1987.

11. Gotoff, S. P., Amirmokri, E., and Liebner, E. J. Ataxia-telangiectasia. Neoplasia, untoward response to X-irradiation, and tuberous sclerosis. Am. J. Dis. Child., *114*: 617–625, 1967.

12. Morgan, J. L., Holcombe, T. M., and Morrissey, R. W. Radiation reaction in ataxia-telangiectasia. Am. J. Dis. Child., *116*: 557–558, 1968.

13. Cunliffe, P. N., Mann, J. R., Cameron, A. H., Roberts, K. D., and Ward, H.W.C. Radiosensitivity in ataxia-telangiectasia. Br. J. Radiol., *48*: 374–376, 1975.

14. Abadir, R. and Karami, N. Ataxia telangiectasia with cancer. An indication for reduced radiotherapy and chemotherapy doses. Br. J. Radiol., *56*: 343–345, 1983.

15. Taylor, A.M.R., Harnden, D. G., Arlett, C. F., Harcourt, S. A., Lehmann, A. R., Stevens, S., and Bridges, B. A. Ataxia-telangiectasia: A human mutation with abnormal radiation sensitivity. Nature, *258*: 427–429, 1975.

16. Paterson, M. C., Smith, B. P., Lohman, P.H.M., Anderson, A. K., and Fishman, L. Defective excision repair of gamma-ray damaged DNA in human (ataxia-telangiectasia) fibroblasts. Nature, *260*: 444–447, 1976.

17. Paterson, M. C., McFarlane, S. J., Gentner, N. E., and Smith, B. P. Cellular hypersensitivity to chronic gamma-radiation in cultured fibroblasts from ataxia-telangiectasia heterozygotes. In; R. A. Gatti and M. Swift (eds.), Ataxia-telangiectasia: Genetics, Neuropatholgy and Immunology of a Degenerative Disease of Childhood, pp. 77–87, Alan R. Liss, Inc., New York, 1985.

18. Paterson, M. C. and Smith, P. J. Ataxia-telangiectasia: an inherited human disorder involving hypersensitivity to ionizing radiation and related DNA-damaging chemicals. Annu. Rev. Genet., *13*: 291–318, 1979.

19. Inoue, T., Yokoiyama, A., and Kada, T. DNA repair enzyme deficiency and *in vitro* complementation of the enzyme activity in cell-free extracts from ataxia telangiectasia fibroblasts. Biochim. Biophys. Acta, *655*: 49–53, 1981.

20. Jaspers, N.G.J. and Bootsma, D. Genetic heterogeneity in ataxia-telangiectasia studied by cell fusion. Proc. Natl. Acad. Sci. U.S.A., *79*: 2641–2644, 1982.

21. Murname, J. P. and Painter, R. B. Complementation of the defects in DNA synthesis in irradiated and unirradiated ataxia-telangiectasia cells. Proc. Natl. Acad. Sci. U.S.A., *79*: 1960–1963, 1982.

22. Jaspers, N.G.J., Painter, R. B., Paterson, M. C., Kidson, C., and Inoue, T. Complementation analysis of ataxia-telangiectasia. In; R. A. Gatti and M. Swift (eds.), Ataxia-telangiectasia: Genetics, Neuropathology and Immunology of a Degenerative Disease of Childhood, pp. 147–162, Alan R. Liss, Inc., New York, 1985.

23. Gatti, R. A., Bick, M., Tam, C. F., Medici, M. A., Oxelius, V-A., Holland, M., Goldstein, A. L., and Boder, E. Ataxia-telangiectasia: A multiparameter analysis of eight families. Clin. Immunol. Immunopathol., *23*: 501–516, 1982.

24. Nakamura, Y., Leepert, M., O'Connell, P., Worlff, R., Holm, T., Culver, M., Mar-

tin, C., Fujimoto, E., Hoff, M., Kumlin, E., and White, R. Variable number of tandem repeat (VNTR) markers for human gene mapping. Science, *235*: 1616–1622, 1987.

25.   Botstein, D., White, R., Skolnick, M., and Davis, R. W. Construction of a genetic linkage map in man using restriction fragment length polymorphisms. Am. J. Hum. Genet., *32*: 314–331, 1980.

26.   White, R. and others. Linkage maps of human chromosomes. Human Gene Mapping Workshop, September, Paris, 1987.

27.   Donis-Keller, H., Green, P., Helms, C., and others. A genetic linkage map of the human genome. Cell, *51*: 319–337, 1987.

28.   Painter, R. B. Radioresistant DNA synthesis; an intrinsic feature of ataxia-telangiectasia. Mutat. Res., *84*: 183–190, 1981.

29.   Kojis, T., Schreck, R., Gatti, R. A., and Sparkes, R. S. Cytogenetic comparisons of lymphocytes and fibroblasts in ataxia-telangiectasia. Am. J. Hum. Genet., *41*: A126, 1987.

30.   Bridges, B. A., Lenoir, G., and Tomatis, L. Workshop on ataxia-telangiectasia heterozygotes and cancer. Cancer Res., *45*: 3979–3980, 1985.

31.   Lander, E. S. and Botstein, D. Mapping complex genetic traits in humans: New methods using a complete RFLP linkage map. Cold Spring Harbor Symp. Quant. Biol., *LI*: 49–62, 1986.

32.   Lander, E. S. and Botstein, D. Homozygosity mapping: A way to map human recessive traits with the DNA of inbred children. Science, *236*: 1567–1570, 1987.

33.   Dixon, W. J. and Massey, F. J. Introduction to Statistical Analysis, McGraw-Hill, New York, 1969.

34.   Ferguson, T. S. Mathematical Statistics: A Decision, Theoretical Approach, Academic Press, Orlando, Florida, 1967.

35.   Gatti, R. A., Davis, R. C., Weeks, D. E., Jaspers, N.G.J., Sparkes, R. S., and Lange, K. Genetic linkage studies of ataxia-telangiectasia: phenotypic blood markers. Disease Markers, in press.

36.   Hodge, S. E., Berkel, A. I., Gatti, R. A., Boder, E., and Spence, M. A. Ataxia-telangiectasia and xeroderma pigmentosum: No evidence of linkage to HLA. Tissue Antigens, *15*: 313–317, 1980.

37.   Renwick, J. H. Progress in mapping human autosomes. Br. Med. Bull., *25*: 65–73, 1969.

38.   Jackson, J. F., Currier, R. D., Terasaki, P. I., and Morton, N. E. Spinocerebellar ataxia and HLA linkage: risk prediction by HLA typing. N. Engl. J. Med., *296*: 1138–1141, 1977.

39.   Gatti, R. A., Boehnke, M., Crist, M., and Sparkes, R. S. Genetic linkage studies in ataxia-telangiectasia: Gm markers. *In;* R. A. Gatti and M. Swift (eds.), Ataxia-telangiectasia: Genetics, Neuropathology and Immunology of a Degenerative Disease of Childhood, pp. 163–172, Alan R. Liss, Inc., New York, 1985.

40.   Minghetti, P. P., Ruffner, D. E., Kuang, W-J., Dennison, O. E., Hawkins, J. W., Beattie, W. G., and Dugaiczyk, A. Molecular structure of the human albumin gene is revealed by nucleotide sequence within q11–22 of chromosome 4. J. Biol. Chem., *261*: 6747–6757, 1986.

41.   Kidd, K. K. and Gusella, J. Report of the committee on the genetic constitution of chromosomes 3 and 4. Cytogenet. Cell Genet., *4*: 107–127, 1985.

42.   Lange, K., Boehnke, M., and Weeks, D. E. Programs for Pedigree Analysis, Department of Biomathematics, University of California, Los Angeles, 1986.

43.   Gatti, R. A., Shaked, R., Wei, S., Koyama, M., Salser, W., and Silver, J. DNA

polymorphism in the human Thy-1 gene. Human Immunol., in press.

44. Murray, J. C., Watanabe, K., Tamaoki, T., Hornung, S., and Motulsky, A. RFLPs for the human alphafetoprotein (AFP) at 4q11–4q13. Nucleic Acids Res., *13*: 6794–6795, 1985.

45. Concannon, P., Gatti, R. A., and Hood, L. E. Human T cell receptor V_b gene polymorphism. J. Exp. Med., *165*: 1130–1140, 1987.

Frequency of Multiple Primary Cancers and Risk Factors for Lung and Breast Cancer Patients

Shaw Watanabe,[*1] Hisako Ochi,[*1] Yumiko Kobayashi,[*1]
Shoichiro Tsugane,[*1] Hiroko Arimoto,[*2] and Kikuko Kitagawa[*3]

*Epidemiology Division,[*1] Radiology Division,[*2] National Cancer Center Research Institute, and Administrative Office, National Cancer Center,[*3] Tokyo 104, Japan*

Abstract: Among nearly 50,000 cancer patients at the National Cancer Center, about 2,000 have multiple primary cancer (MPC), and its frequency has been increasing in recent years. MPC is considered to be a reflection of severe exposure to carcinogens or of a predisposition to cancer, or sometimes it is thought to be an individual expression within familial aggregation. To clarify the roles of these proposed mechanisms, case-control studies and chromosome analyses, including fragile sites on chromosomes, were performed focusing in particular on breast and lung cancer patients.

A histology-matched case-control study of multicentric lung cancer revealed a risk of cigarette smoking, which was also recognized in MPC in different sites among breast cancer patients, in addition to the radiotherapy. The frequency of heritable (rare) fragile sites among 87 lung cancer patients was more than double that of the general population, and the rare fragile site, 17q12, was clustered in the adenocarcinoma. The frequencies of heritable fragile sites among breast cancer patients were the same as the general population. MPC occurred in 10 of 87 lung cancer cases, and in 9 of 90 breast cancer patients; these individuals did not have heritable fragile sites. Heavy smoking and hazardous occupations were recognized in MPC cases with lung cancer, and a family history of rather rare cancers was also more common in MPC cases with breast cancer. One of three triple cancer cases had breast cancer as a feature in chromosomal aberrations of the peripheral blood lymphocytes, which may signify predisposition to cancer in these patients.

The occurrence of multiple primary cancers (MPC) was once rare, but has been increasingly recognized in recent years (*1–3*). Early detection of cancer and curable treatment may be among the reasons for this increase. Some hereditary cancers, such as retinoblastoma, colon cancers associated with familial polyposis, bilateral breast cancers, and others have multiple (multifocal or bilateral) occurrence (*4, 5*). However, since cancer chemotherapy has produced the undesirable effect of leukemia as a secondary primary cancer in patients with Hodgkin's disease, it has drawn the attention of both clinicians and basic researchers, because the second leukemia was quite different from the usual and resistant to treatment (6, 7). This experience indicated the importance of follow-up to obtain accurate data about the occurrence of second primary cancers and to clarify the mechanism as a step toward preventing the second cancer.

The mechanisms leading to second primary cancer are considered to be heterogenous: first is multiple carcinogenic stimulation of different cells with resultant multiple occurrences; second is the influence of the initial cancer in activating resting transformed cells; and third is chemotherapy-induced malignant transformation of normal cells (3, 8). Some sorts of predisposition to cancer may also affect the occurrence of second cancers. In this paper, we report the results of analyses of patients with second primary cancers in the National Cancer Center Hospital during the last 25 years, from 1962 to 1986, and a case-control study seeking factors related to the occurrence of second cancers. Recent results concerning fragile sites on chromosomes are also described in terms of their use to predict the risk of second cancers in particular individuals.

Frequency of Multiple Primary Cancers and Risk Factors for Lung and Breast Cancer Patients

At the National Cancer Center, 49,163 cancer patients were treated during the 25 years from 1962 to 1986. Among them, 1,740 were clinically diagnosed as having second primary cancers. The number of cancer patients by sites and the occurrence of second primary cancers are shown in Table 1. In this paper, patients with lung and breast cancer were the focus of the study, because both have been increasing in frequency recently in Japan and are considered to be related to both genetic predisposition and environmental exposure to carcinogens.

The number of second cancers among lung cancer patients was 132 among 3,845 males (9,069 person-years) and 23 among 1,211 females (3,197 person-years). The most frequent sites of second cancers were lung in both males and females (signi-

TABLE 1. Number of Cancer Patients by Site and Occurrence of Second Primary Cancer

Site of first cancer	No. of cancer patients	No. of person-years	No. of MPC	O/E ratio
Oro-pharynx	2,924	14,338.2	136	1.33*
Esophagus	1,816	3,905.2	119	1.90*
Stomach	10,297	45,388.5	319	0.88
Colon	1,272	6,237.8	87	2.00*
Rectum	1,680	7,801.6	73	1.24
Liver	1,142	2,378.9	7	0.17
Larynx	1,215	8,053.0	97	2.32*
Lung	5,056	12,266.2	155	0.87
Breast (females)	7,369	49,694.1	322	1.24*
Uterus	6,016	37,776.5	194	0.92
Hemato-lymphoid	2,005	6,747.7	19	0.27
Others	8,371		213	0.72
Total	49,163		1,740	

* $p < 0.05$ by Student t-test.

ficantly high O/E (observed/expected) ratio), and then larynx, oropharynx, and hematolymphoid tissue in males (Table 2). The greater association with second cancers in the upper gastrointestinal and respiratory tract was also reported by Harwood (9). The number of second cancers among 7,335 breast cancer patients (person-years 49,694.1) was 322, and the sites of second cancer were significantly high in the opposite breast and hematolymphoid tissue.

Multifocal lung cancer cases and bilateral breast cancer cases were the focus of epidemiologic work, because they were considered to reveal risk factors influenced by genetic predisposition and/or environmental exposure in a more exaggerated form as compared to MPC involving other organs. A relationship between the histologic types of first and second cancers revealed that the histologic coincidence of two cancers of Kreiberg type I or II was observed in 72% of the cases (Table 3) (10). Squamous cell carcinoma, however, accounts for 65% of first cancers, and 33% of second cancers.

A histologically matched case-control study to detect the risk factors for a second multifocal lung cancer was conducted. The cases were 72 patients with multifocal lung cancer, and the controls were 114 sex, age (± 5 years), and histologically matched patients with one (unicentric) lung cancer and having longer survival than most cases. From the hospital charts information was obtained about the smoking history, drinking history, previous illness, residential area, occupation, and familial history. Tobacco smoking was the only risk factor detected by the case-control study. The statistical significance is marginal; the odds ratio, however, shows a dose-dependent increase (Table 4). Other factors, such as familial history of cancer, past illness, drinking history, and occupation were not significantly related to the occurrence of second cancer. However, a few cases were at increased risk of cancer, such as chromate workers and one atomic bomb survivor from Hiroshima.

TABLE 2. Multiplicity of Second Cancers among Lung and Breast Cancer Patients

Primary site	Sex	No. of patients	Person-years	No. of MPC	O/E Ratio by Site of Second Primary Cancer								
					Larynx	Lung	Oro-phx.	Esoph-agus	Stom-ach	Colon-rectum	Breast	Uterus	Hemato-lymph
Lung	M	3,845	9,069.1	132	6.50**	4.62**	5.60*	1.54	0.71	0.96	—	—	4.49*
	F	1,211	3,197.2	23	0	8.18**	0	0	0.56	1.78	0	1.26	0
Breast	F	7,335	49,694.1	322	2.78	0.85	0	1.47	0.48	0.76	6.74**	1.14	3.37**

* $p<0.05$, ** $p<0.01$ by the method of Bailar (18).
Expected number of MPC was calculated by multiplying cancer incidence of Japan (19) by person-years.

TABLE 3. Histology of Multifocal Lung Cancer Cases

Initial cancer	Second cancer					
	Squamous	Small	Adeno	Large	Other	Total
Squamous	23 (1)	6 (1)	13 (1)	2	3	47 (3)
Small					1	1
Adeno		4	14 (4)	4	1 (1)	23 (5)
Large				1		1
Total	23 (1)	10 (1)	27 (5)	7	5 (1)	72 (8)

TABLE 4. Influence of Smoking to Multifocal Lung Cancer (Histology-matched Case-control Study)

Brinkman index	Multicentric cases $n=72$	Unicentric cases $n=143$	Odds ratio
0– 399	16.7	25.9	1.00
400– 799	25.0	24.5	1.59
800–1,599	43.1	38.4	1.75
over 1,600	15.2	11.2	2.16

S^* (Amirtage)$=1.52$ $(p=0.06)$.

TABLE 5. Risk Factors for Second Primary Cancers among Breast Cancer Patients

	No. of MPC	Cigarettes 40/day		Alcohol $+/-$		Family history present/absent		Radiation therapy present/absent	
		X^2	OR	X^2	OR	X^2	OR	X^2	OR
Bilateral	117	0.12	0.89	0.04	0.92	1.92	1.48	3.10	1.79
Multiple	99	4.8*	0.43	3.13	0.52	3.13	1.70	5.44*	2.27

* $p<0.05$.

A matched case-control study on breast cancer patients did not reveal significant risk factors, except for radiation therapy to the initial cancer in cases of second cancer other than of the breast. A family history of breast cancer was not a risk factor even in cases with bilateral breast cancer (Table 5). This lack of significance may be due to overmatching the controls; or as Lynch (11) described, genetically determined breast cancer is only 5% of cases, and statistical power is insufficient to show this influence.

Fragile Sites of Lung and Breast Cancer Patients

Fragile sites on chromosomes are significantly associated with various cancer breakpoints and sites of oncogenes (12). If the frequency and location of fragile sites could serve as indexes for the risk of second cancer, such observations would be useful for prevention. Peripheral blood was obtained from consecutive patients with lung or breast cancer before surgery and the following method was applied: (1) folic acid and thymidine depleted medium for group 1 fragile sites, (2) addition of distamycin A for group 2 fragile sites, (3) addition of bromodeoxyuridine for group 3 fragile sites, (4) addition of aphidicholin for common fragile sites, and (5) control RPMI1640 medium after phytohemagglutinin (PHA) stimulation (13–15).

Eighty-seven lung cancer patients have been analyzed so far, among them 9 had heritable fragile sites (Table 6). Five of 40 adenocarcinoma patients showed a fragility at 16p12, 16q22, and 17p12. Three of 28 squamous cell carcinoma patients showed fragility at 11q13 and 16q22. The frequency compared with that for the general population, reported by Takahashi et al. (13), was more than double in both adenocarcinoma and squamous cell carcinoma. It is interesting that 17p12 aggregated in adenocarcinoma cases.

Among these 87 lung cancer patients, 10 had double primary cancers (Table 7). Such a high frequency was due to our hospital specializing in cancer treatment; patients come with some selection bias, because all had initial cancer in other organs

TABLE 6. Frequency of Heritable Fragile Sites among Lung Cancer Patients

Histology	No.	Folate sensitive		Distamycin A		Total	%
		11q13	16p12	16q22	17p12		
Adeno	40	—	1	1	3	5	12.5
Squamous	28	1	—	2	—	3	10.7
Large	9	—	—	—	—	0	0
Small	3	—	—	—	—	0	0
Other	5	—	—	—	—	0	0
Carcinoid	2	—	—	—	1	1	50
Total (%)	87	1 (1.14)	1 (1.14)	3 (3.45)	4 (4.59)	9	(10.20)
General population (%)		(0.20)	(0.00)	(1.42)	(3.08)		(4.70)

TABLE 7. Multiple Primary Cancer Cases among 87 Lung Cancer Cases

	Histology	Risk factor	Cancer in family[a]
a: Multifocal			
1) Y.M. 56 M	Adeno+large	Tobacco (40/day×30 yrs)	
2) C.O. 58 M	Adeno-4Y[b]-adeno	Tobacco (20/day×40 yrs)	Brain, breast
3) K.S. 67 F	Adeno+carcinoid	Radioisotope	Breast
b: Double primary			
1) S.T. 44 M	Bladder-19Y-adeno	Tobacco (30/day×16 yrs)	
2) K.M. 50 F	Parotid-9Y-adeno		
3) T.T. 53 F	Thyroid-2Y-adeno		
4) S.T. 59 M	Larynx-18Y-Sq	Tobacco (40/day×30 yrs)	
5) D.K. 65 M	Prostate-1Y-Sq	Tobacco (80/day×35 yrs)	
6) M.A. 65 M	Colon-7Y-adeno	Tobacco (15/day×40 yrs) Smelter worker	
7) S.N. 67 M	Stomach-8Y-adeno	Tobacco (10/day×33 yrs)	

[a] within the first generation.   [b] interval between the two cancers.

TABLE 8. Frequency of Heritable Fragile Sites among Breast Cancer Patients

Histology	No.	Distamycin A			BrdU	Total %
		8q24	16q22	17p12	10q25	
Adenocarcinoma	90	0	1	1	1	3 3.3
Benign lesions	10	1	1	0	0	2 20
Total (%)	100	1 (1.0)	2 (2.0)	1 (1.0)	1 (1.0)	5 (5.0)
General Population		(0.71)	(1.42)	(3.08)	(0.29)	(5.5)

except for 3 multifocal cases. None was a carrier of heritable fragile sites, but they revealed risk factors such as heavy tobacco smoking, hazardous occupation and many years of handling radioactive iodide. It is interesting that the family history of brain tumor and breast cancer was recognized only in one multifocal case.

Heritable fragile sites were rare among 90 breast cancer patients. Although 5 carriers were detected in this study, 2 had benign lesions. The overall frequency is the same as that in the general population: the sites were 10q22 in one, 16q22 in 2, 17p12 in one, and 8q24 in 2 (Table 8).

TABLE 9. Multiple Primary Cancer among 90 Breast Cancer Patients

		Sites	Risk factor	Cancer in family[a]
a:	Bilateral			
	1) M.T. 40	Breast+breast		Breast, lung
	2) J.N. 42	Breast+breast	Myoma ut. ope.	Lung
b:	Double primary			
	1) C.Y. 28	Kidney-8Y-breast	Radiation	
	2) K.A. 38	Ovary-18Y-breast	Chemotherapy	Leukemia, breast, lung
	3) H.S. 40	Uterus-23Y-breast		Breast
	4) T.K. 60	Anal-9Y-Paget		Leukemia
c:	Triple primary			
	1) T.F. 48	Paget-6Y-bilateral breasts	Chromosomal aberration	Breast
	2) Y.K. 52	Breast-20Y-stomach+rectum	Tobacco (10×50yr)	Rectum
	3) M.I. 62	Breast-5Y-colon-2Y-breast		Colon, GI tract

[a] Within the first generation.

Double primary and triple primary cancer cases in this study are shown in Table 9. Second breast cancers in two heterochronous cases are considered to be related to the treatment. However, family history revealed leukemia in 2, breast cancer in 4, and lung cancer in 3, in addition to the more common gastrointestinal tract cancers in one generation. Three triple cancer cases were further analyzed for karyotype, and all of them revealed some kind of abnormal karyotype. One patient was operated on for an ovarian cyst at age 28, for genital Paget's disease at age 48, and for bilateral breast cancers at age 54. The karyotype from this patient revealed a reciprocal balanced translocation between 5q15 and 19q13 (Fig. 1). A second patient with triple cancer also revealed translocation between 10q and 13p, but it seemed not to be clonal, so it is thought that this remained long after the chemotherapy. A third patient showed normal karyotype.

The frequency of autosomal chromosomal aberration in the Japanese population is 0.13% for trisomy, 0.19% for balanced rearrangements and 0.02% for unbalanced rearrangements (unpublished data). Hence, it may be concluded that individuals with autosomal aberrations even in the chromosomes of peripheral lymphocytes are at high risk of multiple cancers.

The involvement of common fragile sites is still under study. However, our preliminary data showed that the frequency and the site were influenced by certain host factors, such as age of menarch (unpublished data). Further study is necessary to clarify the relationship between common fragile sites in lymphocytes and neoplastic cells *per se*. Many cancers have shown reduction to homozygosity of genes (*16, 17*), so a more sensitive detection system for chromosome fragility should become one of the indexes of genetic susceptibility to cancer.

Conclusions

MPC involving the lung seemed to be related to environmental exposure. Tobacco smoking was a risk factor for multicentric lung cancer. Genetic factors for

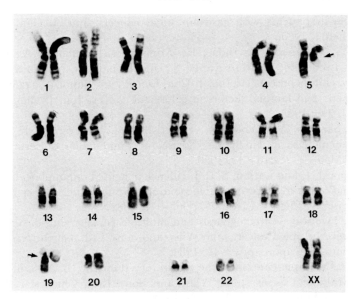

FIG. 1.   Karyotype from the patients with triple cancer. Translocation $t(5; 19)$ (q15; q13) is present.

bilateral breast cancer patients were not significantly detected by our matched case-control study, probably due to overmatching or insufficient statistical power.

The frequency of heritable fragile sites was different for lung cancer patients than for breast cancer patients. The former was more than twice normal, but the latter was the same as that of the general population. Multiple cancer cases in this series did not have heritable fragile sites and showed risk factors, such as cigarette smoking and/or hazardous occupation for lung cancer cases, but not for breast cancer patients. The latter group seemed to be more influenced by genetic factors, because rare cancers such as leukemia, brain tumor and breast cancer were more common in siblings, parents or children.

The presence of chromosomal aberration in two of three triple cancer cases should call attention to chromosomal abnormality as a possible indicator of high risk for multiple cancers and the need for some intervention to prevent these secondary cancers.

REFERENCES

1. Watanabe, S., Kodama, T., Shimosato, Y., Arimoto, H., Sugimura, T., Suemasu, K., and Shiraishi, M. Multiple primary cancers in 5,456 autopsy cases in the National Cancer Center of Japan. J. Natl. Cancer Inst., 72: 1021–1027, 1984.
2. Boice, J. D., Jr., Storm, H. H., Curtis, R. E., Jensen, O. M., Kleinerman, R. A., Jensen, H. S., Flannery, J. T., and Fraumeni, J. F., Jr. Multiple primary cancers in Connecticut and Denmark. National Cancer Institute Monograph 68, U.S. Department of Health and Human Services, NCI, Bethesda, 1985.
3. Watanabe, S., Kodama, T., Shimosato, Y., Arimoto, H., and Suemasu, K. Second

primary cancers in patients with gastrointestinal cancers. Jpn. J. Clin. Oncol., *15* (Suppl. 1): 171–182, 1985.

4. Tsunematsu, Y., Watanabe, S., Inoue, R., Minowa, K., Tsuchida, A., Bessho, F., Tsukimoto, I., Imashuku, S., Matsuyama, S., and Kobayashi, N. Multiple primary malignancies in childhood cancer. Jpn. J. Clin. Oncol., *15* (Suppl. 1): 223–234, 1985.

5. Ushio, K. Genetic and familial factors in colorectal cancer. Jpn. J. Clin. Oncol., *15* (Suppl. 1): 281–298, 1985.

6. Valagussa, P., Santoro, A., Kenda, R., Fossati-Bellani, F., Franchi, F., and Banfi, A. Second malignancies in Hodgkin's disease: a complication of certain forms of treatment. Br. Med. J., *1*: 216–219, 1980.

7. Pedersen-Bjergaard, J. and Larsen, S. L. Incidence of acute nonlymphocytic leukemia, preleukemia and acute myeloproliferative syndrome up to 10 years after treatment of Hodgkin's disease. N. Engl. J. Med., *307*: 965–971, 1982.

8. Berenblum, I. Two-stage carcinogenesis and multiple cancers. *In;* B. A. Stoll (ed.), Risk Factors and Multiple Cancer, John Wiley and Sons, Ltd., Chichester, New York, Brisbane, Toronto, Singapore, pp. 3–12, 1984.

9. Harwood, A. R. Multiple cancers of the respiratory tract. *In;* B. A. Stoll (ed.), Risk Factors and Multiple Cancer, John Wiley and Sons, Ltd., Chichester, New York, Brisbane, Toronto, Singapore, pp. 279–299, 1984.

10. Sugimura, H., Watanabe, S., Tsugane, S., Morinaga, S., and Yoneyama, T. Case-control study on histologically determined multiple primary lung cancer. J. Natl. Cancer. Inst., *79*: 435–441, 1987.

11. Lynch, H. T., Albano, W. A., Danes, B. S., Layton, M. A., Kimberling, W. J., Lynch, J. F., Cheng, S. C., Costello, K. A., Mulcahy, G. M., Wagner, C. A., and Tindall, S. L. Genetic predisposition to breast cancer. Cancer, *53*: 612–622, 1984.

12. Sutherland, G. R. and Hecht, F. Fragile Sites on Human Chromosomes. Oxford Monogr. Med. Genetics, Oxford Univ. Press, New York, Oxford, 1985.

13. Takahashi, E., Hori, T., and Murata, M. Population cytogenetics of rare fragile sites in Japan. Hum. Genet., *78*: 121–126, 1988.

14. Le Beau, M. M. Chromosomal fragile sites and cancer-specific rearrangements. Blood, *67*: 849–858, 1986.

15. Yunis, J. J. and Soreng, A. L. Constitutive fragile sites and cancer. Science, *226*: 1199–1204, 1984.

16. Knudson, A. G. This volume, pp. 221–231.

17. Ali, I. U., Lidereau, R., Theillet, C., and Callahan, R. Reduction to homozygosity of genes on chromosome 11 in human breast neoplasia. Science, *238*: 185–188, 1987.

18. Bailar, J. C., III and Ederer, F. Significance factors for the ratio of a Poisson variable to its expectation. Biometrics, *20*: 639, 1964.

19. Segi, M., Tominaga, S., Aoki, K., and Fujimoto, I. (eds.) Cancer mortality and morbidity statistics. Japan and the world. Gann Monogr. Cancer Res. *26*: 1–274, 1981.

UNUSUAL OCCURRENCES AS CLUES TO CANCER ETIOLOGY, R. W. MILLER ET AL. (EDS.),
JAPAN SCI. SOC. PRESS, TOKYO/TAYLOR & FRANCIS, LTD., PP. 283–294, 1988

Strategies to Control Cancer through Genetics

Kåre BERG

Institute of Medical Genetics, University of Oslo, Oslo 3, Norway

Abstract: Although genetic factors may be essential in only a fraction of common
cancers, it is important to identify individuals who merit genetic evaluation. The occurrence of cancer in an individual under one of the following circumstances may
indicate an increased susceptibility to malignancy as a result of predisposing factors:
cancer in both of paired organs, thought not to be the result of metastasis; more
than one focus of cancer in a single organ (multifocal tumors); histologically similar
malignant neoplasms in different parts of the same organ system; two histologically
distinct cancers (multiple primary malignancies); cancer at an atypical age; at an
atypical site; in the usually less often affected sex; associated with birth defects; associated with precursor lesions; in a person with immunodeficiency; or in a patient
with one of the 200 Mendelian disorders where cancer is part of the clinical picture
or a frequent complication. At risk are first-degree relatives of people who meet any
of the above criteria. Also, a person should be considered at risk if two first-degree
relatives had any form of cancer.

A strategy to control cancers utilizing genetic knowledge should include such
measures as: genetic counseling of individuals at risk for specific cancers because of a
congenital or genetic disease in themselves or their relatives, or because of the pattern
of cancer occurrence in the family; prenatal diagnosis for families with genetic conditions that predispose to cancer and are amenable to prenatal testing; surveillance of
high-risk individuals to detect early manifestations of new or recurrent disease; prophylactic removal of the target organ or tissue in appropriate cases; limiting exposure
of high-risk individuals to known carcinogens or supplementing diets of high-risk individuals with anticarcinogens; and educational and administrative measures to pro-
mote practical application of genetic knowledge and to increase awareness of genetic
factors in the etiology of cancer.

Far from all individuals who are exposed to carcinogenic factors contract cancer,
and in another common disease, atherosclerosis, it is well known that there is genetically determined variation in response to environmental or lifestyle factors that can
cause disease. The emerging fields of human ecogenetics and predictive testing together with research progress in medical and molecular genetics are likely to improve
greatly the possibilities for utilizing genetic knowledge to control cancer.

Early Studies of Cancers in Families

An early, major effort to study the genetics of cancers was made by my mentor and supervisor for my Ph.D. thesis, the Norwegian Professor Georg H. M. Waaler, University of Oslo, who in 1931 published his monograph "Über die Erblichkeit des Krebses" (*1*), shortly after he had worked out his famous two-locus inheritance principle for colour vision anomalies. Examining the families of 616 males and 786 females with cancer, Waaler found increased cancer frequency in the parents, brothers and sisters of cancer patients. One might have expected that this monograph would create an immediate keen interest in the area of cancer genetics but only scattered reports on familial clustering of cancers continued to appear in the literature.

It slowly became an established fact that certain tumor disorders, particularly bilateral retinoblastoma and polyposis of the colon aggregate in families because of the segregation of autosomal dominant genes. By the mid-1970's about 200 conditions known or believed to be monogenic were on record as having neoplasia as a characteristic or a frequent complication (*2*). In approximately one third of the conditions was the mode of inheritance considered definitely proven (*2, 3*). The catalogue (*4*) of Mendelian traits in man has continued to grow and its computerized version comprised 4,159 items by August 15, 1987 as opposed to 2,336 in the mid-1970's. Whether or not the percentage (8.6%) of conditions exhibiting propensity to neoplasia is changed, it may safely be assumed that the genetic repertory of human neoplasia is even larger than the impression arrived at by the analyses conducted in the mid-1970's.

Although the number of Mendelian conditions exhibiting susceptibility to neoplasia is large, it is important that each of them is rare. Therefore, the genes causing these disorders cannot have a major impact on the great majority of cancers.

Early twin studies, summarized by Nance (*5*) seemed to argue against a major effect of genes, since low concordance rates were found in monozygotic (MZ) as well as dizygotic (DZ) pairs. The small numbers in each of the series examined as well as several shortcomings of the classical twin method makes it difficult to interpret some of the early twin data.

Fortunately, important information on familial aggregation of common cancers in relatives other than twins has been reported in recent years although such information is not easily available. Family analyses of diseases occurring late in life are difficult since usually only one affected generation can be studied and since several members of that generation may have died earlier from diseases other than that under study.

Genetics of Common Disorders

The size of the effect from strategies to control cancer will depend on the importance of genetic factors in cancer etiology. The problem is intimately related to the genetics of common disorders in general. It may be helpful, therefore, to examine briefly another common disorder, coronary heart disease (CHD), for which we may soon develop strategies for control through genetics.

Müller (*6*) discovered in 1937 that the triad of CHD, xanthomatosis and hyper-

TABLE 1.   Estimates of Heritability (h^2) of Serum Lipid and Lipoprotein Levels

Parameter	Heritability (h^2)
Total serum cholesterol	0.68
Fasting triglycerides	0.46
Apolipoprotein B level	0.64
Apolipoprotein A-I level	0.55
Apolipoprotein A-II level	0.68
Lp(a) lipoprotein level	1.00

(From ref. *11*)

cholesterolemia segregated as an autosomal dominant trait with a population frequency of about only 1 : 500. This triad accounts for only a small fraction of the total number of cases of CHD. It has, however, become widely realized over the past 20 years that genetic factors are important in the etiology of CHD more generally, particularly when the disease occurs at a relatively young age (reviewed in refs. *7–9*). For example, Nora and his co-workers (*10*) uncovered a heritability of 0.56 for CHD prior to the age of 55 even after monogenic hyperlipidemias had been excluded.

Several biochemical or "anti-risk" factors for atherosclerosis exhibit a high level of heritability (*11, 12*) as summarized in Table 1. Thus, the effects of genes account for about two-thirds of the population variation in the risk factor, apolipoprotein B (apB), as well as in the presumed "anti-risk" factor apolipoprotein A-II (apoA-II).

In 1974 a direct association between the genetically controlled Lp(a) lipoprotein and CHD was detected (*13*), an observation later confirmed by other workers. Rhoads and his associates in 1986 (*14*) found that the attributable risk in a population was 28 percent for myocardial infarction prior to age 60 in men whose Lp(a) lipoprotein levels were in the top quartile. The allotypic Ag(x) system in low density lipoprotein (LDL) is associated with cholesterol as well as triglyceride levels (*15*), and genetically determined isoforms of apolipoprotein E (apoE) are associated with myocardial infarction as well as the cholesterol level (reviewed in refs. *9, 11, 12*). Finally, restriction length polymorphisms (RFLPs) at apolipoprotein loci are associated with risk factor levels or overt atherosclerotic disease (*16–19*). Such information may be utilized in attempts to control CHD (and cancer) by adding a strategy that focuses on individuals at high risk rather than on the total population (*9, 20*).

How Can Both Genetic Factors and Environmental Factors Be of Importance in the Etiology of a Common Disorder?

There are two frequent misconceptions that may have delayed the development and implementation of strategies to control common disorders through genetics. The first is that if environmental, lifestyle or dietary factors are of importance for the development of a disease, genetic factors cannot be so. This misconception may be based on an outdated "nature or nurture" thinking and is at variance with important new information. In reality, there are now many examples of inherited variation in susceptibility or resistance to environmental agents and the term "ecogenetics" is used for this interaction between environmental factors and genetic factors (*3*). Mulvihill (*21*) lists several ecogenetic interactions in human malignancy including sarcomas caused by ionizing radiation in retinoblastoma patients; skin cancer or melanomas caused by ultraviolet radiation in patients with xeroderma pigmentosum or dysplastic nevus syndrome, and urinary bladder cancer caused by N-substituted aryl compounds in people with variant N-acetyl transferase activity. Most likely, tumors caused by cigarette smoking in people with specific genotypes can in the future be added to the list.

In CHD it is clear that lifestyle or dietary factors contribute together with genetic factors to the development of disease. Cigarette smoking clearly increases the risk of CHD and dietary or lifestyle factors as well as genetic factors are known to contribute to the level of the risk factors for hypercholesterolemia and hypertension.

The unifying concept for any common disease where environmental, lifestyle or dietary, as well as genetic factors appear to be of etiological importance, is that environmental factors primarily cause disease in those who have a genetic predisposition. The new ecogenetics of human diseases have taught us that we must think in terms of genes *and* environment, not in terms of genes *or* environment.

The second widespread misconception is that diseases that are completely or partially genetically determined cannot be treated or modified. This misconception may perhaps be based on the situation that prevails for most of the simply inherited disorders of childhood where in most cases the therapeutic possibilities are indeed limited. This line of reasoning is not valid for common disorders where genetic as well as environmental factors are of importance. This is illustrated by the variations in this century in frequency of atherosclerotic disease. Thus, the frequency of myocardial infarction dropped impressively in Norway and other European countries during the greatly changed living conditions of World War II, only to increase again after the war, and the United States and several other countries have experienced a significant decline in myocardial infarction mortality in recent years. These changes in frequencies cannot be caused by genetic changes since it would take several generations for the necessary changes in gene frequencies to take place. The explanation must be that even people with a significant genetic predisposition to CHD may avoid disease if environmental, lifestyle and dietary factors are favourably changed.

The above misconceptions together with difficulties of communication between medical specialties have undoubtedly delayed developments in the area of CHD. Some traditional epidemiologists may fear that the "high risk strategy" which geneticists want to add to the prevailing "total population strategy", could distract attention from the efforts to change everybody's lifestyle in a favourable direction. However, such a worry cannot justify neglecting the possibility to provide those at the highest risk with the best possible opportunities to improve their prognosis by starting efficient preventive efforts at a young age and continuing them throughout life. A growing mutual understanding between the adherents of a total population strategy exclusively and medical geneticists with their additional high risk strategy may now be developing in the area of CHD control. It is important that the mistakes made in the CHD area are not repeated in the area of cancer control.

Aims of Strategies to Control Common Disorders through Genetics

The central purpose of strategies to control common disorders through genetics is to favourably modify the environmental, lifestyle or dietary factors so as to diminish the effect of genetic factors predisposing to disease. Whereas changes in these three factors may be advantageous to the population at large, they are particularly important in people with a genetic predisposition to disease. The capacity to identify people who have such a genetic predisposition is instrumental in the development and implementation of strategies to control disease through genetics. There are two main advantages in identifying those who are genetically at risk. Firstly, detection early in life of a genetic predispositon to a serious common disorder makes it possible to initiate preventive measures as early as possible, and this by itself should greatly increase the possibility to avoid or delay diseases that may develop over a great number of years.

Secondly, the knowledge of being especially at risk because of one's genetic predisposition will in all likelihood strongly motivate people to adhere throughout life to preventive measures. A comparable level of motivation would be very difficult to achieve if only a total population strategy were to be applied.

The hope of successful disease prevention depends on availability of truly efficient preventive measures. For people at risk of CHD such measures are indeed available and include lifestyle and dietary changes, cessation of cigarette smoking and, if necessary, the use of drug treatment to reduce levels of lipids and blood pressure. The situation is more difficult with increased cancer risk since preventive measures with a comparable degree of efficiency are not easily available. However, for certain specific cancers appropriate measures are known such as the avoidance of ultraviolet radiation in people at risk for melanoma or skin cancers. Furthermore, cessation of cigarette smoking would probably be useful for many people at increased cancer risk. Occupational as well as leisure time avoidance of exposure to other known carcinogens would also be reasonable measures. Hopefully, the knowledge of useful preventive measures will increase significantly over the next several years.

An additional, important purpose of strategies to control common disorders through genetics is to secure early diagnosis and treatment with the aim of limiting the consequences of disease. With the present state of knowledge, this would be a central aim for efforts to control cancer through genetics.

The Tools of the Medical Geneticist

The central activities of the medical geneticists are pedigree analyses, genetic counseling, prenatal diagnosis, cytogenetic examination of born individuals, tests aimed at detecting the presence of a given gene either directly or by the use of closely linked loci, and risk computations. These activities may all be useful in efforts to control common diseases through genetics if combined with preventive advice to people at risk and examinations to uncover early signs of disease.

Outline of a Strategy to Control Cancer through Genetics

The above considerations together with research progress too extensive to summarize here make it important to consider which elements should be included in a strategy to control cancer through genetics, given present knowledge and realistic expectations concerning future developments. As a Scholar-in-Residence at the Fogarty International Center for Advanced Study in the Health Sciences, National Institutes of Health, I, together with Drs. Robert W. Miller, John J. Mulvihill and their co-workers was given the opportunity to conduct a workshop on strategies for controlling cancer through genetics, bringing together the knowledge of a number of experts from the U.S. and Canada. A report of the workshop has recently been published (*22*). In this outline of a practical strategy, I have drawn heavily on consensus and conclusions reached at the workshop. In developing the workshop the organizers perceived that more practical use could be made of existing knowledge of human cancer genetics to control cancer in the population, and that future advances in understanding cancer genetics are likely to yield additional insights relevant to cancer control that should be promptly brought to the public. The workshop considered "cancer control" in the broadest sense (*22*).

A review of cancer genetics leads to the conclusion that genetics is of importance for several cancers, including those of the breast, colon and skin, melanoma, retinoblastoma, Wilms' tumor, leukemia, other childhood cancers, and cancers of endocrine organs, particularly those occurring in the multiple endocrine neoplasia syndromes (*23–39*). For the portion of cancers attributed to genetic factors (*e.g.*, 30–40% of all bilateral retinoblastomas, 10% or less of breast or colon cancer) the preventive measures are mainly:

1. *Genetic counseling* of individuals considered at increased risk for specific cancers because of a congenital or genetic disease in themselves or their relatives, the pattern of cancer occurrence in the family, or because they carry a known genetic marker for cancer susceptibility. Adequate risk estimates can be made not only for monogenic diseases, but also in cases where a multifactorial disorder such as breast cancer aggregates in families (*40*).

2. *Prenatal diagnosis* for families with genetic conditions that predispose to cancer and are amenable to prenatal testing, *e.g.*, xeroderma pigmentosum, Fanconi's anemia.

3. *Surveillance of high risk individuals* to detect early manifestations of new or recurrent disease, *e.g.*, development of adenomatous colonic polyps in suspected carriers of the autosomal dominant gene for polyposis coli, production of increased levels of calcitonin in response to pentagastrin stimulation in possible carriers of the gene for multiple endocrine neoplasia syndrome (type II), development of dysplastic nevi in persons with the familial dysplastic nevus syndrome or the appearance of a prostate-specific antigen in serum of men at risk for adenocarcinoma of the prostate (*41*).

4. *Prophylactic removal* of the target organ or tissue in appropriate cases, such as a colon with polyps, a dysplastic nevus, or breast tissue in women at high risk for breast cancer.

5. *Limiting exposure* of high risk individuals to known carcinogens (*e.g.*, use of

sunscreens and sun avoidance in patients with xeroderma pigmentosum, dysplastic nevi or albinism).

6. *Supplementing diets* of high risk individuals with anti-carcinogens (*e.g.*, β-carotene in albinism).

7. *Future approaches* to cancer prevention may include *vaccination* against cancer-causing viruses (*e.g.*, against hepatitis B virus in the areas in which the virus is endemic, or in infants born to carrier mothers), the use of *gene therapy* for genetic immunodeficiencies amenable to cure through bone marrow manipulations (*e.g.*, adenosine deaminase deficiency), and systematic predictive screening for genetic markers indicating cancer susceptibility.

Identification of Individuals Who Merit Genetic Evaluation

The occurrence of cancer in an individual under any of the following circumstances may indicate an increased genetic susceptibility to malignancy that warrants genetic evaluation:

1. Cancer in both of a pair of organs that is thought not to be the result of metastases, *e.g.*, in both breasts, both adrenal glands, both kidneys.

2. More than one focus of cancer in a single organ (multicentric tumors), *e.g.*, multiple retinoblastomas in one eye.

3. Two or more distinct cancers (multiple primary malignancies), *e.g.*, breast and ovarian cancers, endometrial and colon cancers.

4. Cancer that has occurred at an atypical age, at an atypical site or in the sex that is usually far less frequently affected, *e.g.*, lung cancer in a nonsmoking woman.

5. Cancers associated with other conditions such as birth defects, one of the 200 single gene disorders known to be complicated by neoplasia, or with precursor lesions.

6. Unusual or rare cancers, *e.g.*, pheochromocytoma.

Guidelines for Identifying a Family That Might Benefit from Genetic Evaluation

A person with a family history of cancer may benefit from genetic evaluation even if the person is not affective. A family history of cancer may also be significant in evaluating a patient with cancer who does not meet any of the criteria listed above. Two guidelines that incorporate knowledge of the family history are proposed for identifying high-risk situations:

1. One first-degree relative (brother, sister, parent or offspring) who has cancer and meets any of the criteria above.

2. Two first-degree relatives with any cancer at a relatively young age or a rare cancer at any age. Further evaluation is not necessary, however, if the sibship is large and the tumor types are common for the sex and age at diagnosis of the patient in question. Several initiatives to improve clinical practice in this regard are listed in the report from the workshop (*22*).

Research Needs

A strategy to control cancer through genetics should also focus on research needs that would be likely to yield practically useful results in the foreseeable future. Some of these needs are:

1.   Establishment of regional or national repositories for storage of DNA from population-based samples as well as from families, perhaps with links to existing cancer registries. The population-based studies would be of unrelated individuals, collected prospectively in defined populations. DNA from families would be collected retrospectively on individuals with cancers caused by single genes and on their unaffected spouses and first degree relatives (*22*).

2.   Collection of population-based data on the incidence of genetic and familial cancers.

3.   Confirmation or rejection of the hypothesis that heterozygosity for rare recessive disorders with deficient DNA repair (*42*) causes cancer susceptibility.

4.   Further elucidation of the relevance to tumor development of chromosomal rearrangements (*43*), loss of heterozygosity (*44*) and oncogene activation (*45, 46*).

5.   Cloning of genes that predispose to cancer. Candidate genes are, for example, those involved in aryl hydrocarbon hydroxylase inducibility (*47*).

6.   Identification and quantitation of genetic risk factors for cancer.

7.   Development of screening tests to detect cancer susceptibility in high risk individuals. In studies of families this would include genetic linkage studies of DNA polymorphisms to identify markers useful as preclinical indicators of risk status, and screening for deletions (for example, in polyposis coli families).

8.   Development of studies to identify genetic components of environmentally induced cancers (ecogenetics) and to determine the mechanisms of susceptibility.

9.   Chromosomal mapping of cancer-related genes. The gene for neurofibromatosis was mapped earlier this year (*48*) and linkage data on many cancer-related genes were presented at the recent 9th International Workshop on Human Gene Mapping in Paris (*49*). Research to make this new knowledge useful for the assessment of cancer risk should be given high priority.

10.   Development of clinical methods to detect oncogene activation. In view of new evidence that oncogene activation may be an important event in the development of some human tumors (*45, 46*), clinically useful methods to detect oncogene activation *in vivo* could become very useful.

Studies of twins could provide information concerning several of the above research needs. Genes contributing to cancer risk may be identified by comparing the health experiences of dizygotic twins who by descent share 0, 1, or 2 genes at a given locus (partitioned twin analysis) (item 6 above). The genetic components of environmentally induced cancers may be identified by comparing disease concordance in monozygotic pairs who possess *versus* those who lack a given candidate gene (item 8 above). Finally, environmental causes of cancer may be identified by in-depth study of monozygotic twins who are discordant for cancer.

Concerning the Prospects for Identifying At-Risk Individuals

The new DNA technology holds great promise that individual genes contributing to a person's susceptibility or resistance to cancerogenic stimuli will be identified. Several years ago the suggestion was made that genes involved in the inducibility of aryl hydrocarbon hydroxylase contribute to lung cancer susceptibility, and that inducibility in man follows simple inheritance. The latter issue is, however, more complicated. We have shown a high level of heritability of such inducibility in man, but also that environmental factors are of significant importance (*47*). The recent cloning of genes for enzymes related to aryl hydrocarbon hydroxylase function gives hope that influential single genes will be identified.

A report that appeared in 1985 created hope that an RFLP at the Ha-ras locus on chromosome 11 could become useful for detection of cancer susceptibility. However, other workers have had problems in confirming the original findings and at present it is uncertain if any RFLP at or near an oncogene locus will be helpful for risk prediction.

The finding that heterozygotes for ataxia-telangiectasia have increased cancer risk is potentially significant (*42*). If confirmed, and if a useful screening test for ataxia-telangiectasia heterozygosity could be developed, a new possibility of detecting cancer susceptibility would become available.

The linkage information that has recently become available on many tumor-related genes (*49*) may lead to several new possibilities for following the segregation of cancer susceptibility in families and for screening the general population with respect to cancer risk.

Doubtless a variety of new information that will increase the possibility for efficient predictive testing of cancer risk can be expected. The candidate gene approach seems particularly promising as illustrated above, and one should work on the assumption that useful predictive genetic testing will soon become widely available. Much of the progress to date and prospects for the future in the use of genetics for cancer prevention depends on research into rare events in oncology that apply to cancer in general.

Ethical Issues in Predictive Genetic Testing for Cancer Risk

When appropriate methods for predictive genetic testing becomes available, such testing should be offered on a voluntary basis to young people for the purpose of instituting as effective protective measures as possible, for those who need it the most. It is important that the right to abstain from testing be respected and that no pressure to undergo tests is put on any individual or group.

For tests to be ethically acceptable, it must be possible to offer some protective advice to people who are at increased risk of cancer. Even in the absence of highly specific advice, cessation of cigarette smoking would be useful to enough people at risk that this advice by itself may justify predictive testing for cancer risk. It is essential that protective advice be offered at the same time as information about increased risk is given. Thus, one cannot accept a system where laboratory results are handed out without adequate counseling.

For predictive testing to be widely used to prevent disease, it is important that the public feels certain that test results will not be used to their disadvantage. Accordingly, the results of predictive tests should be considered as the individual's private property and it should be explicitly forbidden for insurance companies, employers, pension funds, educational institutions and the military to ask questions about predictive genetic testing or to require such tests to be performed.

The strict rules proposed concerning protection of data from predictive genetic tests should be supported by explicit laws.

REFERENCES

1. Waaler, G.H.M. Über die Erblichkeit des Krebses. Monograph. A. W. Bröggers Boktrykkeri A/S, Oslo, 1931.
2. Mulvihill, J. J. Genetic repertory of human neoplasia. In; J. J. Mulvihill, R. W. Miller, and J. F. Fraumeni, Jr. (eds.), Progress in Cancer Research and Therapy, Vol. 3, pp. 137–143, Raven Press, New York, 1977.
3. Berg, K. Inherited variation in susceptibility and resistance to environmental agents. In; K. Berg (ed.), Genetic Damage in Man Caused by Environmental Agents, pp. 1–25, Academic Press, New York, 1979.
4. McKusick, V. A. (ed.), Mendelian Inheritance in Man, 7th ed., Johns Hopkins University Press, Baltimore, 1986.
5. Nance, W. E. Relevance of twin studies in cancer research. In; J. J. Mulvihill, R. W. Miller, and J. F. Fraumeni, Jr. (eds.), Progress in Cancer Research and Therapy, Vol. 3, pp. 27–38, Raven Press, New York, 1977.
6. Müller, C. Xanthomata, hypercholesterolemia, angina pectoris. Acta Med. Scand., 89 (Suppl.): 75, 1938.
7. Berg, K. Inherited lipoprotein variation and atherosclerotic disease. In; A. M. Scanu, W. W. Wissler, and G. S. Getz (eds.), The Biochemistry of Atherosclerosis, pp. 419–490, Marcel Dekker, Inc., New York, 1979.
8. Berg, K. Genetics of coronary heart disease. In; A. G. Steinberg, A. G. Bearn, A. G. Motulsky, and B. Childs (eds.), Progress in Medical Genetics, pp. 35–90, W. B. Saunders Co., Philadelphia, 1983.
9. Berg, K. Genetics of atherosclerosis. In; A. G. Olsson (ed.), Atherosclerosis. Biology and Clinical Science, pp. 323–337, Churchill-Livingstone, Edinburgh, 1987.
10. Nora, J. J., Lortscher, R. H., Spangler, R. D., Nora, A. H., and Kimberling, W. J. Genetic-epidemiologic study of early-onset ischemic heart disease. Circulation, 61: 503–508, 1980.
11. Berg, K. Genetic risk factors for atherosclerotic disease. Proceedings of the 7th International Congress of Human Genetics, Berlin, September 1986, in press.
12. Berg, K. Twin studies of coronary heart disease and its risk factors. Proceedings of the 5th International Congress on Twin Studies, Amsterdam, September 1986, in press.
13. Berg, K., Dahlén, G., and Frick, M. H. Lp(a) lipoprotein and pre-beta$_1$-lipoprotein in patients with coronary heart disease. Clin. Genet., 6: 230–235, 1974.
14. Rhoads, G. G., Dahlén, G., Berg, K., Morton, N. E., and Dannenberg, A. L. Lp(a) lipoprotein as a risk factor for myocardial infarction. JAMA, 256: 2540–2544, 1986.
15. Berg, K., Hames, C., Dahlén, G., Frick, M. H., and Krishan, I. Genetic variation in serum low density lipoproteins and lipid levels in man. Proc. Natl. Acad. Sci. U.S.A., 73: 937–940, 1976.
16. Law, A., Wallis, S. C., Powell, L. M., Pease, R., Brunt, H., Priestley, L. M., Knott,

T. J., Scott, J., Altman, D. G., Miller, G. J., Rajput, J., and Miller, N. E. Common DNA polymorphism within coding sequence of apolipoprotein B gene associated with altered lipid levels. Lancet, *i*: 1301–1303, 1986.

17. Berg, K., Powell, L. M., Wallis, S. C., Pease, R., Knott, T. J., and Scott, J. Genetic linkage between the antigenic group (Ag) variation and the apolipoprotein B gene: Assignment of the Ag locus. Proc. Natl. Acad. Sci. U.S.A., *83*: 7367–7370, 1986.

18. Ordovas, J. M., Schaefer, E. J., Salem, D., Ward, R. H., Glueck, C. J., Vergani, C., Wilson, P.W.F., and Karathanasis, S. K. Apolipoprotein A-I gene polymorphism associated with premature coronary artery disease and familial hypoalphaproteinemia. N. Engl. J. Med., *314*: 671–677, 1986.

19. Hegele, R. A., Huang, L.-S., Herbert, P. N., Blum, C. B., Buring, J. E., Hennekens, C. H., and Breslow, J. L. Apolipoprotein B-gene DNA polymorphisms associated with myocardial infarction. N. Engl. J. Med., *315*: 1509–1515, 1986.

20. Berg, K. Predictive genetic testing to control coronary heart disease and hyperlipidemia. Proceedings of International Symposium on Familial Hypercholesterolemia, Oslo, August 1987, in press.

21. Mulvihill, J. J. Clinical ecogenetics of human cancer. *In;* Genes and Cancer, pp. 19–36, Alan R. Liss, Inc., New York, 1984.

22. Parry, D. M., Berg, K., Mulvihill, J. J., Carter, C. L., and Miller, R. W. Strategies for controlling cancer through genetics: report of a workshop. Am. J. Hum. Genet., *41*: 63–69, 1987.

23. Albano, W. A., Lynch, H. T., Recabaren, J. A., Organ, C. H., Maillard, J. A., Black, L. E., Follet, K. L., and Lynch, J. Family cancer in an oncology clinic. Cancer, *47*: 2113–2118, 1981.

24. Bloomfield, C. D. and others. Chromosomal abnormalities identify high-risk and low-risk patients with acute lymphoblastic leukemia. Blood, *67*: 415–420, 1986.

25. Friend, S. H., Bernards, R., Rogeli, S., Weinberg, R. A., Rapaport, J. M., Albert, D. M., and Dryja, T. P. A human DNA segment with properties of the gene that predispose to retinoblastoma and osteosarcoma. Nature, *323*: 643–646, 1986.

26. Josten, D. M., Evans, A. M., and Love, R. R. The cancer prevention clinic: a service program for cancer-prone families. J. Psychosoc. Oncol., *3*: 5–20, 1985.

27. Knudson, A. G., Jr. and Kelly, P. T. Genetics and cancer. *In;* R. C. Hickey (ed.), Current Problems in Cancer, Vol. 7, No. 12, pp. 1–41, Year Book Med. Publ., Chicago, 1983.

28. Koufos, A., Hansen, M. F., Copeland, N. G., Jenkins, N. G., Lampkin, B. C., and Cavenee, W. K. Loss of heterozygosity in three embryonal tumors suggests a common pathogenetic mechanism. Nature, *316*: 330–334, 1985.

29. Miller, R. W. Genes, syndromes and cancer. Pediatr. Rev., *8*: 153–158, 1986.

30. Muller, H. and Weber, W. (eds.), Familial Cancer, Karger, Basel, 1985.

31. Mulvihill, J. J., Miller, R. W., and Fraumeni, J. F., Jr. (eds.), Genetics of Human Cancer, Vol. 3, Raven Press, New York, 1977.

32. Schwartz, A. G., King, M.-C., Belle, S. H., and Satariano, W. A. Risk of breast cancer to relatives of young breast cancer patients. J. Natl. Canc. Inst., *75*: 665–668, 1985.

33. Ottman, R., Pike, M. C., King, M.-C., Casagrande, J. T., and Henderson, B. E. Familial breast cancer in a population-based series. Am. J. Epidemiol., *123*: 15–21, 1986.

34. Parry, D. M., Mulvihill, J. J., Miller, R. W., and Spiegel, R. J. Sarcomas in a child and her father. Am. J. Dis. Child., *133*: 130–132, 1979.

35. Mulvihill, J. J. The frequency of hereditary large bowel cancer. *In;* R. F. Ingall and A. J. Mastromarino (eds.), Prevention of Hereditary Large Bowel Cancer, pp. 61–75,

Alan R. Liss, Inc., New York, 1983.

36. Anderson, D. E. and Badzioch, M. E. Bilaterality in familial breast cancer patients. Cancer, *56*: 2092–2098, 1986.

37. Ghadirian, P. Familial history of esophageal cancer. Cancer, *8*: 2112–2116, 1984.

38. Mulvihill, J. J. Research vistas in the multiple endocrine neoplasia syndromes. Henry Ford Hosp. Med. J., *32*: 277–282, 1984.

39. Mulvihill, J. J. Cancer in families. N. Engl. J. Med., *312*: 1569–1570, 1985.

40. Mulvihill, J. J., Safyer, A. W., and Bening, J. K. Prevention of familial breast cancer: counseling and prophylactic mastectomy. Prevent. Med., *11*: 500–511, 1982.

41. Stamey, T. S., Yang, N., Hay, A. R., McNeal, J. E., Freiha, F. S., and Redwine, E. Prostate-specific antigen as a serum marker for adenocarcinoma of the prostate. N. Engl. J. Med., *317*: 909–916, 1987.

42. Reitnauer, P. J., Morrell, D., Chase, C., and Swift, M. Retrospective analysis of cancer incidence in 110 U.S. white families with ataxia-telangiectasia. Am. J. Hum. Genet., *37* (Suppl.): A36, 1985.

43. Mitelman, F. Clustering of breakpoints to specific chromosomal regions in human neoplasia. A survey of 5,345 cases. Hereditas, *104*: 113–119, 1986.

44. Schroeder, W. T., Chao, L.-Y., Dao, D. D., Strong, L. C., Pathak, S., Riccardi, V., Lewis, W. H., and Saunders, G. F. Nonrandom loss of maternal chromosome 11 alleles in Wilms' tumors. Am. J. Hum. Genet., *40*: 413–420, 1987.

45. Rodenhuis, S., van de Wetering, M. L., Mooi, W. J., Evers, S. G., van Zandwijk, N., and Bos, J. L. Mutational activation of the K-ras oncogene. N. Engl. J. Med., *317*: 929–935, 1987.

46. Slamon, D. J. Proto-oncogenes and human cancers. N. Engl. J. Med., *317*: 955–957, 1987.

47. Børresen, A.-L., Berg, K., and Magnus, P. A twin study of aryl hydrocarbon hydroxylase (AHH) inducibility in cultured lymphocytes. Clin. Genet., *19*: 281–289, 1981.

48. Barker, D., Wright, E., Nguyen, K., Cannon, L., Fain, P., Goldgar, D., Bishop, D. T., Carey, J., Baty, B., Kivlin, J., Willard, H., Waye, J. S., Greig, G., Leinwand, L., Nakamura, Y., O'Connell, P., Leppert, M., Lalouel, J.-M., White, R., and Skolnick, M. Gene for von Recklinghausen neurofibromatosis is in the pericentromeric region of chromosome 17. Science, *236*: 1100–1102, 1987.

49. Proceedings of the Ninth International Workshop on Human Gene Mapping, Paris, September 6–11, 1987.

Author Index

295

Subject Index

A-bomb *see* Atomic bomb
A-T, AT *see* Ataxia telangiectasia
ABCC *see* Atomic Bomb Casuality Commission
Acquired cyst in dialysis patients
  cyst fluid chemical composition 83
  lectin-peroxidase conjugate reactivity 83
  natural history 83
  sex difference 83
Acquired hypogammaglobulinemia 149, 154
  survivors of infectious mononucleosis 151
Acquired immunodeficiency syndrome 143, 144,
    149, 159–167, 173, 176
  analogy with known disease 177
  initiation-promotion hypothesis 177, 178
  natural history 178
  possible factor 177
  -related complex 164, 165
Activated N-ras gene
  DNA from atomic bomb survivors 125, 128, 129,
    131, 132
  leukemogenesis 131
Acute lymphocytic lymphoma
  age distribution 88, 89
  Arab population of the Gaza Strip 87–91
  association between HLA types and 90
  children
    ataxia-telangiectasia 90
    Bloom's syndrome 90
    Down syndrome 90
  socio-economic circumstances 89, 90
  spontaneous mutation 90, 91
  subtypes 88
Adult T-cell leukemia 5, 181, 185

AGR *see* Aniridia, genito-urinary abnormalities and
  mental retardation
AIDS *see* Acquired immunodeficiency syndrome
ALL *see* Acute lymphocytic lymphoma
Androgenic-anabolic steroids
  cause of hepatic angiosarcoma 39, 42, 43
Aniridia
  associated with Wilms' tumor 10, 221, 224, 225,
    244
Aniridia, genito-urinary abnormalities and mental
    retardation 238, 239
Anorectal cancer
  associated with homosexuality 166
  relation to human papilloma virus 160
Arsenic 42, 45
  cause of hepatic angiosarcoma 39
  effect, lung cancer in miners 106–109
Aryl hydrocarbon hydroxylase 290, 291
Asbestos
  lung cancer 5, 9, 13, 14
  mesothelioma 9, 14
At the time of bombing
  age 117–119
  age- and risk of death 120
  sex and age- 121
Ataxia telangiectasia 6, 291
  abnormality of DNA repair 236
  association with leukemia 236
  chromosome aberration 236
  complementation group 261, 262
  deletion mutation model 268
  genetic model 261, 264–270
  heterozygote assignment 264, 265, 270

297

302

N-CWS *see Norcardia rubra* cell wall skelton
Nasal cancer
  cigarette smoker 17
  mortality rate 16
  workers in textile industry 17
Nasopharyngeal cancer 149, 178
  association with Epstein-Barr virus 149
National Cooperative Diethylstilbestrol Adenosis Project 70, 72
National Institute of Occupational Safety and Health 43, 44
Neuroblastoma 224
  Japan 7
  U.S. whites 7
Neurofibromatosis 8
NHL *see* Non-Hodgkin's lymphoma
NIOSH *see* National Institute of Occupational Safety and Health
Nitrites
  volatile 178
    possible cofactor for Kaposi's sarcoma 177
Non-Hodgkin's lymphoma 149, 159–167
  exposure to herbicides 13, 21
  occurrence
    heterosexual 164
    homosexual 163, 164
  renal transplant patients 163
Norcardia rubra cell wall skelton 95, 99–101
NPC *see* Nasopharyngeal cancer

Oil disease *see* Yusho
Oncogene
  anti- 222, 228, 229
  myc 155
  proto- 228
  recessive 222, 228
Opportunistic infection 159, 160, 167
Opportunistic malignancy 159–167
Oral cancer
  elevated rate in Florida 13
  relation to alcohol consumption 17
  risk factors for 17
  snuff-dipping 10, 13, 18
Oral contraceptives
  carcinogenicity 54
  cause of benign liver neoplasm 4, 7, 47–55
  mutagenicity 54
  promoter activity 54
Ore dust
  effect, lung cancer in miners 103–114
Osteosarcoma
  radium-dial painter 5

Pancreas cancer
  dietary factors 19
  smoking effect 19
Paralytic poliomyelitis 174–176
PCBs *see* Polychlorinated biphenyls
PCDFs *see* Polychlorinated dibenzofurans
PCQs *see* Polychlorinated quaterphenyls
PIC *see* Polymorphic information content
Pneumocystis carinii 159, 160, 177
Poison gas
  chloracetophenone (tear gas) 96
  diphenyl-chlorarsine (sneezing gas) 95
  diphenylcyanarsine (sneezing gas) 96
  hydrocyanic acid (asphyxiating gas) 95, 96
  Lewsite (erosive gas) 95–97
  lung cancer in—worker 97–99
  phenacylchloride (tear gas) 95, 96
  phosgene (asphyxiating gas) 95, 96
  Yperite 95, 96
Polychlorinated biphenyls 61, 62
Polychlorinated dibenzofurans 61, 62
Polychlorinated quaterphenyls 61–63
Polymorphic information content 263, 270
Polyvinyl chloride 39–41
Predictive genetic testing
  ethical issues 291, 292
Prostate cancer
  ethnic factors 21
PVC *see* Polyvinyl chloride

Radiation
  dose-response for mortality 118, 119
  -induced cancer
    in-utero exposed children 122
    cumulative rate 121
    latent period 119, 120
    sex difference 122
    site 118
    temporal incidence 119
  -related excess cancer risk 118
Radiation Effects Research Foundation 117, 118
Reed-Sternberg cell
  Hodgkin's disease 189, 191
Renal cancer
  dietary factors 19
  ethnic associations 19
  schematic illustration for development 84
Renal transplantation
  immunosuppression 165
  induction of melanoma 256
  occurrence of non-Hodgkin's disease 163
  relation to Kaposi's sarcoma 161
RERF *see* Radiation Effects Research Foundation